Andreas R. Dombret / Holger J. Kern

European Retail Banks – An Endangered Species?

Andreas R. Dombret / Holger J. Kern

European Retail Banks —
An Endangered Species?

Survival Strategies for the Future

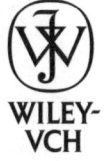

WILEY-VCH GmbH & Co. KGaA

Written in collaboration with Sibylle Pollehn

1. Auflage 2003

Bibliografische Information Der Deutschen Bibliothek
Die Deutsche Bibliothek verzeichnet diese
Publikation in der Deutschen Nationalbibliografie;
detaillierte bibliografische Daten sind im Internet
über <http://dnb.ddb.de> abrufbar.

Printed in the Federal Republic of Germany

Gedruckt auf säurefreiem Papier.

Satz   Kühn & Weyh, Freiburg
Druck und Bindung   Ebner & Spiegel GmbH, Ulm
Umschlaggestaltung   init GmbH, Bielefeld

ISBN   3-527-50064-2

Table of Contents

1
Executive Summary

Structure

Looking at the current retail banking landscape (Chapter 3), increasing levels of competition and innovation are originating from new entrants to the market, the so-called »non- and near-banks«. The objective of this book is to understand what the appearance and success of these »non- and near-banks« mean for the traditional retail banking landscape and what can be learned from their examples.

In order to better understand the capabilities of both incumbents and new players, a value chain of retail banking is defined and each separate step analysed in detail (Chapter 4.1). Case studies from both inside and outside the financial services industry are used to illustrate specific challenges, capabilities, successes, and failures. After understanding the challenges and success factors at each step of the value chain, successful players' approaches are then combined to yield an »ideal retail bank for the future« (Chapter 4.2). While hypothetical, this model points to the areas where improvement is possible and illustrates role models, which – in other industries – have already been successful in optimizing these aspects of their business. To better understand how the *realistic* retail bank of the future might look, several specialized business models are defined and described. Finally, the viability and possible limitations of these business models are discussed (Chapter 4.3).

Chapter 5 looks at the transition from today's broader organizations to tomorrows more focused players, covering the selection of a new business model, the design of the underlying business system, and the process to transform the organization. Chapter 6 gives a brief outlook into possible future developments.

Content

Today's retail banks are facing a less rosy future than they might be expecting. Several trends – each one alone perhaps easy to disregard, but together posing a sizeable challenge – are facing the industry. Most importantly, competition is increasing: between the existing market players (as technology extends their reach), from large, international players entering local markets, and from new entrants such as supermarket banks. Not only are more players competing for business, but more specialized players are emerging such as investment advisors, focusing on certain customer groups; on-line brokers, focusing on certain products; and transaction banks, focusing on certain processes. These specialized players concentrate fully on their chosen businesses, displaying cost structures that leave the traditional »universal retail banks« far behind. As a result, cost pressures are rising as well.

At the same time, the market is becoming more transparent and customers are increasingly experienced, demanding, price sensitive, and less loyal. Customers have begun moving away from having only one banking relationship to dealing with several players: for example, one for the standard checking account, another one for brokerage, and possibly several others for various investment needs. As a result, the original retail bank is left with less and less profit potential: on the one hand, it is the better educated, more affluent, and therefore more profitable clients who are most likely to defect and take part of or all of their business elsewhere. On the other hand, it is the unprofitable part of the business, such as the current account, that is likely to be left behind. Defecting clients tend to move their brokerage accounts, fixed term deposits, investments, credit cards, and mortgages. These are the products that predominantly yield relatively stable margins at a relatively low risk. In short, both increased competition and less loyal customers have resulted in significant margin pressures for retail banks.

However, today's retail banks face additional challenges. Only very few players have developed a strong brand that their customers are able to identify with. As long as clients choose their bank according to which branch is closest (rather than walking the proverbial mile for a camel cigarette), brand building in retail banking will be far behind what is already standard in other industries. Instead, banks try to differentiate themselves on technical terms, i. e. through their product offering or through differences in services, terms, or conditions that are often perceived as irrelevant by consumers. However, as the success of new entrants such as the UK's supermarket bank Tesco Personal Finance has shown, clients can be easily won despite a standard product range by offering products through clever channels of access and under a strong existing brand.

In summary, the current focus in retail banking appears to be on the wrong issues. To begin with, banks overdeliver in the sense that customers are offered a variety of product differentiations for which they have little interest. At the same time, banks underdeliver on other important parts of their services. For example, customers do not receive the level of independent, unbiased advice and the personalized treatment they would like. Customers today do not differentiate between brands and have no emotional attachments. Instead of feeling cared for and understood, they are offered a myriad of products, but no solutions for their problems.

In order to cope with these challenges, retail banks will have to stop trying to be all things to all people. Specialization is required, whether it be in specific parts of the retail banking value chain, on certain customer groups, on specific products, or on a particular value proposition. These specialized players will form a network of companies linked by mutual outsourcing / insourcing relationships, and together constitute the retail banking industry of the future.

The retail banking value chain consists of three major steps, which can be split further into six detailed ones (see Exhibit 1: The Overarching and Detailed Value Chains of Retail Banking). First, there is product development. Second, there are the three customer facing activities of branding and marketing (product branding and marketing; corporate branding), sales (including distribution, channel decisions, distribution cooperations, and all customer interaction at the point of sale (POS)), and client management (anything done to sell an additional product to an existing client). In this book, these activities will be referred to as the »customer interface«. Finally, there is infrastructure, which is comprised of the two areas transaction/administration and risk management.

Today, virtually all retail banks cover the entire range of steps themselves. In light of the increasing competitive pressures, which future business mod-

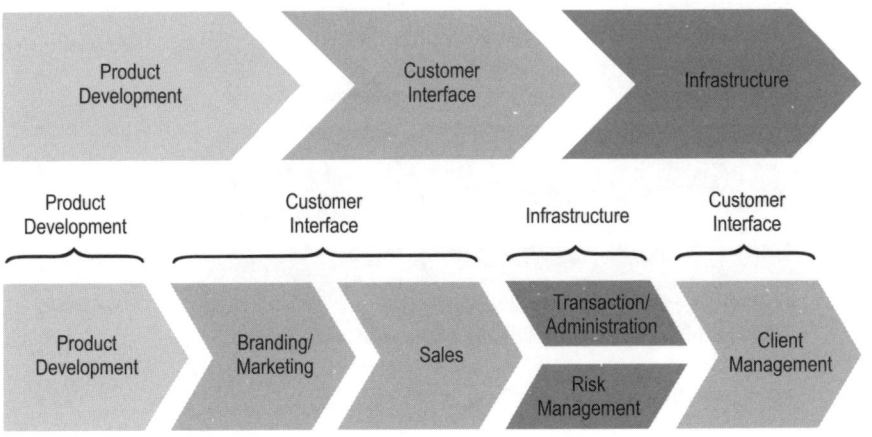

Exhibit 1: The Overarching and Detailed Value Chains of Retail Banking

els exist within the value chain on which today's retail banks could focus successfully? Where are the unique markets, operational efficiencies (including economies of scale or scope), defendable niches, or convincing value propositions?

Seven general business models can be constructed within this equally general three step value chain (see Exhibit 2: The Seven General Business Models of Retail Banking).

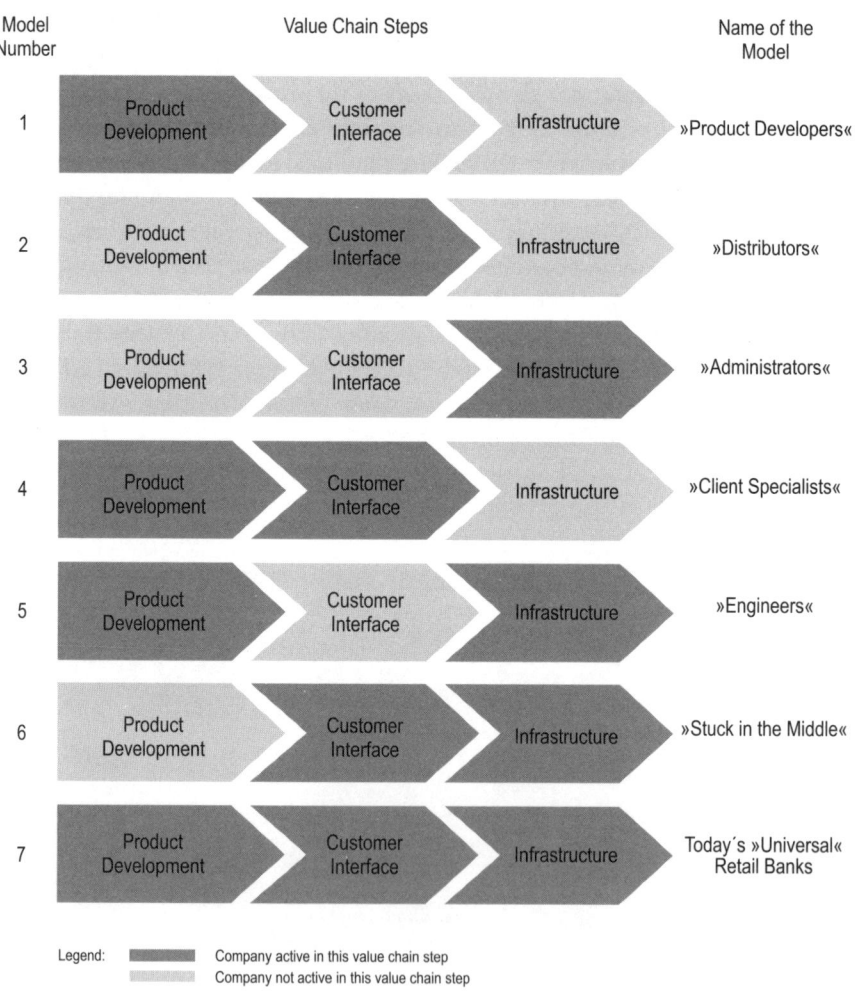

Exhibit 2: The Seven General Business Models of Retail Banking

Not all of these combinations yield viable future business models. However, some of these models may actually leave room for several innovative differentiation scenarios.

Model 7 describes today's »universal retail banks«, a model which we assume to be viable only for very few players on the long run. Model 6, which is the combination of customer interface and infrastructure activities, is unlikely to become relevant, as there are too few synergies between the two sets of activities to warrant a combined business model. Neither can the customer interface serve its customers better due to anything done on or learned from the infrastructure side nor vice versa. Those players would be stuck in the middle, as their lack of focus on one core activity only would always make them inferior to a combination of models 2 and 3. For the remaining five models, future players are easy to imagine (see Exhibit 3: Detailed Future Business Models in Retail Banking). What might their business models look like?

Exhibit 3: Detailed Future Business Models in Retail Banking

Model no.	Name	Specialization
1	»Product developers«	• Specialist product developers (»Rocket Scientists«)
2	»Distributors«	All focusing on the customer interface and seeking differentiation through: • Price (»Aldi Banks«) • Convenience (»McDonalds Banks«) • Quality (»Delicatessen Banks«) • Niche (»Fur-Hats-Are-Us Banks«) The »real« banks behind the Aldi and McDonalds Banks (»Gray Eminences«)
3	»Administrators«	Focusing on various aspects of Infrastructure: • Transactions (»Assembly Line«) • IT or support functions (»IT and Admin Specialists«)
4	»Client Specialists«	Combining a focus on the customer interface with product development
5	»Engineers«	Combining a focus on transactions with product development

Instead of developing all products themselves, retail banks could outsource the development of specialist products (i. e. the more elaborate, engineered investment products like tax driven investments or retirement provisions) to the focused »Product Developers« described in model 1.

Among those retail banks focusing on the customer interface (the »Distributors« in model 2), many areas of specialization are possible. Differentiation can occur via low prices, convenient access, high quality of services, or by focusing on a specific niche of customers or products. In order to be able to fully concentrate on their chosen business, these »Distributors« will have to outsource the non-customer facing processes as far as possible, including product development, and focus on marketing, banding, sales, and client management. Ideally, some of them will not only outsource *parts* of the non-core processes and still be involved in their coordination, but will outsource the *entire* banking processes to another bank who would operate in the background, a so-called »Gray Eminence«.

There are already many examples of the »Administrators« of model 3. Some of these specialized companies, particularly those focusing on transactions, come from within the financial services industry such as State Street, the world's largest custodian. Others, who have a stronger focus on IT or support functions, come from traditionally non-financial services industries. Examples of such players include IBM who managed to insource several large financial institutions' IT operations within the last two years.

In addition to the three business models focusing on one value chain step only, i. e. the »Product Developers«, the »Distributors«, and the »Administrators«, there are another two viable models that combine two value chain steps thus allowing for better offerings or higher efficiencies. Integrating the customer interface activities with product development, as in model 4, could be very interesting for those competitors who specialize on a specific target group to a very high degree. For these »Client Specialists«, developing specific products for their clients would significantly enhance their customer-focused business model. Similarly, a combined focus on transactions and product development can offer economies of scope for the »Engineers« of model 5. The detailed know-how of transactions and underlying customer preferences that these players would gain through their focus on transactions would allow them to develop better products, i. e. products that are more customer-focused, cheaper, or easier to produce.

How should retail banks manage the necessary transition from their current, all-encompassing business model to a future, more focused one? To begin with, a fitting business model must be chosen, i. e. one that is viable and feasible to achieve given their current core competencies. Secondly, the underlying business system must be meticulously designed around the chosen business model. Finally, today's business system must actually be resculpted into the future one through a combination of internal and external transformations. »External transformations« refer to transactions such as acquisitions, mergers, joint ventures, or divestments, while »internal transformations« refer to changing the internal processes, structures, and mindset of the bank.

In this transformation process, the future organization, structures, processes, and focus must not be compromised by the currently existing activities or structures (which can develop into holy cows). Only if the chosen focus is clearly maintained and the entire operations are streamlined around that focus can a player occupy a defendable market position in the network of specialized companies that will form the retail banking landscape of the future.

2
Introduction

Facing ever-increasing competition, the Retail Banking Market in Europe is experiencing constant change. The industry is undergoing concentration on a national and, though to a lesser degree, even on an international level. This concentration has led to many markets being dominated by a few top players. In a move towards even greater efficiency, branch networks have begun to be thinned out and – together with the ongoing streamlining of organizations and processes – this has resulted in the general rise of overall retail banking profitability over the last couple of years. The impact of the Internet has also been felt strongly, with new players entering the market and new channels being established. Influenced by the Internet and its ubiquitous offer of information, customers have changed significantly in their demands, preferences, and level of financial education and sophistication. As a result, customer loyalty is decreasing.

In response to these challenges, most banks have tried to position themselves as broadly as possible. Retail banks started adding insurance products to their product range, thereby also catering to customers' increased needs for old age provisions, by either acquiring, being acquired by, or cooperating with insurers[1]. One level higher, both among larger and smaller financial institutions, the concept of the universal bank was pursued actively. This concept integrates retail banking not only with corporate banking, as has been commonplace for a long time, but also investment banking. During the late nineties, the ever rising stock markets produced such a wave of mergers, acquisitions, IPOs, and venture financing, so that some banks publicly considered getting rid of their – comparatively unprofitable – retail banking arms altogether. The wave subsided, the markets collapsed, and retail banking remained as it had been: a large, relatively recession proof, and nicely profitable part of the banking institutions. The numbers support this: between 1997 and 2001, the cumulated average growth rate of total shareholder return was over 40 percent for private banking, around 30 percent for asset management and investment banking, still around 25 percent for diversified banks, but only 21 percent for retail banking. With only five percent monthly standard deviation in 2001, however, retail banking volatility was about half of the value of the other three areas of specialization[2].

Being active in a nicely profitable and consolidated market, however, is no reason for complacency. Competition is rising – from new entrants, through new channels providing a ubiquitous presence, and through internationalization – and will continue to do so, especially where the margins are high. At the same time, more demanding and less loyal customers are increasingly willing to defect. The potential for the near-oligopolistic players in many large markets to get hurt is certainly there. The species of retail banks is more endangered than a mere glance at double digit return on equities might suggest.

3
The Current European Retail Banking Landscape

Size: The Number of Retail Banks in Europe is Decreasing

Using credit institutions as a proxy for retail banks, 8 022 retail banks were operating in the European Union as of December 2001, with Austria, France, Germany, and Italy accounting for more than two thirds of this number (see Exhibit 4: Credit Institutions in the European Union at the End of 2001). With almost one third of institutions alone, Germany harbors by far the largest share.

Exhibit 4: Credit Institutions in the European Union at the End of 2001

Country	Credit Institutions		
	Number	% of EU	Change vs. 1998 (%)
Austria	836	10.4%	−6.9%
Belgium	112	1.4%	−8.9%
Finland	369	4.6%	6.0%
France	1 050	13.1%	−14.4%
Germany	2 526	31.5%	−22.0%
Greece	61	0.8%	3.4%
Ireland	88	1.1%	12.8%
Italy	843	10.5%	−9.7%
Luxemburg	194	2.4%	−8.5%
Netherlands	561	7.0%	−11.5%
Portugal	212	2.6%	−6.6%
Spain	366	4.6%	−9.0%
Eurozone	**7 218**	**90.0%**	**−13.9%**
Denmark	203	2.5%	−4.2%
Sweden	149	1.9%	0.7%
U.K.	452	5.6%	−13.2%
European Union	**8 022**	**100.0%**	**−13.4%**

Source: European Central Bank, Structural analysis of the EU banking sector 2001, November 2002

Compared with 1998, a significant amount of consolidation has taken place and the number of credit institutions has decreased by more than 13 percent across the EU. With a decrease of 22 percent, despite still having too many, Germany experienced by far the sharpest decline. On the other hand, increases of 13 and 6 percent, respectively, were observed in Ireland and Finland.

With regard to balance sheet volumes, the credit institutions in the European Union had an aggregated volume of more than 24 trillion Euros in 2001, corresponding to about 2.7 times European GDP (gross domestic product at market prices)[1]. The most important countries were Germany (26 percent), the UK (24 percent), and France (16 percent), who together represent two thirds of EU balance sheet totals. Note that with a share of almost one quarter, the UK banks play a much more significant role than the absolute numbers might suggest.

Internationalization is Generally Still Low, but Rising

Despite the ongoing integration of European markets, even in 2001 the level of international interconnectivity was still relatively low. Only 8 percent of all credit institutions were legally dependent foreign subsidiaries. However, this share rose from only 5.5 percent in 1998, thus confirming the trend towards internationalization. Of these 649 (or eight percent of) credit institutions, only 15 percent have a parent company outside of the EU[2]. Therefore, apart from in investment banking, the direct involvement in the European market from outside of Europe (for instance from the United States) is so far limited.

In line with their large balance sheet volumes, Germany and the UK are the main target markets for foreign banks' subsidiaries. Considering the current weak performance of German banks, however, an expansion into the German retail banking market might seem unattractive for foreign banks for the time being, and at least into the near future. As the Financial Times stated in late 2002: if you want to own German banking stocks, it would be Deutsche Bank – but why would you want to own German banking stocks?

Concentration is Highly Advanced in Many Markets, However, Germany is Still Very Fragmented

On average, the largest five banks of each country account for 54 percent of total balance sheet volumes in 2001, compared with 50 percent in 1997. Very high levels of concentration can be found in the Scandinavian countries. Sweden is absolute top with around 88 percent, followed by the Netherlands, Belgium, and Greece, all well above 60 percent (see Exhibit 5: Consolidation: Share of the Five Largest Credit Institutions in Total Assets 1997 and 2001). At the opposite extreme, the German market is still very fragmented with the leading banks accounting for only about 20 percent of the total balance sheet volume.

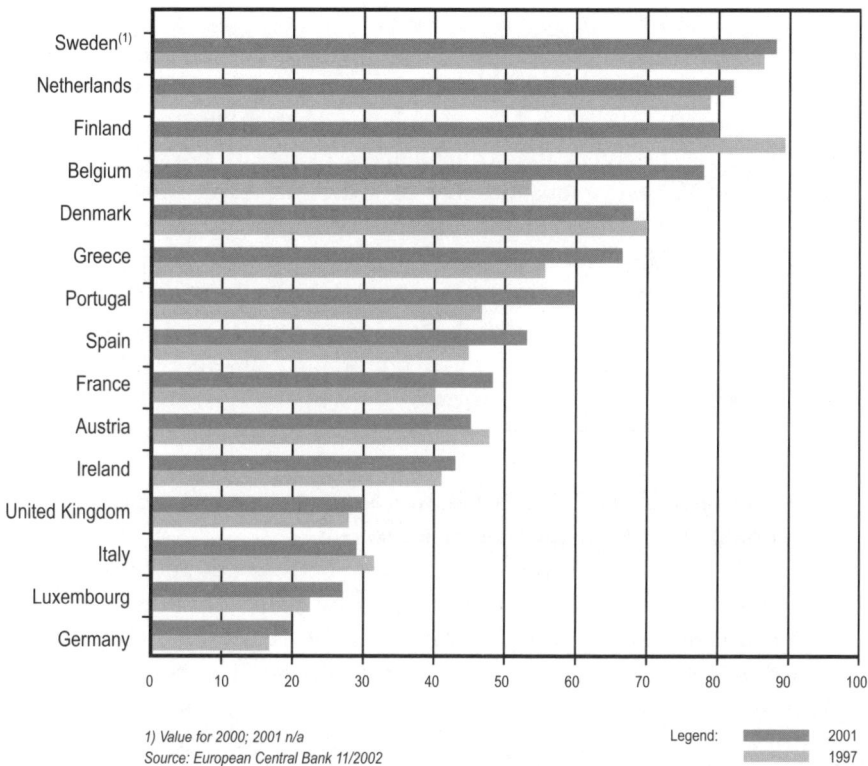

1) Value for 2000; 2001 n/a
Source: European Central Bank 11/2002

Legend: ■■■■ 2001
        ▭▭▭ 1997

Exhibit 5: Consolidation: Share of the Five Largest Credit Institutions in Total Assets 1997 and 2001 (in %)

Private Banks, Savings Banks, Co-operative Banks, and the Need for Consolidation in Germany

The leading private banks in Germany operate in a highly fragmented market. Concerning credit business in 2001, savings banks controlled a market share of 37 percent, co-operatives 14 percent, and private banks only 26 percent. This is due to historic development and the fact that savings and Landesbanks benefit from certain favorable regulations, in particular »Gewährträgerhaftung« (an institutional liability) and »Anstaltslast« (a guarantor liability). These regulations allow them to borrow funds more cheaply due to state-backed guarantees. As a result, these players have been able to offer credits at margins that were hard to match for private banks. However, according to an agreement in 2001, these regulations will be phased out by mid of 2005.

As a consequence, savings banks might need to consolidate, as might co-operatives, in order to increase efficiency and ensure competitiveness in the future. Co-operatives have already begun to do this, as evidenced by recent M&A (mergers and acquisitions) activities. Besides aiming at a reduction of the enormous number of individual banks, both savings banks and co-operatives might also use M&A to facilitate structural change. The savings banks in Austria have shown what such structural changes could look like: The savings banks themselves use their wide branch network to focus on distribution, whereas their central body, the exchange-listed Erste Bank, focuses on product development for the entire sector.

Based on Technological Capabilities and Superior Customer Access, New Competitors Have Entered the Market

As will be discussed in more detail later, many »non- and near-banks« have entered the banking market during recent years. These new entrants have focused on one of two advantages. In the first case, they used the rapidly developing technology to offer new services on the Internet (such as on-line banks). In the second case, they branched off from positions in other industries and used their strong access to clients (at the points of purchase) to offer financial services beyond simple consumer credits as part of the daily shopping routine or as part of other larger financial transactions. Examples of this model include banks affiliated with supermarket chains and car manufacturers.

Customers Have Become Significantly More Sophisticated, Demanding, and Disloyal

In recent years, customer behavior has changed significantly. The Internet has provided customers with both increased convenience – for example transactions can be initiated anywhere and anytime – and information about stock markets and banks' offers. Banks have lost their information advantage versus their customers, offers became more comparable, and the retail banking market as a whole has become more transparent. Customers have not only become more informed and more demanding, but also more independent. Together with higher market transparency, this has led to increased price sensitivity and decreasing customer loyalty. As a consequence, keeping their customers is harder than ever before for European retail banks. One of the ways in which banks have tried to adapt to this challenge is by improving their marketing, sales, and customer relationship management, but with little evidence of success so far.

Retirement Provisions and Other Investments are Becoming Important Issues

Demand regarding products has also changed over the past few years. The first change is due to recent stock market developments: The equity boom some years ago made many customers aware of the possible high returns, the subsequent collapse clearly showed the high risks associated with these investments. As a result, customers are no longer satisfied with mere savings accounts and demand more attractive returns. However, at the same time, they do not want to forego the safety that their equity investments lacked. Secondly, individuals have an increasing need to build retirement provisions. As a consequence, endowment policies and the like are becoming more and more important and are being sold by both insurance companies and – in similar forms – by banks. This offers a significant market potential for banks if they are able to either compete with insurance companies in the sale of own policies or – more likely – team up with insurers to adopt some model of »bankassurance«. This concept has been adopted widely throughout Europe, with all major banks having some kind of partnership with an insurance partner or similar subsidiary.

Branch Consolidation and Increased Use of Technology Lead to More Efficient Distribution

In the European Union, almost 200 000 branches offered services at the end of 2001[3]. This equals, on average, one branch per every 1 960 inhabitants (see Exhibit 6: Branch Density in Europe: Number of Inhabitants per Branch). For an overview of products offered, please refer to the appendix. Due to its size and the inclusion of Postbank branches, Germany accounts for more than one quarter of all branches, over 54 000, and is thus quite »overbanked« with only 1 520 inhabitants per branch. Spain has the densest branch network with one branch per 1 030 inhabitants but counters potential negative effects on profitability by having by far the smallest branches in the EU with an average of 6.3 employees per branch. This compares to an EU and German average of over 14 employees per branch[4]. Finland, Sweden, and the UK are at the other extreme with a relatively low branch density of above 4 000 inhabitants per branch.

Exhibit 6: Branch Density in Europe: Number of Inhabitants per Branch

Country	1997	1999	2001	Change in branch density 1997–2001[3]
Finland	4 000	4 350	4 350	–8%
Sweden	3 130	4 170	n/a	–25%
United Kingdom	3 570	3 850	4 170[1]	–14%
Ireland	3 130	3 450	3 850[1]	–19%
Greece	4 170	3 850	3 570	17%
Netherlands	2 330	2 560	3 030	–23%
Denmark	2 330	2 330	2 270	3%
France	2 270	2 330	2 270	0%
Italy	2 270	2 130	1 960	16%
Portugal	2 080	1 890	1 850	12%
Austria	1 720	1 750	1 790	–4%
Belgium	1 390	1 470	1 670	–17%
Germany	1 300	1 410	**1 520**	–14%
Luxembourg	1 350	1 410	1 470[1]	–8%
Spain	1 030	1 010	**1 030**	0%
European Union	**1 850**	**1 890**	~1 960[2]	–6%[2]

Source: European Central Bank, Structural analysis of the EU banking sector 2001, November 2002
(1) Values for 2000; 2001 not available
(2) Approximate value only; sources: European Central Bank, Eurostat, Bundesverband deutscher Banken
(3) Values for 2000 or 1999 where 2001 not available

However, branches are only one part of a retail bank's distribution system: Today's banks have adopted »multi-channel banking«, the combination of branches, automated teller machines (ATMs), call centers, on-line banking, Minitel (France only), and increasingly WAP or iDTV (interactive digital TV) to distribute their banking products. Being able to offer these channels required retail banks to make considerable investments, and offering a broad choice of channels has become a prerequisite for attracting and keeping customers.

Retail Banking Profitability is Acceptable to Good on Average, but Poor in Germany

Overall retail banking profitability has been rising over the last couple of years. The differences in Europe are striking, however. Of the five largest markets (Germany, UK, France, Italy, and Spain), the UK and Spain are most attractive.

In the UK, profitability has been very high since the mid nineties, especially for traditional retail banks such as Lloyds (now with TSB). As in the entire Anglo-American area, profits mainly stem from consumer finance. This positive situation also constitutes a dilemma, however. Lloyds TSB, for example, has almost exhausted its local growth opportunities and has difficulties further expanding its retail activities through domestic M&A. Any deal would be dilutive due to the lower profitability of potential targets.

Spain has successful and profitable banks both among the focused traditional retail banks, such as Banco Popular, and the big, diversified universal banks, like BBVA and Santander Central Hispano. The success of Banco Popular is especially interesting: They focus on retail banking only, but have been extremely good at it. Judging by the stock performance, the financial community has also taken notice.

France has experienced among the largest changes in retail banking during the last years. The various players have refocused their activities and are pursuing different business models. Huge investments were made to open new markets and develop new products, especially in the profitable credit card and consumer finance businesses. As a result, retail banking profitability has improved markedly. BNP Paribas, for example, saw pre-tax return on equity (RoE) in retail banking increase to some 25 percent, making it the bank's most profitable business unit[5].

Consumer cultures vary, however, and while consumers in France or the UK make heavy use of credit cards and consumer credits, Germans are much more sceptical towards what they regard as »taking on debt«. Here, the demand for deposits is therefore much higher than for the high-margin consumer credits. Together with the high fragmentation of the market and the dominant market position and lack of profit orientation of the savings banks and co-operative banks, this is one of the reasons why German retail banking has shown a very low profitability over the past years (see »Private Banks, Savings Banks, Co-operative Banks, and the Need for Consolidation in Germany« above).

In Italy, profitability has been high recently, mainly due to the brokerage activities during the stock market boom. The difficulty for Italian retail banks now is to manage the change from the asset gathering to the lending side. UniCredito has been very successful at this: After increasing RoE from around 5 percent in 1996 to roughly 20 percent during the boom in 1999, the bank has been able to sustain this high profitability until now.

A comparison of the retail banking activities of the major banks in France, Germany, Spain, and the UK shows this in detail[6]. British banks show the best performance in their retail operations, with the six leading banks earning at least 25 percent and up to 36 percent RoE. Spain is not far behind: Its four largest banks lie in the same range with only one exception of 14 percent. The top six banks in France earn a somewhat lower RoE, with four being in the 15 to 21 percent range, and the other two earning seven and eight percent, respectively. The current situation in Germany is different. Here, the top four banks show RoEs between minus six and plus seven percent only, thus hardly being profitable. Analyzing cost/income ratios in retail activities shows that at least a part of the problem lies in a too high cost base. At 86 to 102 percent, the cost/income ratios of the top German players by far exceeds those of the others, at 39 to 70 percent.

A Challenge for the Future Despite Relatively Good Profitability

Retail banks show different levels of performance and engage in different activities across Europe. Those facing profitability problems primarily seek to lower their costs. At first glance, they may be right, as capital intensity per customer is still high in some countries. However, the real problem lies in the low revenues generated per customer. Banks are not able to sell enough products to one customer, and some are even experiencing decreasing revenues per customer.

At the same time, none of the trends described above show signs of disappearing. All of them are expected to continue or even accelerate in the future. Many of these trends are deteriorating the market environment of the retail banking industry, for example, the increase in internationalization, the entry of new competitors, and the decreasing loyalty of customers. For those retail banks operating in Germany, the situation is not ideal to begin with. But even in other countries, continued cost reductions cannot be the only answer to increasing margin pressures. Rather, as France has shown, a change in focus is necessary.

What, in detail, do the recent developments mean for the retail banking industry, and how is it going to adapt itself in order to continue to successfully cope in the future?

4
The European Retail Banking
Landscape in the Future

The Customer Interface is Becoming More Important

One of the more remarkable changes in the retail banking landscape in the past years is not just the market entry, but rather the success of new competitors.

On one side, there were technology enabled, often specialized Internet brokers and banks. Their key competitive advantage was to use a new channel, the Internet, to offer their services in a more customer friendly way: around the clock, ubiquitous (and especially from home), and often cheaper. By now, this advantage has been lost as it was replicated by the established banks that either bought a new entrant or built their own on-line capabilities. As a result, today on-line banking is just one of several distribution channels and is a must for every bank. It is not a competitive advantage anymore.

On the other side, there are new competitors like Tesco Personal Finance and Virgin Money in the UK, and BMW Financial Services in Germany. Their strategy is a completely different one, but is similarly successful.

Tesco is the UK's largest food retailer with a market share of 16.5 percent. Throughout the nineties, Tesco has focused on developing the brand into non-food areas such as electrical items, home entertainment, toys, sports equipment, clothing, and even lighting and furnishing. In 1997, Tesco teamed up with the Royal Bank of Scotland to offer customers a broad range of financial products. Today, Tesco Personal Finance offers savings accounts, credit cards, loans, travel money (including home delivery of currency and travelers checks), ISA (a UK-specific savings account with certain tax exemptions), and life, travel, motor, pet, and home insurance. Most conveniently, money and checks can be deposited and money withdrawn at the checkout cashiers. By August 2002, Tesco Personal Finance had over three million customer accounts.

Founded in 1971 as BMW Kredit GmbH, BMW Financial Services has, until recently focused on offering leasing and finance solutions for individuals, business customers, and the dealer network worldwide. Since then,

BMW Financial Services has widened its services to offer fleet management, on-line banking, credit cards, and savings and investment to its more than 500 000 customers. Since June 2001, BMW Financial Services offers investment fund products selected by the Frank Russel Company in the US. Almost 5 000 customer securities accounts have been opened for this product during the first six months alone. The latest success has been an on-line, day-to-day money account: In the first four months after its start in June 2002, 22 000 customers deposited over 500 million Euro. Interestingly enough, about two thirds of these clients were previously neither customers of BMW or Mini nor of BMW Financial Services.

Virgin Money is part of Richard Branson's Virgin Group. The Virgin Group includes businesses as diverse as travel, retail, entertainment, and finance, which are kept together by Branson's conviction that if you can run one business well, you can run any business well. The Virgin Group has offered financial services since 1995, first under the names of Virgin Direct, a personal finance business, and Virginmoney.com, an e-broker business. Today all offers are consolidated under the name Virgin Money, which provides deposit accounts, credit cards, personal loans, insurances, trusts, and pensions to more than 500 000 customers in the UK.

Why are these new entrants successful? What niche did they discover, what »holes« in the classic way of doing retail banking did they exploit to establish themselves in the market? While each of them, in line with their different origins as a supermarket, car manufacturer, and consumer goods/services conglomerate, found a slightly different hole to exploit, they all follow a pattern: All of them use their superior skills in addressing the customer, focusing on his needs and marketing to him, and being in the right place at the right time. In short, all of them focus on the customer interface. In addition, many of them use their point-of-sales (POS) advantage: Every purchase involves a financial transaction, large purchases might even require loans. Offering financial transactions at a POS is thus a promising way to catch a customer while he is willing to, or even needs to, think about his finances.

Tesco combines three elements. They use their point-of-sales advantage and their brand, and count on the convenience factor: Once you are out in the supermarket, why not do one-stop-shopping and withdraw money or »buy« a financial product as well? BMW Financial Services started attracting customers simply by catching them at a good moment: Many people need financing when buying a new car. When expanding their product range, BMW used its image and was able to offer attractive financial products. For example, fixed term deposits can be used within the BMW Group as a relatively cheap internal source of financing. Virgin used its strong brand and trendy and successful image to attract specific customers to a new business Richard Branson had spotted as a promising one.

The reason why all of these banks were able to lure away customers from the more established ones is that the established retail banks show significant deficits in managing their customer interface well, for example, in branding, marketing, sales, and customer relationship management. Whereas the retail banking industry has been quick to imitate and absorb the first type of new entrants' competitive advantage – on-line banking – they have been remarkably unaware of, or at least slow to respond to the intruders who use professional customer interface management as their competitive advantage.

Thus, the overall competitive pressures – especially from new entrants, but also from existing players – have been rising significantly over the last decades. Looking at both shifting customer preferences and the focus of the new players, the main differentiation between banks, and therefore one of the paramount battlegrounds of the future, will have to be the customer interface. This will lead to significant changes in the entire retail banking industry.

The Vertical Scope of Operations is Only Decreasing Slowly

The success of new entrants into retail banking has been remarkable, as has been the very slow response of the industry to an otherwise ubiquitous trend: outsourcing. Currently, most retail banks still do almost everything themselves. Not only do they offer a broad range of products (see Exhibit 7: Typical Product Offers of »Universal« Retail Banks), they also largely carry out all the corresponding development and transaction processes in-house. Their objective to offer a full product line might be understandable, but is not entirely justified as the success of some of the new entrants has shown. These banks' propensity to cover the entire design, marketing, selling, and manufacturing processes in-house even appears somewhat old-fashioned when compared with other industries.

Exhibit 7: Typical Product Offers of »Universal« Retail Banks

Current account	O	*Current account*
	O	*Debit card*
	O	*Transfers (national/international)*
Savings	O	*Savings account*
	O	*Fixed term deposits*
Credits	O	*Overdraft credit*
	O	*Consumer credit*
Credit cards		
Investments:	O	*Account*
Securities Trading and Brokerage	O	*Shares*
	O	*Bonds*
	O	*Mutual funds*
	O	*Derivatives*
Other Investments	O	*Tax driven investments*
	O	*Retirement provisions*
Services, esp. personal advice	O	*Investments*
	O	*Financing*

Predominantly in the area of physical products, but also within services, other industries have already reduced their vertical scope of integration over the past years and decades. The classic example for this is the automotive industry. In Germany, for example, the vertical range of manufacture in the automotive industry has decreased from 40 percent in 1970 to 37 percent in 1980, 33 percent in 1990, finally plummeting to 22 percent in 2001[1].

Reducing the vertical scope of operations leads to higher efficiency and means the company can focus on what it does best and what their customers value most. However, it is not only interesting to look at what part of their operations companies outsource, but also at what parts they do not. Take the example of passenger cars at BMW: As with many other car manufacturers, BMW has increasingly withdrawn from the manufacturing of components and will continue to do so for all parts that are not seen as strategically important. Even in assembly, outsourcing is not a taboo: The new cross-country vehicle X3 will be assembled entirely in Austria by Magna Steyr Fahrzeugtechnik. Nevertheless, BMW would never think about outsourcing their engine R&D and/or production, at least as far as the 6-, 8-, and 12-cylinder motors are concerned. The company regards this know-how as a key competitive advantage and feels strongly that having these capabilities in-house is an important part of maintaining their brand and image.

Traditionally, the retail banking industry has been slow to adopt this trend. This pattern has started to change only recently as various banks – albeit cautiously – began to outsource some of their activities. One of the more recent and fairly large-scale examples of outsourcing within the retail banking industry has been Deutsche Bank's agreement with IBM in September 2002 to outsource their entire IT operations.

Nevertheless, compared to other industries, European retail banking has lagged behind. To better understand trends, developments, and restrictions in outsourcing (i. e. changing the vertical scope of operations), it is necessary to take a closer look at the value chain of the retail banking industry.

4.1 The Retail Banking Value Chain

Similar to other service industries, the typical retail banking value chain differs from that of traditional manufacturing industries in that banking products are always »produced to order«, that is, the actual »production« of a transaction begins only after the customer has initiated it (see Exhibit 8: The Retail Banking Value Chain, and Exhibit 9: Overview of the Retail Banking Value Chain Steps).

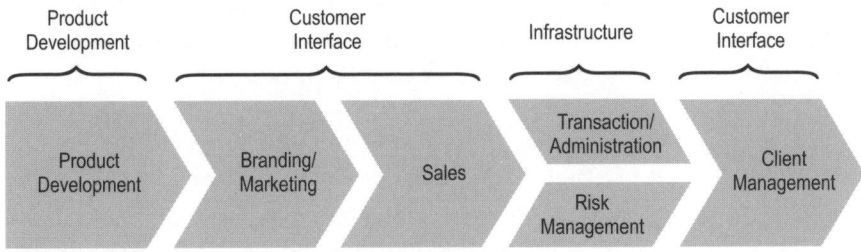

Exhibit 8: The Retail Banking Value Chain

Product Development: First, comparable to traditional R&D, a product and its necessary infrastructure need to be designed. The product design stage includes product philosophy, financial engineering, profitability, and conditions. During the development process, a bank has to make sure that its administration, transaction, and risk management departments can deal with the product. For a new derivative product, for instance, product development would comprise philosophy, target group, pricing, and profitability as well as the fit to accounting standards, a risk/return assessment, and the appropriate transaction mechanisms.

Branding and Marketing: Afterwards, depending on the product's sophistication and complexity, it might be branded and marketed specifically. The customer base would be segmented and the target group selected, and positioning, pricing, POS activities, and possible additional product features would be determined.

Branding includes corporate branding such as all efforts to select the appropriate brand architecture and establish and maintain the corporate brand(s).

Sales: Next, the product needs to be sold. Distribution channels and POS (point-of-sales) must be chosen and the customer interaction and detailed pricing per channel must be defined and prepared. Clerks might also have to be trained. At this point, the actual sale takes place and the customer orders the product, for example, initiating a transfer from his account or buying a complex investment product.

As soon as the sales process itself is over, the banking infrastructure starts to process the order/transaction:

Transaction/Administration: Here, the customer's order has to be carried out: A money transfer must actually take place, a share be bought, a loan screened, interest calculated, and the account administered.

Risk Management: Processes must also be initiated to record the transaction internally and externally. Internally, products and services sold at the front-end must recorded, monitored, and processed. Externally, risk exposure has to be reported to the legal authorities (for instance BAFin in Germany) on a regular basis (mostly daily, weekly, or monthly). At the same time, risk exposure is reduced internally by asset liability management (ALM) or externally by transfer on the interbank or capital markets.

Client Management: Finally, the customer relationship needs to be managed and clients targeted according to their needs. Client management includes anything done to induce cross-selling and make the customer buy additional products, for example mailings, targeted calls, or product ads on the web site.

Exhibit 9: Overview of the Retail Banking Value Chain Steps

Step	Definition
Product Development	Design of the product and the necessary infrastructure/ transaction
Marketing/Branding	Product branding and marketing, corporate branding
Sales	Distribution incl. channel decisions and distribution co-operations, all customer interaction at the POS
Transaction/Administration	Internal process to produce the product: actually carrying out the customers' orders
Risk Management	Processes parallel to the transaction to record it internally and externally. Transfer of risk internally (e. g. ALM) or externally (e. g. on interbank or capital markets)
Client Management	Anything done to sell an additional product to an existing client

To understand the individual steps of the value chain, we will look at each of their trends and drivers, methods of differentiation, key success factors, and opportunities for outsourcing. Most importantly, we will look for best practices and for successes and failures of certain concepts both inside and outside of the financial services industry.

Product Development – Quality is Not as »In« as You Think!

Future challenges:
- *Moving the focus away from differentiation and towards cost efficiency*
- *Continuing to develop better products*

The emergence of new players like supermarket banks has shown that differentiation via products or product quality is not necessary for a bank to be successful. As there are economies of scale and scope, product development is an area where outsourcing can reduce costs. At the same time, bundling product development with fewer specialized players (insourcers) can lead to a deeper understanding of the customers and the markets, thus enabling the development of better and more profitable products.

For a long time, product development has not been a major issue for retail banks. »Banking R&D«, if you ever could call it that, has focused on process innovation, new distribution channels (for example on-line banking), or complex corporate banking products. The standard product spectrum of retail banking has remained largely unchanged over the years.

This has changed recently due to three main factors. First, life expectancy is growing continuously, and – together with some state-run pension systems in Europe that are almost expected to break down before today's payers become receivers – this has prompted old age provisions to become more and more of an issue. Second, more people are now becoming wealthy enough, especially through inheritance, to become interested in affluent retail banking and are expecting corresponding products and services. Third, the average retail customer has also become increasingly sophisticated and expects to invest in more than just a savings account. As the Internet bubble has burst, thereby abolishing expectations of continuous double-digit annual returns, the focus has now shifted toward safety and the risk/return profiles of investments.

Today, banks still develop all their products in-house, the rationale being that »better products«, i. e. those with better performance, lower prices, or both, will help to attract and keep customers. Looking at the success of the new entrants who are focusing on the customer interface – for example Tesco Personal Finance and Virgin Money – begs the question of whether this hypothesis needs to be re-evaluated, if not set aside altogether. These new competitors have managed to attract new clients despite offering only standard, off-the-shelf products.

If the quality of products is not what attracts and retains customers and if – as we are going to argue in the remainder of this chapter – customers feel more attracted by brands, clever client management, and convenient distribution channels than they do by products, then product development loses the importance it is implicitly given today through being carried out in-house. This means product development could be sourced out if it makes the process more cost efficient, provided that viable business models for product-development companies exist.

Cost advantages of outsourcing usually result from the economies of scale (decreases in per-unit cost as a result of increases in output, for example, lower prices for purchased goods or lower administration costs per product) and/or economies of scope inherent in the outsourced process (the costs of producing products are interdependent, such that producing one good lowers the cost of producing another). Product development is not a mass production like many banking transactions. Nevertheless, economies of scale and scope exist in that experienced players have an advantage in virtually everything that makes a good product developer. Product development differentiates itself primarily along two dimensions. The first way is through more innovative ideas, connections, or partnerships to combine the building blocks needed to form more attractive offerings. The second way is through better capabilities to calculate the conditions of the products in order to offer cheaper prices while still making a profit. The preciseness with which product conditions can be calculated depends on how well the future can be predicted and therefore on the quality of the underlying risk tables. What is required is a better macroeconomic understanding, earlier detection of trends, and a better understanding of customers and their preferences, histories, and risks. These key success factors favor experienced players, who have had time to develop tools, build connections, and understand both the products and the market. Thus, as economies of scale and scope do exist, outsourcing product development to an external company should reduce costs while yielding at least the same if not better quality.

In particular, small and medium-sized banks can gain from outsourcing product development. Significant differences also exist between European countries regarding the efficiency of product development. In France, for example, product development cycles are reported to be four times faster than in Germany. In such a case, outsourcing the process to a more experienced, and more efficient, specialist can help to bring less efficient players up to speed.

Outsourcing, with its consequence of concentrating processes in fewer players, will also result in opportunities to develop more attractive products, that is, with better performance or lower prices. Consider the case of one specific reinsurance company. Reinsurers reinsure primary insurers against their losses. In this way, the risk of financial burden from loss events can be spread throughout the market and borne by many shoulders. Reinsurers can live with lower margins than the primary insurers – and therefore are able to make money out of their deals – because their business is less risky. This lower risk stems from their wider exposure across businesses, target groups, and geographies, the fact that they have better ratings and therefore lower refinancing costs, and because they have more experience and a better understanding of the market.

The specific reinsurer we would like to use as example focuses on the area of property and casualty reinsurance and, like any reinsurance, covers risks for many different primary insurers. Recently, the company has started to aggregate their customers' anonymous data, i.e. information about the insured risks and the occurring loss events, while respecting client confidentiality. Having access to a much wider and more diverse sample of data than the individual primary insurers, the company is able to achieve a better understanding of the underlying mechanisms and risks, and uses this deeper understanding to design specific *primary* insurance products, i.e.

catered to its own customers' customers. These products are offered to the primary insurers to sell to their mass-market clients. Using its possibility to aggregate data across various primary insurers, the company was therefore able to develop better products than its own clients, despite the fact that it is not active in the market of primary insurances.

Transferring this to the retail banking market reveals a vast untapped potential. Wherever outsourcing happens on a larger scale – be it in product development or transactions/production – the insourcer gains access to information that enables him to develop products from a much better understanding of the underlying patterns, risks, and developments. Even though the »quality« of the products will be of lesser concern within the overall retail banking operations of the future, innovation, even beyond today's possibilities, will be granted in this new world of outsourcing.

Branding and Marketing – Do (Retail) Banks Really Have a Brand?

Future challenges:
- *Branding a retail bank*
- *When and why to introduce product brands*
- *Aligning brand and customer experience*

Most banks have a weak brand which is built on technical rather than on emotional differentiation. As a technical brand message is easy to overstretch and does not yield strong customer loyalty in a business with as few tangible differentiations as banking, banks will have to learn to build emotional brands. To achieve more specific positioning, product brands can be used for specific services. In addition, banks will have to pay attention to aligning the actual customer experience with their brand message.

People buy Evian instead of Volvic, or vice versa; they swear by The Gap, Benneton, or Calvin Klein; they purchase expensive sneakers from Nike, even if they have no money at all; they smoke Marlboro, Gauloises, or walk an extra mile to buy Camels; they refuse to switch to Pepsi, even if they preferred it to Coca-Cola in the blind test. But they still choose their bank according to which branch is the closest: 60 to 65 percent quote the proximity of a branch as the main factor to chose a bank, five to ten percent are looking for a large national or international network and cash availability, and the remainder wants good on-line or telephone accessibility plus the ability to withdraw cash nearby free of charge[2]. Seemingly, compared to many other industries, banks do not have a strong brand to attract customers, and customers feel little loyalty towards their bank. It is largely the switching costs that keep clients where they are. The only part of a bank's brand that seems to instill the necessary trust is the word »bank«. Is it a matter of banking services being too similar? About there being no room for differentiation? Think about mineral water: yes, Perrier is decidedly different from Evian. But Evian from Volvic? Still, each has its loyal customer group.

Banks, differently than all other products mentioned above, have sold themselves mostly on the basis of technical competence and reliability. A slightly different product, slightly better access, slightly better conditions, these are the messages on which bank marketing seems to focus. Despite the efforts to point out the differences, to the customers the products are too similar so that banks have to seek differentiation via price, increasing the already existing margin pressure. In comparison, how often have you heard Marlboro, Coca-Cola, or Evian focus on the performance, the objective differentiation of their product? Instead, all of them have tried to build a feeling around their products and portray a lifestyle with their brand. For example, the rough Marlboro cowboy versus the unconventional Gauloises rebel. Customers rarely choose one taste over the other. In the example of cigarettes, they choose the image of freedom over rebellion or vice versa.

Is it possible at all to create brands around a product as vague as retail banking? Even less tangible and accessible products have been successful, as Intel has shown. Intel processors are about as inaccessible as today's products go. For the final user, they are a complete black box, one where it is not even clear what exactly it does. You cannot see it, you do not really know how it functions or what it looks like, and you do not even really understand how it is manufactured. As far as the user is concerned, it is there, and it works. Yet, with its »Intel Inside« campaign, introduced in 1991, Intel has managed to create a powerful brand and strong consumer awareness. In 1998, Ashton Brand Group reported that the brand recognition of the Intel name among mainstream consumers jumped from only 22 percent to an astounding 80 percent within two years of initiating the campaign. Market research conducted by the company showed that consumers were willing to spend 300 US Dollars more per chip than on comparable products in the marketplace, roughly a 50 percent premium, for the peace of mind of knowing that they have »Intel Inside«. Intel is now established as the world's number four brand, after Coca-Cola, Disney, and McDonald's[3]. Besides generating consumer awareness and trust, and thus being able to reap this hefty price premium, Intel has succeeded with this campaign in further cementing its position as the undisputed worldwide market leader with a market share of now over 83 percent[4].

Recently, HypoVereinsbank was the first German bank to really try to create an emotionally based corporate brand. »Live. We look after the details« arguably was as good or bad as any retail banking slogan. However, their recent series of TV trailers was clearly aimed at creating a purely emotional response. Different spots of only four to seven seconds in length showed a well known young German actor as a movie projectionist pondering questions that had a somewhat absurd touch – they were completely unrelated not only to banking but often to pretty much everything else including the film that followed: »Why can't the world revolve around *me*?«, »Why does nobody ever notice the madman in the backseat?«, »Why are flashbacks always black and white? I personally remember in color!«, »Which came first? Movies or popcorn?«, »I think they could make a lot of money with movie snacks that don't rustle«, or »What would we align our sofas with if we didn't have TV sets?« are typical lines from the campaign, which left many viewers smiling and with a feeling of sympathy towards the brand.

Brands in retail banking often have an additional weakness. Beyond the overall issue of not having very strong brands, retail banks often tend to try to stretch their brand to include all targeted customer groups and business segments. In addition, the chosen marketing attributes are usually not very unique, leading to even less differentiation possibilities. As a result, the brand becomes unfocused, or even overstretched, and many target groups cannot relate to it.

On a company-wide international level and across business units, this is a classical question of brand architecture. Brand architecture requires significant attention especially in M&A scenarios and will therefore be covered in depth in Chapter 5. The individual local retail customer, however, cares little about brand architecture, as he is exposed to a small fraction of the overall concept only. He cares about a company and products and services he can relate to, whether or not the retail businesses in the rest of the world or the investment banking operations have the same brand[5].

Deutsche Bank has recently given an example of not brand-, but »campaign-overstretch«. In September 1999, Deutsche Bank introduced »Leading to results« as the slogan for the entire business: wholesale, i.e. corporate, and institutional customers, retail, private banking, and asset management. As a bank's results for its clients are highly dependent on the development of the markets, Deutsche Bank's – as any other bank's – results were devastated when the stock bubble burst. Whether their results were comparatively better than the market or not was not important anymore. The clients were angry. Since then, the campaign has been limited to private banking only, where a limited number of affluent clients valued Deutsche Bank's services and could be managed in a more personal way. Having one brand or positioning for the entire business need not be a problem – as long as it is an emotional and not a technical positioning. However, stretching a technical message too far can become problematic.

Although retail banking makes up only a small fraction of the overall banking world, the various customer groups to be catered to are almost invariably too diverse to feel attracted by the same, often somewhat vague positioning. Two routes can be taken. In the first approach, described in Monitor's »center of gravity« concept, the brand is focused explicitly towards one main customer segment, but »docking areas« are provided for a handful of other customer groups. For example, while Nike focuses its campaigns on serious athletes, clever emotionally oriented ads and diverse but easily recognizable product designs allow a plethora of other users to identify with the concept: Many customer groups relate to the brand, from image conscious teenagers and everyday comfort wearers to urban youths and male baby boomer weekend athletes.

In the second approach, product brands can be used to create a focused positioning towards a specific customer group. Especially in consumer goods, the corporate brands almost vanish behind the much more visible product brands: Philip Morris markets 74 cigarette brands in 180 countries, among them brands as well known as Marlboro, Philip Morris (yes, that is a company name *and* a product brand), and Virginia Slims. Similarly, British American Tobacco sells Lucky Strike, Dunhill, Rothmans, Peter Stuyvesand, and others. The two competitors even share one product brand, Benson & Hedges, which they distribute in mutually exclusive regions. In all cases, the marketing focuses exclusively on the product, not on the companies. This allows for differentiated positioning, target groups, point-of-sales activities, and the like. However, in retail banking only few efforts have been made so far in this direction. We predict this to change, especially as product brands offer an additional valuable advantage. As innovative and non-traditional distribution channels become increasingly important, a branded product (or service) allows a bank to distribute this one branded, recognizable product through a new channel without having to introduce its entire offer into that channel (or a subset of products, streamlined to the channel and its customers). Again, this allows for more focused, more specific positioning and easier handling of the distribution channels from an organizational point of view.

One example of this strategy are the efforts of the Dutch company Aegon, one of the world's largest listed insurance companies. Instead of trying to enter Germany with its entire product spectrum, Aegon introduced only one product range under the brand name »MoneyMaxx« in 1995. Combining life insurance with mutual fund-based savings, MoneyMaxx offers a regular savings product and specialty savings concepts tailored to education or retirement provisions. Aegon focused on direct distribution and some selected partners like book clubs. The concept has been very successful, and similar product ranges are also available in Italy, Belgium, Spain, and Hungary under the same brand. By introducing one branded product range only, Aegon was able to focus its efforts on a specific positioning, product offering, and distribution channel, avoiding any unnecessary costs. Introducing the concept in other countries is comparatively simple, as – again – the message is simple and the marketing and distribution highly focused.

Other industries have already been using product brands for a long time, but often for a different reason. Product brands can limit or even avoid possible spillover effects in case a product »goes wrong«, i. e. the product flops or somehow causes damage to customers. Back in 1989, when alcohol-free beers were not yet a standard product, the German brewery König Brauerei introduced its first alcohol-free beer under the new brand name Kelts in order to avoid potential negative spillovers. The beer was accepted, and since then all subsequent manufacturers have dared to associate their own brand names with their alcohol-free beers.

Bayer, on the other hand, has learned the hard way what happens if a product is linked to the manufacturer too closely. In 2001, problems occurred with Bayer's blockbuster drug Lipobay, branded Baycol in the US. Both names clearly show the link with the manufacturer. Taking the product, which is prescribed to people with high cholesterol levels, together with certain other drugs – something strictly forbidden in the directions – caused the death of some patients. In August 2001, Bayer took the product off the market worldwide. In a spillover effect, sales of other products plummeted as well.

Finally, branding an (otherwise often dry) banking product also can make it more accessible to clients. For instance, while a checking account usually would not be given a lot of attention, HypoVereinsbank in Germany nevertheless introduced, branded, and marketed a special »3D-account«. This checking account could be accessed in the branch/via paper, by telephone banking, and on-line. In the end there was nothing special about this product. However, by giving it a name and a campaign, clients could relate to it and were made more aware of the offer.

Besides having to catch up both in establishing strong brands and product branding, retail banking faces a third challenge in this area: to establish consistency between the branding message and the customer experience. This is a problem all brand intensive industries face: Unless the customer experience – including product purchase, product design and use, service, and complaint handling – reinforces the brand message and positioning, the brand will not be successful with customers. The consequences range from a somewhat diminished customer loyalty to instant product switching at the next purchase. Such a disappointed customer will be very hard, if not impossible, to win back.

For most retail banks, losing customers is devastating. For years, competition has been about redistributing the market, not about growing it. As a consequence, the costs of acquiring new clients are especially high. Traditional brick and mortar banks are estimated to have customer acquisition costs of usually between 300 and 1 000 Euros[6]. For on-line banks, costs can be as low as 20 US Dollars[7], but can reach up to over 600 Euros as well[8]. Many players quote values of around 200 to 300 Euros. Therefore, for most banks, the loss of a customer is very expensive to compensate.

United Airlines' (UAL) marketing campaign »United Rising« was a good example of how not to do branding. In 1997, UAL started its new campaign, announcing plans to put the customer at the center of attention and to surpass other airlines, particularly in the areas of punctuality, service, and customer care. The US Department of Transportation's analyses of 1998 and 1999 airline performance reveal the reality behind the campaign. Concerning on-time arrivals for these two years, UAL was in places seven and six out of the ten US airlines with at least one percent of total domestic scheduled-service passenger revenues. Regarding customer complaints per 100 000 enplanements, United came in seventh and fifth, again out of ten. In both measures and both years, their performance was below average. From October 20 1998 to November 15 2001, roughly three years United had received a total of 3 842 passengers complaints, the vast majority of which had been copied to either the Director of Customer Relations or the Chairman and CEO. A mere 58 of these complaints ever received a reply. Public reactions referred to the campaign as full of hot air and as the biggest joke of 1999. United abandoned this campaign, some say abruptly, in October 1999. This was probably for the better, as by end of 2000 UAL had fallen back to tenth and ninth place respectively for punctuality and number of customer complaints.

Some companies get it right. The Swedish furniture company IKEA International has shown how to establish a clear positioning and support it with both consistent marketing and an authentic customer experience. Prepared by the advertising, customers are very aware of the Swedish origin of the company and thus expect – and get – furniture and accessories of a typically Nordic design. The high »do it yourself« portion of the experience is supported by the young, hip, and unconventional positioning and reinforces it. Overall, all parts of the customer experience form a consistent picture that people can relate to and that has been successful worldwide. Interestingly enough, this strong brand managed to generate and then maintain IKEA's popularity despite the relatively low product quality, and sometimes even quality problems, that the company experienced for many years. In 2000, IKEA was the world's largest retailer in home furniture and furnishings with twice the market share of their nearest competitor[9]. Thus, a strong brand built by intelligent branding and marketing can act as an insurance against mishaps, whether it is a somewhat persistent one, as with IKEA, or a short-term, but well-handled one, as with the former Daimler-Benz's new, unstable A-Class in 1997.

Lufthansa offers another example of an interesting and – especially recently – successful positioning. At a time when other airlines for years have marketed their superior services – wider seats or rows in economy class, bigger and better designed seats in business or first class, better food, better in-flight entertainment, larger screens, or just a more friendly service level among staff – Lufthansa focused on safety and reliability. Fly Lufthansa once, and you will see that on transcontinental routes, their service is very similar to that of the competitors. However, being a German company, they were aware of what the customers would believe and, especially, what they would not. The positioning aimed at a niche the company knew it could not only deliver but also market in a believable way.

More generally, the similarities between the retail banking and the airline industry are striking. Both sell highly comparable products with the possibility to differentiate only via add-ons and service. Different from retail banking, however, airlines started to consciously focus on brand building and differentiating via service levels a long time ago – to such a degree, in fact, that differentiation is much less clear than the industry would like it to be.

The key point of these examples is as follows: branding, marketing, and positioning must be both believable and supported by a coherent customer experience. If building the brand has been successful, it can be a powerful aid in weathering storms of misfortunes.

Regarding consistency, however, retail banking faces an even greater challenge than other industries. Compared to other industries, retail banking uses a wider range of distribution channels to distribute a more diverse range of products. On the product side this includes everything from physical cash, account statements, or traveler's checks to transactions like transfers or securities trading to advice concerning investment strategy or retirement provisions. In addition to branches, ATMs, telephone banking, and on-line banking, there are third party distributors who are entirely beyond control. Nevertheless, customers expect the bank's performance to be not only consistent in itself, but also consistent with the brand positioning across the entire spectrum of products and channels.

To give an example, several US American and German on-line banks have overpromised and underdelivered when it came to adding »bricks to the clicks«. Promising a »real, living« customer interface to give advisory services and to thus complement their web-based offer, the outlets were seen as impersonal and uninviting. Employees seemed to be hiding behind their desks rather than approaching the clients and actively addressing their needs. Both compared to the promises made, as well as to the competence, comfort, and user friendliness on the web sites, the customer experience in the outlets was disappointing. While expected to help penetrate the growth barriers experienced by the on-line banks when the Internet bubble burst, the branches were unable to deliver. For lack of success, some on-line banks even have decided to close their outlets again.

HSBC provides a good example of a bank with a strong brand image. In 1998, the company made the strategic decision to create a unified brand for the entire company, using the HSBC name and the red hexagon symbol. This effort, which was estimated to cost approximately 50 million US Dollars (excluding advertising) in changes to branch signage and interiors, checkbooks, credit cards, forms, stationery, and marketing materials, sought to position the bank as a global firm with a local footprint. Since that time, HSBC has maintained a consistent look and feel to its operations around the world, comprising a total of 7 000 offices in 81 countries. A recent international ad campaign stresses the company's international coverage and suggests that HSBC's intimate local knowledge gives them an advantage over outsider institutions. HSBC maintains a policy of staffing offices with local people in order to promote this intimate local knowledge. Marketing efforts stress the international scope of operations as a competitive advantage in today's global marketplace, calling the organization »the world's local bank«. HSBC claims to have local banks in more countries than anyone else, exemplifying its success in becoming a truly global bank.

Whether one is referring to an entire banking brand or to a product brand, a brand can be successful only in reaching its intended target group(s) if the customers receive the treatment they were led to expect. In this case treatment refers to all activities carried out towards the customer: products, services, communication, and marketing. The brand acts as a visible figurehead for everything a retail bank wants to offer to its client. Conversely, every action has a direct influence on a bank's image and therefore the brand itself. Especially in banking, where differentiation along tangible dimensions is so difficult, and where differentiation through emotional brand messages has not been utilized much so far, the active alignment of brand and customer experience is imperative to support the building of strong future retail banking brands.

Looking ahead, if banks do not want to risk losing customers – less to each other but increasingly to the wave of new entrants – they will have to face the challenges in branding just described. These challenges are building a robust brand that is able to attract customers and create customer loyalty, adding product brands where necessary in order to enable focused positioning, and supporting all branding efforts with well-aligned processes and customer interactions. Branding will have to be at the heart of any retail bank that chooses to compete actively on the customer interface.

Sales – Do (Better) or Die (Slowly)

Future challenges:
- *Building and using new channels: how and where to sell banking products*
- *Managing channels profitably*
- *Focus on solutions rather than products*

Over the last years banks have opened new channels and changed their branch concepts to make access to banking and banking itself easier and more appealing. As the success of, among others, supermarket banks has shown however, customers seem to like banking to be inserted into their daily routines more seamlessly than any stand-alone bank can ever achieve. Distribution cooperations will fill this gap.

In order to maximize profitability while not losing valuable customers, the various channels need to be managed intelligently, for example by introducing price spreads between channels. In addition, as part of a truly customer focused organization, the focus has to be shifted from selling products to selling solutions and truly addressing the clients' needs.

Doing sales well, i.e. providing the customer with a positive purchase experience, is not an easy task. The right product needs to be distributed through the right channels, where »right« means »in line with customer needs and preferences«. Potential purchasers need to be given as much information about the product as they require, and the purchase itself must be easy and hassle free. Especially for standard purchases, customers want to solve a particular problem rather than to acquire a particular item. When it comes to providing a positive purchase experience, luxury items have a good position as their margins are large enough to make personalized service possible. But what about standardized products? Starbucks and Amazon, the on-line retailer, show the way.

If you ever tried to buy just a coffee at Starbucks, you know what happens: »Would you like a flavor in this?«, »Would you like some cream on top?«, or »Would you like a croissant with that?« are the standard responses. Many customers hesitate for a moment and then answer yes, obviously having been convinced to add something to their purchase that they had not thought of purchasing originally. In a convenient channel that solves the problem of having a good coffee without having a lot of time, Starbucks sells their products in a quick and efficient way – and manages to sell the customer more than he might have wanted. In addition, in their stores they display – and, obviously, one can purchase – everything from Starbucks cups, coffee, and the CDs they are playing to Starbucks-branded coffee machines. Amazon, on the other hand, is excellent at offering potential buyers advice about the products. For their products – including books, CDs, Videos, DVDs, and Computer programs – they not only publish their own review, they also invite the customers to contribute their personal reviews which are then made public for everyone to read. Admittedly, this is an easy task in the efficient world of the Internet. Nevertheless, it makes shopping at Amazon a pleasant experience. Retail banks, however, have not become very good yet at making their customers' purchasing experience a pleasant one.

For the last two decades, retail banks have been mainly concerned about and working on opening new channels: first the emergence of ATMs and service terminals during the eighties, plus Minitel in France, then the addition of telephone access via call centers, and finally the emergence of on-line banking during the late nineties. The next channels banks are getting into include WAP access, 3G/UMTS, and interactive digital TV (iDTV), which has been a success mainly in the UK already[10], where the penetration of iDTV is estimated to reach over 40 percent of all households in 2003. All these innovations are increasingly catering to the technologically literate. However, many customers still rely predominantly on the traditional branch network and ATMs.

To cater to these customers, some traditional retail banks have started to think about radically new branch concepts – but mainly in response to the new entrants at the customer interface, such as Tesco Personal Finance and Virgin Money.

Washington in the US, the sixth largest banking company and largest savings institution, has decided to introduce a new branch concept under the name of »Occasio« in order to offer clients a more relaxed and customer-centric atmosphere. Having their stores designed by Dayton-based Design Forum, which designed the Disney stores as well, Washington Mutual has created a true retail experience, even referring to their locations as Occasio »stores« rather than branches. Instead of teller windows there are computer kiosks where employees and customers can jointly view account information and withdraw cash. Tellers have been eliminated entirely, and employees work on the retail floor to help customers and sell products. A »store within a store« approach allows separate products such as investments or home loans to have specialized areas for customers to learn and purchase.

Washington Mutual reports that Occasio branches have a higher loan production than traditional branches, are signing up new checking accounts at double the rate, and have deposits running at about triple the rate.

There are currently over 200 Occasio locations in the US, and Washington Mutual plans to make all of its retail centers Occasio stores.

Abbey National, the 6th largest bank in the UK, has also worked on their branches in a variety of ways. In July 2000, Abbey National teamed up with Costa Coffee to offer cafes inside some branch locations. At the end of 2002, the company had 25 branches with in-store cafes. While this concept is aimed at changing the customer experience profoundly, Abbey National also started a new program that targeted customer satisfaction in a more subtle way and at the same time improved internal efficiency and productivity. In 2000, Abbey National launched a scheme to begin franchising its branches. Initially, the program involved »internal franchising« to employees, without a transfer of ownership. This produced impressive results, with a sales increase pre-to post-franchising of on average 28 percent[11]. In 2001, the bank extended the model to »external franchising«: Managers are given a 49 percent ownership stake and the respective branches are made wholly owned subsidiaries, i. e. autonomously operating businesses. The sales increase amounted to another eight to 38 percent in comparison to »internal franchises«. The bank estimates it will generate up to an additional 30 million British Pounds a year in increased sales and cost savings[12], and by end of 2002 had extended the model to roughly 50 percent of its branch network.

Obviously, other banks can learn a great deal from these examples on how to attract new customers and more volume through unconventional new concepts. Whether the cost-benefit ratio of these new concepts is as high as that of traditional branches, however, remains open, as no separate data is publicly available.

ING Direct Makes Retail Banking Easy

ING Direct is ING's fully owned subsidiary for direct banking, that is on-line and telephone banking. ING Direct started business in Canada in 1997. Since then, six countries have been added: Spain, Australia, France, US, Italy, and Germany (in cooperation with DiBa and now Entrium). Currently, ING Direct Cafés exist in the US, Canada, Spain, and Italy.

Arkadi Kuhlmann is President and CEO of ING Direct USA. The first statement you hear from him when asking about ING Direct is »high volume, low margin«. And »We make banking easy, as easy – and as much fun – as having a cup of coffee«. During the interview, these viewpoints are repeated several times, and this is intentional. All banks claim to aim at the same objectives: good service, high cross-selling rates, long customer relationships. For Kuhlmann, the difference lies in the execution: »You have to be evangelic about this, like Apple was in the eighties« he claims. »It is all about creating a new culture in the company«. Success proves him right. ING Direct entered the US only in 2000 and already has over one million customers. ING Direct is the US's fastest growing retail bank with new accounts opening at a rate of 60 000 per month and savings deposits growing at 500 million US Dollars per month.

The philosophy behind the concept is simple: ING Direct wants to be the »take-away fast-food place« of retail banking. The product line is standardized and limited, with a focus on savings products, but the quality of the product is excellent: The interest rates on the savings accounts are high, there are no fees, the value proposition is good. ING Direct can afford to give good rates due to their uncompromising focus on easy processes and easy to handle customers. »Easy to handle customers« means no discussion about terms or interest rates, very limited use of the telephone hotline, no extra services, and no extra costs. Customers who do not fulfill this profile are politely asked to close their accounts. Three quarters of the »sinners« pout and leave, one quarter change behavior and stay. »Two telephone calls a month eat up our entire margin on an average account«, Kuhlmann justifies this strategy. »You cannot expect the service of a gourmet restaurant in a fast food place. Our business model is not designed to deliver that. *We* deliver excellent *fast-food* service!«

The system seems to work. 38 percent of ING Direct's US customers come through word of mouth. Together with very targeted marketing, this leads to customer acquisition costs of only 70 US Dollars. The competition has around 300 US Dollars acquisition costs for standard products such as checking accounts.

The four ING Direct Cafés in the US are an important part of the system. Here, customers can enjoy a coffee in a relaxed atmosphere and do their banking at the same time. The cafés are designed to be bright and clean, and to give a fresh and crisp feel. Corporate orange is ubiquitous. The waiters act as »bank salesmen« as well – to call them clerks would be misleading. »We don't hire bankers for this job, we hire from retail businesses. It is much easier to train a retailer in banking products than make a banker think retail«, Kuhlmann remarks. Internal processes are also streamlined for cost efficiency. The waiters focus on servicing and selling and the administration is done centrally.

The cafes act as a physical interface to the customers, and, together with the merchandise operations, provide additional marketing for ING Direct: Customers experience the »living« brand. »We sell 50 000 US Dollars worth of coffee and merchandise a month.« Kuhlmann points out. Currently, 800 to 1 000 visitors come to the cafés each day. Place your bet how high this figure will rise once the new location in Coconut Grove, Florida is open ...

The central question is, however, whether this answer to the new »customer interface-competitors« aims at the right level, that is at the source of the

The European
Retail Banking
Landscape in the
Future

threat. What is the root cause of success of these new entrants? Is it just about providing the customer with a more relaxed and casual environment for his banking transactions? Is it about giving him a more familiar and more emotional brand to identify with? The rationale may lie deeper: Ultimately, virtually no one really wants a banking product. People want a car, not a loan. They want to access their cash virtually anytime, but they do not want an ATM. They buy a house, not a mortgage. Perhaps the only banking products that really satisfy a deep human need and that people are fundamentally interested in, because of the large potential impact on their future are long term investments, retirement provisions, and certain fundamental insurance products. Such products satisfy a need for security. Everything else is just »necessary hassle«, something which is essential to enable other transactions in today's world. The new entrants at the customer interface, probably without even being aware of this paradigm, have put retail banking where it is emotionally for most people – in the back seat.

This is not to say that retail banking is not important and that it does not have a fundamental role to play in today's economies, both from an economic and a client's point of view. It just raises the question how customers want to be addressed, where, how, and in which environment they want to do their banking, and ultimately what shape the future sales and distribution environment will take.

There is no question that there will be many, and many successful, forms of sales and distribution. Regarding the products that satisfy fundamental needs, only a few, likely technology-literate customers might ever be willing to do without a face-to-face conversation. Most likely, these products will always require branches, service centers, and the like. What we should be looking at are all the other products that require no advice, such as checking accounts, transfers, savings accounts, credit cards, or consumer loans. These products form the backbone of any retail bank and, interestingly enough, the complete product spectrum of most of the new entrants, even if they often add some bread-and-butter, off-the-shelf insurance products. For these »necessary« products, including the basic insurance products mentioned, the new entrants seem to have found a more appealing way to satisfy customer needs. They are simply offering them as one product within a larger product range of daily necessities.

The electronic banking unit of CIBC of Canada has perhaps perfected this approach in its partnership with the Toronto supermarket giant Loblaw Cos. Ltd. Using Loblaw's powerful President's Choice brand for their financial service offer puts them right next to President's Choice cheese, President's Choice crackers, and President's Choice tea. It literally makes banking a product like any other; simple, off-the-shelf, and with a powerful own label denoting good quality at a comparatively low price. Since its launch in 1998, President's Choice Financial has signed up about one million customers and is expected to become profitable in 2003.

Retail banks might have to get used to the thought that one of the best channels for their non-advice products might be one that is not theirs: cooperations with external distributors like retailers, bookshops or clubs, automotive associations, and airlines, which would offer such banking products under the distributor's brand.

In the long term, all of these branch and physical distribution concepts might be regarded as stone age banking. Future technologies might replace all need for physical contact, identification may become electronic, and retail banking as ubiquitous and portable as today's mobile phones. Until then, however, physical locations will continue to be necessary. Customers need to be served, and market shares built and maintained in order to be in a good position for when the new world of retail banking arrives.

Once the retail banks have built their channels and possibly supplemented them with external distribution channels like retailers, the main future challenge in multi-channel banking will be how to combine the various channels to reap the maximum cost benefits. Trying to get the customers to buy the products and services over the respectively cheapest channel while at the same time excelling at fulfilling the customers' demands is a demanding combination of objectives.

Closing certain channels for certain products and offering, for example, transfers just over the phone and on-line, would certainly be a wrong move. Many traditional clients would simply refuse to move to these newer technologies and would rather switch banks. Nevertheless, banks will have to analyze their detailed cost structures by products and by channels well enough to be able to price additional costs for certain product/channel combinations into the single products or the product combinations designed to address specific target groups.

Some banks have already started this as far as money transfers or trading and brokerage are concerned. For example, doing transactions via service terminals or on-line may result in a refund in case of transfers, and lower commissions and account management fees in the case of trading and brokerage. As these are the most transaction focused services a bank offers, it is natural that the efforts to move clients to more cost efficient channels have started here.

However, merely shifting technology-savvy customers between electronic channels is only part of the solution. The hurdles are somewhat higher when it comes to convincing your own grandmother to move away from a face to a machine. Many customers today still use the branches to receive services they could easily get in a more automated fashion, thus wasting valuable manpower. If one were to watch the traffic at a counter, one would see numerous clients withdrawing small to medium-size amounts of cash, well below the threshold level that would prevent them from using the ATM located within the same branch. Others hand in paper slips for money transfers, even though they often do not need the bank's stamp to certify that the transfer has taken place. In some banks, customers can access a standard savings account via a small booklet only, not by a customer service card or the like. The consequence is that many clients show up at the branch at the beginning of each month to have their newly accumulated interest payments recorded in the booklet. This does not even include the several additional visits to withdraw or deposit savings. Some customers even come in and hand their service card to the clerks in order to have them pull out their new account statement, when they could get it themselves at the service terminal located in the same hall. In all these transactions, precious manpower is wasted both during the customer interactions themselves and the administration induced by the manual, paper-based processes. The ratio of administrative work to client interaction and sales is estimated to be 70/30 for the average bank teller[13].

So far, most traditional retail banks are not putting the right disincentives on such behavior. Even though it would be a highly unpopular measure, withdrawing cash, handing in paper based money transfers, or getting one's account statement at the counter should incur extra fees for the customer in line with the extra expenses incurred by the bank. Slowly, some retail banks are starting to introduce such pricing schemes. In addition, bank products should be changed in order to enable clients to manage them without using the capacity of the bank's employees. The original, manual products should either be abolished or should be made more expensive. Ultimately, every bank will have to judge separately whether introducing these tough changes would be worthwhile, due to their positive impact on the cost structure, or rather devastating, as customer losses would be likely to occur. Only an intimate understanding of one's customers and their preferences can prevent making the wrong decision.

In addition, the principle of trying to move customers to more efficient channels can be carried further; for example the pure exchange of information for a credit or credit card application could be done on-line and followed up by a personal meeting, resulting in a one-time refund or cheaper rates. Signatures might be collected by any branch in the network or electronically, once the technology for electronic identification and signature is available. Before that, signatures could also be verified via other, more convenient and ubiquitous channels like, for example, the postal branches. In the German »PostIdent Verfahren«, for instance, post offices are authorized and enabled to certify the identity of a person and his signature. This service is mainly used by those banks that do not have a wide branch network like on-line banks. Mortgage applications could be handled on-line, providing the necessary information about both the applicant and the property, thus resulting in lower rates. And we are not necessarily talking about introducing lower rates, but introducing a price spread, i. e. sometimes increasing the rates for using less efficient channels.

In the end, the challenge of profitable channel management will be met best by those players who know their costs, know their client segments and what they can ask of their customers (and what they cannot), and have built enough incentives (for example a strong brand) to make customers stay, switch channels, or accept higher prices. Being able to combine channels in an innovative and cost-efficient way will be a significant competitive advantage, as it allows retail banks to focus both efforts and financial resources to improved services and the customer interface, exactly those areas where future competition will be most fierce.

Currently, very few banks know their customers well. Virgin Money has provided an interesting example of how beneficial a good understanding of one's customer base can be. Compared to other banks, Virgin's index mutual funds are quite expensive. Of all 62 index funds available in the UK, only seven are more expensive than Virgin's, six are priced equally, and 34 are cheaper[14]. For the remaining 14, either no charges were given or the given charges were not comparable due to a combination of higher initial and lower annual charges. Nevertheless, Virgin's mutual funds are a success. Not only does the strong Virgin brand lead specific client segments to accept the higher pricing, the company also knows its customer base well enough to be able to exploit this brand strength and transform it into higher, but still acceptable, prices.

After setting up all required sales channels and having managed these in the most cost-effective way, banks finally need to adapt their offers to the changing demands of their customers. Customer loyalty today is not based on client satisfaction and product or service benefits, but on a lack of better

The European
Retail Banking
Landscape in the
Future

alternatives. Banks have tried to understand their customers better and cater to them by increasing market research, widening the product offer, accelerating development cycles, and introducing customer relationship management (CRM). Nevertheless, whether in the general approach to product development or the individual sales interaction, most banks are still trying to fit the client's problem to their products rather than their products to the client's problem; they still sell products rather than solutions, and are product-driven rather than demand-driven.

This is surprising, as banks know rather well how to sell solutions to their wealthier clients. Active asset management today is a standard offer of private banks catering to high net-worth individuals. On the retail side, similar solutions should be found – and they need not be as expensive as personnel-intensive asset management.

One such solution might be to offer a truly open architecture when it comes to selling investment products. Especially during the recent share price bubble, retail banks were very keen to sell the client their house-made mutual funds. The performance of these funds disappointed many customers, not only during the stock market crash, but also because many banks simply could not offer the same performance as competitors' funds. Regarding mutual funds and investments more generally, the trust in retail banks was eroded significantly. Realizing their mistakes, many retail banks claimed to change their strategy towards a more open architecture. While you can get most mutual funds at most banks today, even though they are not actively sold, the architecture becomes rather less open when it comes to selling high-margin products such as structured investments. As a result, the bank's advice is seen as biased and therefore not trustworthy. The winners of this have been the independent financial advisors, who were able to secure a significant and seemingly permanent market position for themselves despite sometimes not even being truly independent and unbiased.

Similarly, after-sales service often leaves much to be desired. After purchasing an investment product (be it an internal product or that of a competitor), banks often fail to deliver on the technicalities of owning such assets, for example, offering advice on how to fill in tax returns. Note that this could easily be automated, which means that its cost structure would be well below that of active asset management based on human intelligence. In this area, a positive example is the US American Templeton Growth Fund, which regularly sends out clear and useful support on how to fill in respective local tax forms.

Another solution for which a market most definitively exists is long-term investing and retirement provisions. Despite their sales forces' reputation, which is often poor, life insurers have very effectively positioned themselves to make their offers appear personal and valuable. Their corresponding products can therefore command comparatively higher pricing to include the higher advisory costs. Banks, on the other side, often complain that they cannot charge for their advisory services. As long as their perceived value added is as low as it is today, they will not be able to change that.

More generally, retail banks will need to systematically understand their customers' problems and demands and develop their offers from there. They need to adapt their processes and interfaces to cater to their clients' circumstances. They need to deliver their solutions in the most flexible and personalized way possible. They need to gain trust by making the customer feel that his problems have been discussed, understood, and solved. Otherwise, banks will lose their most valuable clients. It is the educated and wealthy who have the most funds to invest or use for retirement provisions. It also is the educated and wealthy who are most willing to switch banks entirely or move parts of their business to other suppliers.

Not losing or – to begin with – acquiring those promising customers must be at the heart of any retail banking strategy. Amazingly, however, most do not specifically address the topic of winning promising customers at the beginning of their retail banking lives. Models of future customer value would need to be used to detect such future high potentials early. Instead of treating these customers according to their current business volume, i. e. with no special focus at all, targeted programs or products could be developed to account for the future potential and offer those clients specific incentives to stay. Germany's MLP used this idea of accounting for future business potential when deciding to acquire students and grow with them into their professional careers.

Overall, retail banks have lost their importance in the customers' lives and, as an article phrased it two years ago, have been reduced to the »financial equivalent of doing the laundry«[15]. Regaining customers' trust (and business) will require a lot of hard work at the sales processes. Retail banks will have to find new ways of distributing their products and services, whether it be through different branch concepts or external distributors. They will also have to manage their channels better so as to work more cost efficiently and have more time for the customers. Finally, they will have to increase their value added for the customers.

Transaction/Administration – Buy Rather Than Make!

Future challenges:
- *Focusing on increasing efficiency: outsourcing, insourcing, and merging*
- *Selecting the appropriate processes to outsource*
- *For specialized players: building a viable insourcing business*

In retail banking, there are many back-office and administrative processes that display economies of scale but are not necessarily sources of competitive advantage. For these processes, increasing efficiency, for example through bundling volumes, must become the main focus. Outsourcing will become the most prominent solution, but works only if the insourcer is not suspected of competing with its clients or of channeling sensitive information to a parent company that might be a competitor.

Generally speaking, customers buy a product because they like its appearance, brand, price, or the service with it. They do not care about what it is made of (except where image or questionable ingredients are concerned) and in general they do not care about where, or by whom it was manufactured (again, as long as the image is not concerned).

Retail banking products are no different. The reliability of the product itself matters, but – similar to other »commodities« – not much else. The rest is branding, image, pricing, service, and accessibility. Once this is clear, the rest becomes obvious: What matters in the transaction, i. e. the actual carrying out of the client's orders, is reliability and cost efficiency. Reliability has to be ensured through high quality processes and control mechanisms. Regarding cost efficiency, at some point the end of the potential benefits of trimming organizations and processes is reached. After that, the answer lies most often in increased volume.

There are three ways of increasing efficiency by bundling volumes; these include buying additional volume (M&A), contracting it in (insourcing volume from other companies to add it to your own), or contracting volume out (outsourcing processes to a more efficient player). The relevant difference between the three is whether the process is kept in-house and the volume enlarged – be it through M&A or insourcing – or whether the process is outsourced to a supplier.

Several criteria must be used to decide which of the strategies is the best (see Exhibit 10: Activity Matrix – Outsourcing Versus In-House Activity). First, only those activities can sensibly be outsourced where the company does not regard the product, process, or know-how in question as a key capability or strategic asset, which provides it with a competitive advantage. Consequently, all other processes where economies of scale can be reaped, but which are not strategic assets requiring tight control, should be sourced out in order to focus critical resources on the more strategic areas. Second, the speed of technological development plays a role. Outsourcing an activity means that the company does not have to worry about keeping pace with technological changes as this responsibility would then be left to the specialist. Third, companies will have to be unusually candid about the level of their capabilities. Are current inefficiencies really caused by subscale operations, or is the organization perhaps not very good at performing that specific activity, in which case outsourcing it to a specialist would increase the efficiency beyond just adding more volume?

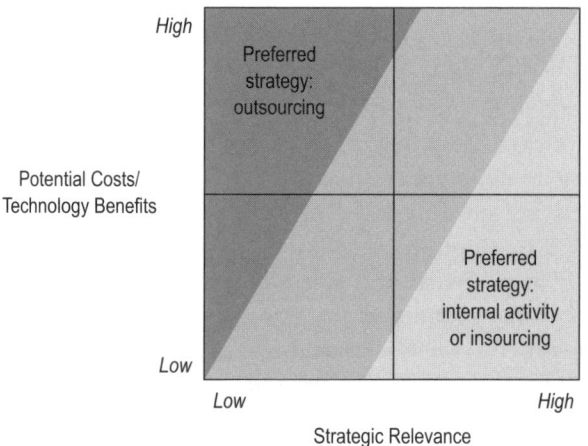

Exhibit 10:   Activity Matrix – Outsourcing Versus In-House Activity

Increasing operational efficiency through larger scale has become commonplace in many industries. As a consequence, outsourcing has grown in scope in recent years from mere »out-tasking« of single components or processes to include strategic alliances in which entire business systems are handed over to an external supplier.

Consider the example of Porsche. Nobody would seriously claim that Porsche builds cars of a lesser quality than average. If anything, it is the opposite. Surprisingly, however, Porsche has a significantly lower vertical range of manufacture than the average car manufacturer: For both the 911 and the Boxster, the vertical range of manufacture amounts to 19 to 20 percent only. For the newer Cayenne, increased outsourcing reduced this figure even further to only between ten and twelve percent. Nevertheless, the company manages to keep its distinct image and high quality standards.

Red Bull, the company which markets the energy drink of the same name, is also a showcase of lean management. Ever since the first sales in 1987, the Austrian company has done nothing in-house except for marketing, communication, controlling, and coordinating production and its (by now enormous) distribution. Red Bull does not own a single bottling plant, warehouse, or truck. Manufacturing is and has been done by only one supplier on three production lines in Austria and a fourth in Switzerland. From there, the small cans are then shipped across most of Europe as well as to Russia, Australia, New Zealand, South Africa, Namibia, Ghana, the United Arab Emirates, Israel, Brazil, the Bahamas, and many other countries. Red Bull is a pure marketing success, pushing its liquid-adrenaline image, which is why marketing is the only major function that will never be outsourced. The sales growth of Red Bull has been astonishing. In its first year of activity in 1987, which was limited to only Austria, Red Bull sold one million cans. In 2001, that number was one billion cans.

For retail banks, the lessons are straightforward. Regarding those back-office and other business processes which are not core competencies, do not offer competitive advantages, and display economies of scale or scope, the focus must be put on increasing efficiency by bundling volume. In retail banking, these conditions appear most evident in the processes of product development and transactions/administration.

Unisys Bets on Outsourcing of Business Processes

Philip Heggie, Unisys Vice President and General Manager UK, Europe and Africa for Global Outsourcing, is certain: The trend towards outsourcing is significant across all industries. In financial services, the major outsourcing field has traditionally been IT. But lately, business processes like check processing, mortgage processing, or account maintenance have been increasingly outsourced as well. So far, Anglo-Saxon countries and the Netherlands have been the fastest to adopt outsourcing, whilst Germany and France have been significantly slower, with the rest of Europe hovering somewhere in between.

»The eighties and early nineties were about systems integration, the late nineties and the early 21st century are about outsourcing. With outsourcing clients shift their investments to us, and we get it back per transaction«, Heggie notes. »In the past decade, this has significantly shifted our business model.«

Apart from financial services, Unisys is also active in communications, transportation, commercial, media, and the public sector. Outsourcing is happening everywhere, and the rate is accelerating. Heggie is sure: »Financial services may be somewhat of a late starter in this, but once it takes off, they will display an even faster rate of adoption than the rest, and if it is only for the cost pressures.« Whenever it happens, Unisys is prepared. In line with the observed trend, the number one strategic objective for 2003 is continued double-digit growth in business process outsourcing.

In banking as in any other industry, little of this is new. Predominantly in the area of transactions, both M&A activities and increased in- and outsourcing are taking place in order to consolidate volumes. The problem with outsourcing is that many have tried – for instance in the areas of transfers, clearing and settlement, and custody – and only few have been entirely successful. What worked, what did not, and most importantly why?

Clearstream International, in Luxembourg, was formed in October 1999 as a 50/50 joint venture through the merger of the clearing and settlement and depository activities of Cedel International and Deutsche Börse. Clearstream offers a comprehensive service covering equities and bonds both domestic and cross-border. The intention was to form a European clearinghouse through successive pan-European mergers and cooperative agreements. As no international partners could be found, however, Deutsche Börse took over the remaining 50 percent by acquiring Cedel and is now the sole shareholder of Clearstream International. Even though Clearstream could not reach its initial targets, it was successful in building a viable business. By year-end 2001, the company served more than 2 500 customers in 94 countries, most of whom were banks and investment companies. Only 24 percent of Clearstream's revenues of about one billion Euros were generated in Germany, 18 percent in Northern Europe, 35 percent in Southern Europe, twelve percent in the UK, seven percent in Asia/Pacific, and six percent in the Americas. Over the past four years, Clearstream grew on average 29 percent per year, currently has over 7.4 trillion Euros worth of assets under administration, and is expected to handle in excess of 150 million transactions in 2002.

Commerzbank of Germany has had mixed results with its spin-off »Ebase«, the »European Bank for Fund Services«. Ebase offers depot services, IT services, and Marketing&Sales services to financial services providers and asset management companies. The company sees itself as a single point of contact for securities administration and custody. While being expected to break even in 2003 and being the largest and most successful outsourcing platform of its kind in Germany, Ebase was not able to attract nearly as much external business as originally planned. Only two cooperation partners use the Ebase platform to fully outsource their account management, one of which is the original in-house client, Commerzbank's asset management subsidiary Cominvest. Another 13 cooperation partners do not offer brokerage services themselves, but simply channel those of their customers who want to be active in securities trading and brokerage to Ebase. With a current total volume of over one million accounts and 4.6 billion Euros under management, the spin-off into a separate company is estimated to have created an additional volume of less than ten percent of Commerzbank's original volume only. Currently, Ebase is attempting to improve its positioning in order to attract additional external business.

In general, particularly large retail banks seem to be cautious when it comes to outsourcing a process to a direct competitor or an independent provider who is a spin-off from a direct competitor. This is, for example, Commerzbank's case with Ebase. Any suspicion of a competitive threat seriously endangers the chances for the success of an external transaction provider. Often it is long-built animosities, sometimes pure vanities, sometimes simply the fear that the competitor – or the newly established »independent« spin-off that might channel data back to the competitor – will use the original data to learn more about customer structures, preferences, or even the individual customers themselves.

Success is much more likely when no competitive threat to the outsourcing company is evident. For example, the supplier might come from within the industry, but is so specialized on a particular transaction or process that he is no competitor to the regular business. Alternatively, several competitors might come together and build a joint venture focused on one specific process and, most importantly, jointly supervised by all partners such that no uncontrolled flow of information to any one of the partners can take place. Lastly, the supplier might come from an entirely different industry in which case the question of competitive threat is irrelevant.

This might be the reason for Clearstream's success: Neither the company itself nor its owner, Deutsche Börse, is competing directly with possible clients. Clearstream is too specialized to be a competitor and Deutsche Börse is simply in another business. This is also one of the reasons why Clearstream was able to build as international a business as it has done.

State Street is Building a Successful Business by Focusing on and Expanding its Key Capabilities

With roughly 15 percent of total capitalized fungible securities under administration, State Street is the world's largest custodian. State Street's main clients are institutional investors with large asset pools such as mutual funds, pension plan sponsors, insurance companies, banks, corporations, collective investment fund managers, and not-for-profit organizations. For its clients, State Street can provide custody only, or can add fund accounting, the entire middle office services, or additional value added services like lending securities, managing cash or currencies, performance measurement and analytics, or can offer trade support products like transition management and commission recapture programs, and so forth. The most complex service State Street offers is to insource the entire asset servicing and then do everything after the trade is completed. Being able to pick from such a wide range of offers, clients can choose exactly to which degree they would like to outsource aspects of the asset management processes and what they would prefer to do themselves. Parallel to this business area, State Street supports clients with research during the pre-trade phase, offers execution for the trade itself, and is active in passive asset management, with market leadership in this area.

Thomas A. Bergenroth, Senior Vice President and Managing Director of State Street and General Manager of State Street Bank GmbH, points out: »The insight we get from our position of administering massive capital about where the market is going is enormous. When investors have executed their trades and we have captured them, we can assess immediately where the markets are going, for example into or out of the Yen. This is how we can provide our clients with the most up to date and real transaction based research: we simply see it happen. It comes right out of our custody and accounting engine.«

In addition, State Street has focused on passive asset management, in other words managing index funds. This area of specialization fits the business model very well: Being able to mirror indices – particularly

---

large, global ones – requires highly developed IT capabilities and processing power. That is exactly what State Street is good at.

With great professionalism, State Street has managed to build one of the largest insourcing businesses in the financial services industry. Fine-tuning their portfolio of businesses until today, the company makes sure to offer the clients everything they need to be successful in managing their investments – but within the scope of their limited and specialized business areas only. These are likely to be two of the reasons for State Street's overwhelming success. By meticulously avoiding sensitive markets and activities, the company poses no threat to its customers, and it focuses clearly on only those activities it is good at.

To illustrate the case of several competitors establishing joint external capabilities, look at Barclays', HSBC's, and Lloyds TSB's check processing unit in the UK. Originally, in 2000, a joint venture between Lloyds TSB, Barclays, and Unisys was formed to create a new company called Intelligent Processing Solutions Limited (iPSL), which would handle all check processing functions for the two banks. HSBC was the third of the four major retail UK banks to join the venture. In addition to the three shareholders, other banks as well use iPSL and its advantages of scale to handle their checks; by now, the company processes approximately 67 percent of all checks in the UK or 13 million items a day. iPSL is planning to extend its value-added service offers into image-based archival services which will allow clients to retrieve web-based images of processed checks.

iPSL: Compete During the Day, but Collaborate at Night, and – Trust Each Other!

For Lloyds TSB and Barclays, both long-standing Unisys clients, the issue was clear. Check volumes in the UK are falling, while high reinvestments are required to stay in business. The solution was obvious: outsourcing. Rather than outsourcing to Unisys' existing check processing company UPSL, however, the two wanted to use their combined volume – and therefore economies of scale – to build a separate company. And they wanted a stake in it to participate in the likely success of the business. Intelligent Processing Solutions Limited (iPSL) was born. Later, HSBC joined as well.

Philip Heggie, Unisys Vice President and General Manager UK, Europe and Africa for Global Outsourcing, sees the topic of non-competitiveness as crucial for an insourcer's success. »If one bank just builds capabilities and wants other banks, as a matter of fact competitors, to outsource their business to them, it simply doesn't work. There will always be too many suspicions in the air. You need at least two companies to join forces, and even then they will not be successful unless they have an independent third party, a catalyst, to facilitate the partnership.« Heggie sees the existence of this third party – Unisys – as key factor in the success of iPSL. He points to the company's three shareholders Lloyds TSB, Barclays, and HSBC. »Remember, during the day, these companies are still competitors, even if they collaborate during the night. You *need* an independent moderator.«

For Heggie, Unisys' majority stake in iPSL is also crucial. »The reason these banks wanted to outsource check processing is that it was not one of their core competencies. For us, this *is* our core business.« Unisys knows the underlying business very well: Half of all checks worldwide are processed using Unisys payments solutions.

Heggie is certain: »We would never have been able to do this if we hadn't had long-standing relationships with Lloyds TSB and Barclays already. This is all about trust.«

Some of the most prominent examples of successful outsourcing arise from IBM, who has been able to secure several large players of the financial industry as clients. In 2000, the Royal Bank of Scotland (RBoS) announced a strategic alliance with IBM under which it would outsource its entire IT infrastructure, thereby transferring the employment of more than 500 staff and leasing its purpose-built IT center in Edinburgh to IBM. The alliance is reported to be worth 700 million British Pounds and RBoS estimates it will save 150 million British Pounds as a result of the agreement. In February 2002, American Express announced plans to outsource its entire IT to IBM in a deal worth four billion US Dollars over seven years. This will include transferring management of transaction processes, web operations, network servers, storage, and its help desk, as well as 2 000 American Express IT workers who will continue to operate out of AMEX data centers. In September 2002, Deutsche Bank (DB) and IBM announced that they were in final negotiations over an agreement to outsource DB's entire IT function to IBM for 2.5 billion US Dollars over ten years. As part of the deal, 900 of DB's IT employees will be transferred to IBM. In November 2002, DBS, the largest bank in South

East Asia, announced a similar agreement worth 679 million US Dollars over ten years. IBM will consolidate and enhance DBS's data centers in Singapore and Hong Kong, provide an integrated 24/7 customer helpdesk, and manage many of DBS's current applications. DBS's IT group will continue to be responsible for IT services not included in the outsourcing, namely, IT strategy and architecture, IT security, and strategic projects. JPMorgan Chase followed suit in December 2002, outsourcing a portion of its data processing technology infrastructure, including data centers, help desks, distributed computing, and data and voice networks, to IBM for seven years in a deal worth five billion US Dollars. As part of the agreement, JPMorgan Chase will transfer approximately 4 000 employees and contractors to IBM in the first half of 2003. Application delivery and development as well as desktop support will be retained inside JPMorgan Chase. The vision is to create a »virtual pool« of computing resources to be accessed and deployed as needed.

»The financial services industry has always had a very good IT infrastructure, both regarding security and the quality of services« says Gerald Münzl, head of Marketing and Sales Support Central Region of IBM Global Services – Strategic Outsourcing. »Consequently, the main driver for outsourcing is not an improvement in quality or security, it is cost. Technology is improving ever more quickly, and the banks want to avoid having to build the skills and make big investments. Besides, they simply want to get assets off their balance sheet and people off their pay roll.« Münzl compares this to the manufacturing industry in the nineties: The more the cost pressures increase, the more open companies grow toward the idea outsourcing.

The Three Levels of IT Outsourcing

According to Gerald Münzl, head of Marketing and Sales Support Central Region of IBM Global Services – Strategic Outsourcing, there are three levels of IT outsourcing: The first level is infrastructure hosting, where the supplier manages data centers, the client server infrastructure, or the wide area network. In a more advanced form, companies outsource all of this infrastructure management in one large deal. The second level is application hosting, including the development and maintenance of standard and legacy applications plus the respective infrastructure. Lastly, there is business process outsourcing, where the supplier is responsible for *managing* an entire process, or parts thereof, including the underlying IT infrastructure.

Münzl observes the typical geographical pattern of adoption: In the Anglo-Saxon countries, banks are beginning to think about business process outsourcing, and application hosting is beginning to really take off. In other countries, like Germany, the »one-bid-deal« form of infrastructure hosting is gaining ground quickly, partly due to (for Germany) the groundbreaking deal with Deutsche Bank. Outsourcing parts of the IT infrastructure has already been the norm for many years. Application outsourcing is starting very slowly, but business process outsourcing is not yet an issue at all. »It will happen«, Münzl says. »The Anglo-Saxons are always a couple of years ahead, but margin pressure and focus on the core business will make the others move in the same direction as well.«

Other processes often outsourced to third parties from outside the financial industry include call centers, card processing (particularly for credit cards), and check processing.

The general pattern thus becomes clear: Understandably, retail banks are willing to outsource strategically non-relevant, but still sensitive, processes only if they can be absolutely certain that no competitor will gain access to this data and that confidentiality will be preserved. Consequently, only those insourcers or service providers that clearly put themselves above any suspicion of competitive threat, i. e. are not active in their customers' remaining business areas and are not closely affiliated with another bank or other company which is, can attract business.

The topic of outsourcing will be central to the future of retail banks. Whether they choose to focus on the customer interface or in the back-office, whether they see their strength in selling products, developing or producing them, they will end up either at the giving or the receiving end of outsourcing relationships.

Risk Management – No Worries for Future Retail Banks

Future challenges:
- *For corporate banking: adapting to IAS, Basle II, and probably MAK*
- *For retail banks: also adapting to IAS, Basle II, and MAK, which are likely to have a lesser impact due to the significantly lower importance of risk management*
- *No outsourcing possible*

Generally, risk management will not be important for retail banks due to their comparatively lower exposures. However, as part of a larger universal bank, retail banks will feel the effects of the reorganizations demanded largely from their corporate banking siblings. Even stand-alone retail banks, theoretically »free« from the bounds of a universal bank parent, have little room to maneuver in risk management: Legislation prevents them, as virtually all banks, from outsourcing this activity.

Risk management is not, and will not be, top priority for retail banks or, to put it more realistically, the retail arm of today's financial institutions. For today's European banks almost all operate in the three business areas of retail banking, corporate banking, and investment banking. The exceptions are mainly the new entrants, such as on-line banks or those at the customer interface like Tesco Personal Finance or Virgin Money.

In general, risk management is more of an issue for corporate banks than for retail banks. However, developments in corporate risk management will affect retail banking where the retail part of a universal bank, rather than a stand-alone retail bank, is concerned. This is because risk management for both is sometimes – and increasingly will have to be, as we will discuss later – performed by the same unit within the umbrella of the universal bank.

Over time, the sources of risk have increased as banks enter foreign markets, offer different products, and address new customer groups. In addition, the complexity of financing structures, derivatives etc. has increased. Regarding the two main risk categories – market risks and credit risks – market risks are less of a threat these days. Structured products, such as derivatives and the like, are well developed and banks are able to cover market risks effectively. As the case of Barings proved, using these tools unwisely will always be able to fell a bank. In general, however, the market risks are largely under control.

Credit risks, on the other hand, have arguably never been less under control than they are now. As the cases of Enron and WorldCom demonstrate, even large and publicly quoted companies can become so good at providing unclear or partially wrong information about their financial status that they are able to fool both banks and investors alike and bring out massive bankruptcies almost out of the blue. The result is huge credit losses, for example in the case of Enron amounting to more than eight billion US Dollars for JPMorgan Chase, Citigroup, Credit Suisse First Boston, and other banks and 1.9 billion Euros for Bayerische Landesbank in the case of Kirch. Europe and, more specifically, Germany are taking their toll on the current economic downturn as well. Bad loan provisions for the period of January to September 2002 have approximately doubled compared to 2001: For Deutsche Bank, the figure rose from 468 to 1 611 million Euros, for Commerzbank from 571 to 998 million Euros, and for HypoVereinsbank from 1 335 to 2 476 million Euros, to name just a few[16]. Instruments for dealing with credit risks are still being developed and not yet used widely. Asset-backed or mortgage-backed securities are making credit risks tradable.

For years, European legislation has been busy changing the way credit risks must be handled. The introduction of IAS accounting principles until 2007 will force banks to assess their risk positions in a new way. This may not seem at the outset to be a big issue, but in order to account for those positions, complex and – needless to say – very expensive risk management systems are necessary. These systems must either now be reconfigured or bought anew.

Secondly, »Minimum Requirements for the Credit Business of Credit Institutions« (»Mindestanforderungen an das Kreditgeschäft«, MAK) are being introduced – initially in Germany only – as a joint project by the German regulator BaFin and the German Central Bank. The MAK are process-oriented and aim at improving the organization and management of the credit business within banks, which have often been inadequate in the past. As a result of this inadequacy, numerous banks have got into trouble and sometimes even become insolvent. Right now, the MAK are a draft only, but are rumored to be introduced in Germany in 2005. So far, MAK is only a German initiative, but discussions to make it European law are already underway.

For most banks, meeting MAK requirements means a substantial restructuring of their credit processes from customer-based to process-based. At present, many banks are organized around customer groups, for instance corporate customers, private customers, and affluent customers. Usually, each division is headed by a different member of the management board. Within each segment, the functional tasks of the credit business – ideally »Market« (credit issuance etc.), »Post-Market« (third party assessments, ratings etc.), and »Monitoring« – are performed more or less separately from those of the other divisions. Processes and procedures differ across the bank in the same way as the responsibilities. MAK will require banks to perform these functional tasks across all of their business units, rather than within each one separately, in order to achieve consistency. This will require significant reorganizations, as a »Market« unit, a »Post-Market« unit, and a »Monitoring« unit will have to be created, each performing their specific tasks for all customer groups. The implementation of the internal changes required

The European
Retail Banking
Landscape in the
Future

by the MAK regulation is likely to take one or even two years. If the law is passed in 2003, banks will have to show significantly altered organizational structures by the end of 2005.

Finally, the Basle capital accord (»Basle II«), which will be finalized in the fourth quarter of 2003, also deals with credit risks and requires implementation in each country by year-end 2006. Basle II does not address internal processes, but rather the procedure for capital allocation, and forces banks to match their employed capital to the risk of the respective credits or credit portfolios. Again, significant changes in processes and organizations will need to happen for Basle II to be implemented.

All of this will impact on the traditional retail banking divisions, first indirectly, as the organizationally neighboring corporate banking units will be forced to adapt, and later directly, as reorganizations will have to happen in order to comply with MAK.

What about the stand-alone retail banks, of which we predict there will be many at the customer interface in the future? Obviously, these banks will have to do risk management by themselves, but for them, like for the retail operations within universal banks, risk management will not be a big issue as the exposures are relatively small. Will it be possible for them to outsource this task?

Early examples of outsourcing risk management exist. In the German co-operative sector, banks are not only merging and consolidating but also outsourcing their credit management task, including risk management. »Kreditwerk«, a joint venture between DGHyp and Schwäbisch Hall, handles credit management and IT for its two parent companies. Other co-operative banks are welcome to join, but have not yet done so. The same development is likely to happen in the savings bank sector, where a »Kreditfabrik« has been set up, albeit lagging behind the developments in the co-operative sector.

Unfortunately, two issues will prevent this from becoming more than an exception: Perhaps most importantly, in most countries legislation does not allow banks to outsource activities that are an integral part of their business as a bank or as a financial institution (for example in Germany KWG (German Banking Act) § 25a, Sect. 2). Credit Management certainly falls in this category. Only in some pockets of the market, like savings or co-operative banks, might legal exceptions exist. Unfortunately, this does not leave many opportunities to outsource risk or credit management. Secondly, for the few legal exceptions that are possible, many individual banks are quite unwilling to grant other institutions insights into their credit and loan book. This, however, is a necessary prerequisite for the outsourcing of credit management.

Ultimately, risk management is unlikely to give future retail bank managers many sleepless nights. Where the retail bank is part of a larger operation, both market and credit risk management will be comparatively less important than for the corporate part of the business. As a result, reorganizations will have to be endured, but will not change much for the retail banking part. If we are talking about a stand-alone retail bank, legislation is likely to forbid the outsourcing of credit management and risk management from the start. This leaves only a few exceptions, whose efforts will be interesting to follow, but cannot be generalized to the entire market.

Client Management – Only Better Client Know-How Can Increase Revenues

Future challenges:
- *Understand customer needs better and cater to them*
  - *Use existing information better to induce cross-selling: Customer Relationship Management (CRM) is not the sole answer*
  - *Segment the customer base better and focus on target groups*
  - *Personalize offers to target customers according to their needs*
  - *Gain (back) clients' trust by offering competent and especially unbiased advice*

Currently, retail banks are not very good at client management, i.e. treating their customers in the right way to generate repeat purchases. Large investments in CRM might have increased data transparency, but have not improved client management. To increase customer loyalty, retail banks will have to understand their clients' needs and act accordingly. Existing data must be used to tailor offers to specific customers or customer groups. Trustworthiness has to be improved by giving better and more objective advice, which also means including competitors' products into the offer. Overall, the customer needs to feel taken care of personally and in accordance with his specific needs.

Ask anybody who regularly does on-line shopping about who has the best client management. The answer you will invariably get is »Amazon«. What is it they are doing and why is their way of treating the customer regarded as so special?

Apart from the fact that their website is well organized, simple to use, and quick (which is a matter of sales more than of client management), they use the information they have gathered about their customers in a perfect way. Every time a person visits the web site he is greeted personally and a range of products are offered according to his past purchases. What makes this special is that one does not have to log in for this, this is Amazon's homepage, but parts of it are personalized to the individual customer. Every time a customer orders a product or puts it onto his wish list, Amazon learns about that customer's interests and preferences. They then match it according to other customers' purchases and provide a selection of results: »Customers who purchased this article, also bought: ...«. While giving the customer their suggestions, they even tell him which of his interests (orders, wish list entries) it is based on. By design, this is a learning system that improves both its breadth and its accuracy automatically over time.

In addition to fostering cross-selling within the category both via the personalized offers described above and via special vouchers, for example for Christmas, Amazon also offers incentives for cross-selling into other categories. In-category vouchers are mailed for special occasions only, but out-of-category vouchers arrive regularly, for instance for audio books, CDs, DVDs, or computer programs/software.

Amazon is even cannibalizing part of their business in order to prevent customers from defecting to other suppliers. Recently, Amazon also started offering used books. Private and other independent book sellers can put books into the system, which will then be offered on the same website right next to Amazon's own new book offering. Both the order process (including personal pre-settings) and the payment take place via Amazon to guarantee process quality and trustworthiness. The book itself is shipped by the independent seller. With this offering, Amazon certainly cannibalizes its regular business. At the same time, however, it prevents its customers from defecting to used books sites, Ebay, and other similar channels to find cheaper alternatives. Moreover, this system allows Amazon to fill »empty spots« where books are out of print and can only be found in second-hand bookshops.

In addition to all this, Amazon's processes work beautifully: Customers are informed of each step of the mailing process (»order received«, »order mailed and closed«) and order cancellations, returns, and complaints are handled quickly and in an unbureaucratic way. As a result, at any point during an order process or while just browsing around, the customer feels taken care of, understood, and catered to in a personal way.

This example can be used to define client management. In the context of this book, »Client Management« will refer to everything done to sell additional products, i. e. all types of client specific marketing (as opposed to product-specific marketing, see above). More specifically, client management includes, first, using customer knowledge to tailor offers specifically towards the client's need (the right offer at the right time) and, second, doing everything possible to fulfill the customer's needs, even if it means a slight cannibalization of your original business. In view of the maturity of the retail banking market and the extremely high costs of acquiring new customers, the loyalty a bank would receive in return for such efforts would more than make up for the lost business.

Admittedly, client management is harder in some industries than in others. However, consider the case of BAA plc, the British Airport Authority, which manages seven airports in the UK including Heathrow and Gatwick, and is involved in twelve airports outside the UK as well. BAA manages all the commercial facilities at their airports including shops, restaurants, pubs, bureaus de change, car hires, and car parks. When one thinks about the running of the duty free shops, it might seem impossible to cater to specific target groups. BAA, however, found a way: They manage to redecorate the shopping windows so quickly that they are able to adapt to the origin of incoming airplanes, i. e. the nationality of arriving customers. In doing so, BAA specifically targets, for example, the needs and tastes of Japanese, Saudi, or US American visitors.

What does all this mean for retail banking? Banks must learn to cater to their clients more specifically by using their existing information better, to give better incentives for cross-selling, and to offer optimal service – including being willing to cannibalize existing business to a certain degree if it benefits the customer.

Today's retail banks are not very good at using the information they have about their clients. Like many information-intensive industries, banks have become aware of this deficit and spent millions over the last years to introduce CRM tools and data mining. Two problems remain, however. First, regarding CRM, retail banks have the specific difficulty of working with many layers of legacy systems, whose structures often do not allow for the use of modern CRM systems. The data exists, but the analysis is made close to impossible by the layered structure of the databases. Secondly, once this consolidation of data is fulfilled, banks unfortunately face the issue of still not being able to use the knowledge about their clients well. The problem has only been shifted to a different level. Again, banks have this problem in

Customer Segmentation as a Prerequisite for Success

Market segmentation is known to be one of the most powerful tools to help develop marketing strategies and allocate scarce resources. However, the segmentation approaches typically applied in the financial services industry, including retail banking, produce results, which although »interesting« are far from being perceived as useful by the organization and the individual employees.

As summarized in Exhibit 11, traditional segmentation concepts are often problematic for three reasons. First, the existing segmentation schemes are either too simplistic to lead to any real insights into market behavior (for example income, age and gender as the main variables) or they yield interesting, but useless, results. More specifically, they do not predict customer behavior or describe the levers the banks need to address in order to stimulate growth (not »meaningful«), nor are they easily observable, measurable, and translatable into immediate actions (not »actionable«). Second, key stakeholders are not committed to, nor do they understand, the segmentation (for instance, bank clerks at the POS are unable to use the segmentation to support the selling process). Third, top-management does not share a common view of what drives market behavior.

Outside the financial services industry, many companies have started to use innovative segmentation approaches that cope with the drawbacks of traditional techniques. Particularly consumer goods companies, including some of the world's largest and best-known ones, use concepts that help them to understand their customers not only statistically but also individually, thus generating double-digit top line growth rates. The basic characteristics of this approach are outlined in Exhibit 11. The main output of this methodology is a segmentation map, which defines meaningful and actionable segments by grouping customers according to their common behavior and motivations. As described above, such a segmentation map is »meaningful« in that it predicts key behavior the banks need to address in order to stimulate growth and is »actionable« in that it is easily observable, measurable, and translatable into immediate actions by sales and marketing as well as other levers available for retail banks.

The segmentation process itself is highly important as well and must be managed carefully. The process serves not only for management to learn about the market, the customers, and their preferences, it also aims at aligning management behind the final outcome so that this shared understanding can be used to generate focused and mutually supporting and enhancing activities.

Having identified meaningful and actionable customer segments, retail banks need to take actions to improve cross-selling rates, customer retention, service levels, and so forth. Here, all activities need to be targeted towards the identified segments, and an in-depth understanding needs to be developed for each of them. The »average consumer« is not buying any products, so pure statistics are insufficient for this process. It is a real person with all his individual traits and quirks who decides whether or not to buy a financial services product in a bank.

Exhibit 11:   Traditional Versus Innovative Customer Segmentation

Innovative Segmentation	Traditional Segmentation
Actionability is the primary criteria for building segments	**Actionability is considered after the analysis** of the research and often requires proxies
Utilizes a **wide range of market data** from multiple points in time including qualitative and quantitative research, management experience, market anecdotes, databases, etc.	Based on a **single research instrument** (typically quantitative) fielded at a point in time which attempts to capture all potential segmentation dimensions at one time
Creates **actionable output early** in the process based on informed hypotheses	**Output only at completion** of the project - after fielding quantitative research
Designed to build on management intuition based on their participation in the process	**Limited use of management intuition**, typically utilizes market research hypotheses about potential segmentation dimensions
Results are internalized by senior management and implementers as part of the process	**Results are »explained«** and sold to senior managers who then sell it to implementers
Senior management learning about the market is a key benefit of the process – their market intuition improved	**Senior management does not participate** in the learning process and therefore has limited learnings – their market intuition remains largely unchanged
Delivers an **adaptable market frame** that can be updated as any new information surfaces	Delivers a **stagnant market frame** which requires repeating the process to update the segmentation

common with many other information-intensive industries. As a result, the clients themselves have not benefited from these efforts. However, retail banks generally seem to be unaware of this new deficit. Instead, they should think about better segmenting their customer base and offering more targeted services.

Retail banks might observe a client making substantial annual payments to his life insurance, and even though the bank offers life insurance products as well, nobody will ever approach the client in order to try and win this business. The same is true for any other insurance product, even though the sums involved are substantially smaller. Retail banks observe a customer paying his monthly credit card bill to an external provider. If they made him a good offer, he might be willing to switch. They also observe customers paying off their mortgages with another financial institute. Why do they not use times of low interest rates to offer an attractive refinancing? Why not do the same for a substantial consumer credit? Retail banks observe large bonus or termination payments arrive in their customers' accounts – and see them leave again, most likely to be invested elsewhere. Why don't they offer advice? And even if they offer it, why does it feel so impersonal? On the other hand – would customers view such behavior as a violation of privacy and therefore oppose it?

As retail banks know their clients' income patterns and sources, spending patterns and preferences, and debt levels, they now need to get better at inferring tailor-made offers from their knowledge of these transactions.

Looking at the information credit card companies have about their customers, client management becomes more detailed and more oriented towards relationship building than towards business generation. The customer buys a lot of concert or theater tickets? Cooperate with a specialized agent and keep him informed about future events in his home city. The client keeps flying from A to B every couple of months? Cooperate with a travel agent, keep him informed if a new and cheaper fare comes up, and offer him a discount on repeat purchases. The client repeatedly makes purchases at the same boutiques? Inform him about fashion shows and special sales at these locations. Why should a credit card company make the effort? Because it will increase customer retention significantly if you can offer the client something he knows he cannot get from the competitor – at least not at once, as the competitor needs some time to profile the client's interests.

Looking a couple of years ahead, more futuristic and more efficient ways of generating customer loyalty might become feasible. Why should clients have to learn how to deal with the system, once the system can be set up to

The European
Retail Banking
Landscape in the
Future

learn how to deal with the client? Through a combination of portable and even wearable computers, voice recognition, identification systems, and intelligent interfaces, banks – or other service providers – could offer their customers an »electronic butler«: A system that not only reminds the client of his mother's birthday, but also understands the order »please send ten pink carnations to Mom« – because the system knows who »Mom« is, knows her address, remembers or finds the closest flower shop, and automatically transmits both the order and the credit card number to pay with. »Transfer 1 000 Euros to my wife« should be equally easy, as all the relevant details are stored in the system. Once a system has been set-up by the bank and filled with the client's relevant information required to perform tasks in this way, customer retention would increase significantly.

In this futuristic model, the companies who get to provide this interface and manage the customer data will be extremely powerful. Like today's food retailers, they will know the customers' behavior and preferences – information and data that today's food industry is unable and has a strong desire to obtain. In food, the channel now owns the customer. Regarding retail banking, the same might happen. Extrapolating the current business, this type of client interface might not be a typical future playground for retail banks. However, unless they make the effort to be present in this market, they too might lose valuable information about their customers.

While using existing information to tailor services to individual customers can be very labor intensive, improving cross-selling rates need not be. Insurance companies have started long ago to offer existing clients rebates on additional products: For example, a second insurance purchased may be subject to a reduction of five or ten percent, a third or fourth of 15 or 20 percent. Hotels, rental car companies, and telephone providers, among many others, have started to cooperate with airlines to offer their customers frequent flyer miles for their purchases. As other similar industries have shown, awarding points or actual miles from other airlines' programs for certain transaction behavior can work as effectively as product bundling or pricing discounts. With few exceptions, like Credit Suisse or Consors, banks so far have not followed this route.

Granting rebates or awarding points can be automated and therefore is comparatively uncomplicated. After that, however, generating cross-selling starts to be a more fundamental issue. What is needed is a detailed customer segmentation, a decision which segments to focus on, and specific products and services to cater to exactly that segment. Repeat purchases are also induced by trust and positive customer experiences. Here, banks need to cre-

The European
Retail Banking
Landscape in the
Future

ate a distinct image and brand that instill trust, align offers and processes to deliver a positive customer experience, and improve their advisory services to better fulfill clients' needs.

Using the existing information better and working harder at creating cross-selling is not enough if the bank is not seen as going out of its way to serve the client best. To achieve the latter, banks must begin to fully live by the concept of open architecture: Customers must be offered comprehensive and transparent information and product packages, even for investments and retirement provisions. Only if competitors' products are included in the offer and actively sold where appropriate, thereby cannibalizing the banks proprietary offer, will the customer feel well advised and well taken care of. We have argued that products will become less and less important when it comes to attracting clients. Here, products are not assumed to regain importance. Quite the contrary, it is the quality of the advice that will win customers, and that in turn depends on being viewed as unbiased and therefore including competitors' products as well.

Here, perhaps, another of Amazon's »gimmicks« may be worth copying: Might there be a demand for clients being informed about the status of some of the more important or more complicated transactions? For being informed when an order has been carried out – for example, receiving an e-mail when a certain share or fund has been bought or sold? Or perhaps that a transfer – particularly the more error-prone international transfers – has reached its destination? Or for an SMS with the current account balance? Detailed market research will be necessary to answer questions such as these.

All in all, retail banks have a lot to learn when it comes to client management. They need to learn about their customers' needs and possible sales opportunities from information they already have. They need to personalize their offers to the targeted customer (groups). They need to improve the quality of their advice and the range of products offered, including competitors', to regain their customers' trust and therefore build customer loyalty. Only at that point when the client feels understood and regards his bank as a competent and unbiased partner for his financial transactions and plans, will he feel comfortable in his banking relationship, increase his business with his retail bank, and feel no incentive anymore to defect and switch to a competitor.

4.2 The Ideal Retail Bank of the Future

In discussing the respective trends, restrictions, and examples for success or failures, the future challenges of the single value chain steps have become clearer. How can retail banks respond to these challenges? What do they mean for the structure of future retail banks and the future of the retail banking industry as a whole?

If an »ideal bank« could be patched together freely from different companies from different industries, it might look like the example described below (see Exhibit 12: The Ideal Retail Bank of the Future). Such a company would have its products developed by two types of companies. For the »mass products«, the product developing reinsurer described earlier would be used and would be able to gain additional insights about products, customers, and markets by bundling the processing of transactions, like account management, money transfers, or stock brokerage. For the specialty products, a range of specialized players would be used. Focusing on the customer interface entirely, the ideal retail bank of the future would use IKEA to develop a strong brand and back it up with the appropriate products, processes, and overall customer experiences. For the task of sales, the ideal retail bank might resort to Starbucks, which manages to deliver the right product through a highly convenient channel – and makes customers buy more than they originally planned to by simply posing a few friendly questions. Transactions and Administration would be handled by Porsche, which is very good at managing a network of external companies to which the various components and modules, in this case the transaction processes, are outsourced. State Street would take on the custody part, IBM the entire IT, and the product developing reinsurer would take over those transactions upon which he develops his new products, but only if his processing capabilities are excellent as well. Risk Management would not be outsourced, but done in-house. Client management would be handled by Amazon, who not only knows all about the right tools, but also has a lot of experience in processing electronic purchasing data to segment customers and manage the client relationship accordingly.

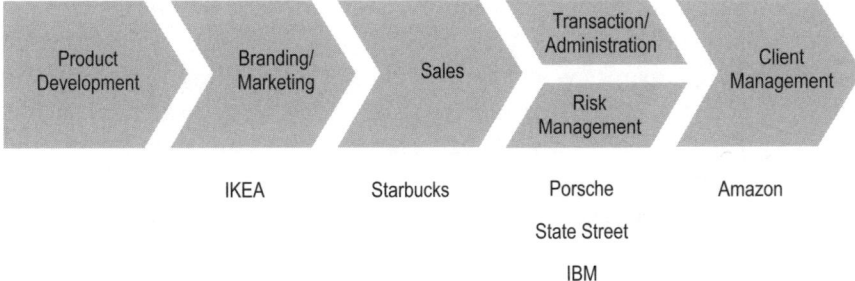

Exhibit 12: The Ideal Retail Bank of the Future

This ideal retail bank might be a nice concept, and it points to the areas where improvement is possible and where companies from other industries have already been successful in optimizing certain aspects of their business. Now let us look at what, exactly, today's retail banks can learn from this, how the future retail banking landscape will look like realistically, and what business models players can adopt in order to position themselves well for the future.

4.3 Realistic Future Business Models and the Network of Specialized Companies

Obviously, there will never be one single bank combining all the companies mentioned above. There will not even be a single bank that is as good a product developer as our reinsurer, as excellent a marketer as IKEA, as good in sales as Starbucks, as good in their transaction and IT as State Street and IBM, and as good a client manager as Amazon. The reason for this is that it is hard enough to achieve excellence in one step of the value chain. It is impossible to do so for all. Those who try will risk being mediocre in all areas.

The solution to this problem is to create a network of specialized companies. Companies, or retail banks, in this case, which focus all their efforts on one chosen area and let other members of the network carry out the other tasks. Outsourcing relationships will link the companies of the network.

In this network, each player will choose an area in which he will build his capabilities, and he will streamline his entire operations accordingly. Which future business models, however, are likely to develop? For which services does demand exist, and which of the corresponding business models are sustainable?

In order to start designing future business models, we will look at the value chain again but at a slightly more aggregated level. Realistically, no two different companies would divide the tasks of branding/marketing and sales; all of the client-related activities are highly likely to remain in one company. For this reason, we will aggregate branding/marketing, sales, and client management into one step – the »Customer Interface«. Product development is an independent activity, which will therefore remain separate as a step of its own. Regarding transaction/administration and risk management, these activities are relatively similar: All of them are carried out in order to process a transaction. Even though transactions, administration, and risk management could very well be handled by different companies, in this case we will view them together as »infrastructure« due to their similarities and for simplification. The result of these considerations is a more aggregated, simplified value chain (see Exhibit 13: The Aggregated Retail Banking Value Chain).

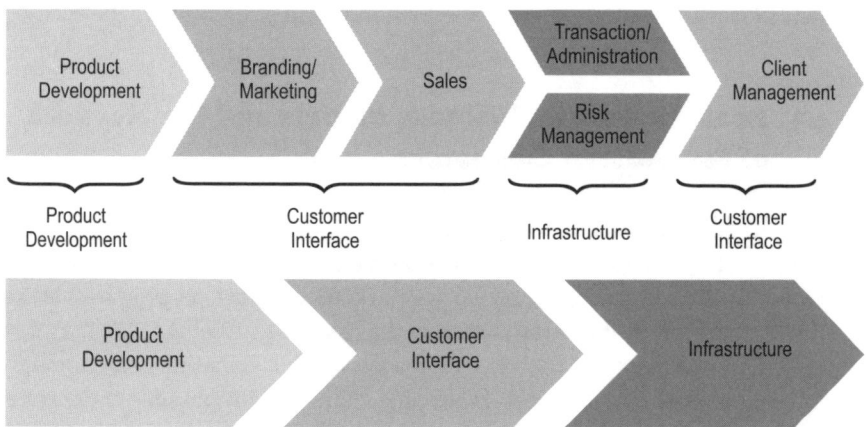

Exhibit 13: The Aggregated Retail Banking Value Chain

In which ways can these activities be performed by various specialized players in order to yield realistic and sustainable business models?

To discuss possible business models, let us take a look at the possible combinations of the three aggregated value chain steps. Theoretically, there are seven combinations (see Exhibit 14: Hypothetical Business Models – the Theoretically Possible Combinations). Every single value chain step could provide a stand-alone business, any two of them could be combined, and all three of them could provide an overall business model, in fact a fair representation of the majority of today's retail banks. Which of these combinations make sense? Which ones offer convincing value propositions and could find enough customers to become viable businesses?

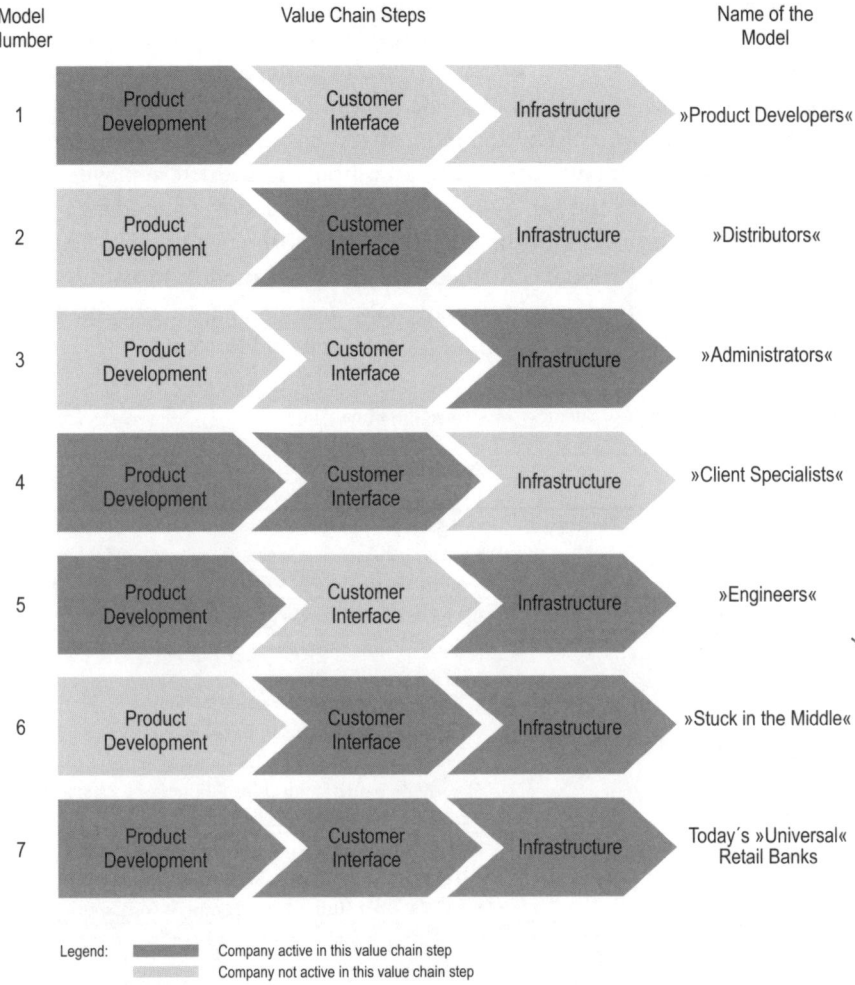

Model Number	Value Chain Steps			Name of the Model
1	Product Development	Customer Interface	Infrastructure	»Product Developers«
2	Product Development	Customer Interface	Infrastructure	»Distributors«
3	Product Development	Customer Interface	Infrastructure	»Administrators«
4	Product Development	Customer Interface	Infrastructure	»Client Specialists«
5	Product Development	Customer Interface	Infrastructure	»Engineers«
6	Product Development	Customer Interface	Infrastructure	»Stuck in the Middle«
7	Product Development	Customer Interface	Infrastructure	Today's »Universal« Retail Banks

Legend: ▆▆▆▆ Company active in this value chain step
░░░░ Company not active in this value chain step

Exhibit 14: Hypothetical Business Models: the Theoretically Possible Combinations

First of all, some of the theoretically possible models need to be eliminated. Model 7, the »universal retail bank«, represents the model by which most retail banks operate today and which we predict will become close to irrelevant. Undoubtedly, there are some very successful players with this business model – for example the Royal Bank of Scotland, but even they are outsourcing some of their processes and starting to use external distribution channels, thereby already beginning to deviate from the traditional model 7. Ultimately, only the best »universal retail banks« will be able to survive. As this model provides no new insights and as we predict today's retail banks to be overtaken by networks of more specialized companies, model 7 will not be discussed further. Also model 6 provides little additional value in our view. There are no economies of scope in being active in both the customer interface and infrastructure: No better offers, cost advantages, or increased differentiation can result from such a combination. Such a player would always be inferior to the far more efficient combination of models 2 and 3 and would thus be »stuck in the middle« between the two models. Thus, we will also not discuss model 6 further. The other five models remain interesting, and some of them might actually take various shapes and forms (see Exhibit 15: Realistic Future Business Models in Retail Banking).

Exhibit 15: Realistic Future Business Models in Retail Banking

Model no.	Name	Specialization
1	»Product developers«	• Specialist product developers (»Rocket Scientists«) • Mass product developers (business model viable as joint venture only)
2	»Distributors«	All focusing on the customer interface and seeking differentiation through: • Price (»Aldi Banks«) • Convenience (»McDonalds Banks«) • Quality (»Delicatessen Banks«) • Niche (»Fur-Hats-Are-Us Banks«) The »real« banks behind the Aldi and McDonalds Banks (»Gray Eminences«) !
3	»Administrators«	Focusing on various aspects of Infrastructure: • Transactions (»Assembly Line«) • IT or support functions (»IT and Admin Specialists«)
4	»Client Specialists«	Combining a focus on the customer interface with product development
5	»Engineers«	Combining a focus on transactions with product development

Let us look at these five models and their respective specializations in more detail in order to understand better their products and clients, which market segments they will occupy, which other players they might need to cooperate with, and what parts of their offer or positioning makes them unique.

Model 1: The ›Product Developers‹ — Companies Focusing on Product Development

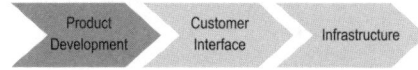

How viable is this concept of external product development? Would an independent product developer be able to survive?

First of all, two classes of products need to be distinguished. On the one hand, there is the standard product range of retail banking: the current account (including account management, debit cards, and transfers), savings accounts and fixed term deposits, overdraft and consumer credits, credit cards, and trading of shares, bonds, mutual funds, and derivatives. On the other hand, there are specialty products, i. e. the more elaborate, engineered investment products, like tax driven investments or retirement provisions.

For the standard product range, little sophistication is required: These are the basics of retail banking, virtually all players offer them – including the new entrants (but often with the exception of trading) – and virtually all offers are more or less identical. Pricing becomes a question of target group and image, not of sophisticated calculations. The market to develop standard products is relatively small. How often does a retail bank introduce »new« current or savings accounts, fixed term deposits, credit cards, or brokerage services? The answer is every once in a while, but not very often. Overall, the demand for developing these products is low.

For specialty products, the story is different. In order to satisfy their various customer groups again and again, retail banks can launch both different products at the same time as well as many products after each other. Each product satisfies slightly different preferences on the risk/performance frontier. As an example of an innovative product, take for example Commerzbank's product »Safe-T«, a product offered in connection with the IPO of Deutsche Telekom 1996. The Telekom shares purchased via »Safe-T« were locked until one day after the 2002 shareholders' meeting. On that day, the investors were guaranteed to receive the original issuing price, even if the current stock price was lower. Price gains could be realized fully. As compensation, Commerzbank would receive all dividends until the due date. The customer was allowed to cancel the agreement anytime beforehand and sell off his shares. In that case, no guarantee for the invested capital was given[17]. With Safe-T, Commerzbank addressed a largely new clien-

79

tele – most Germans did not own stock at that time – with a product tailor-made for those who regarded stocks as too risky an investment.

When we are talking about investments into specific projects, each product, by definition, has a limit as to how much money can be invested. Different from mutual funds, which theoretically can function indefinitely without ever having to be designed anew, these project-linked products can actually sell out, and new ones may need to be developed. The demand for products, and thus for product development, in the specialty sector is therefore significantly higher.

For the standard products, it is difficult to imagine how a stand-alone player could survive. There are few products to develop per type, but quite a few types. The »Mass Product Developer« would have to possess a significant breadth of capabilities in order to be able to satisfy his customers. He would therefore have to acquire many large clients at pretty much the same time for his business to be viable. It is much more likely that a couple of large players – in order to generate scale – would join forces to outsource these product development activities into a common joint venture. Once the entity is up and running, other clients could be served as well.

For specialty products, the picture is different. The more specialized and sophisticated the product, the greater the advantage of highly specialized, focused niche players. Here, a deep understanding of the market, risks, demographic developments, and client preferences is needed. Scale matters as it leads to experience, but it would be sufficient to be active only within the very focused area of one certain type of product. In contrast to potential »Mass Product Developers«, developers of specialty products, or »Rocket Scientists«, could be small and focused, more of a boutique than a larger company.

Model 2: The ›Distributors‹ — Retail Banks Focusing on the Customer Interface

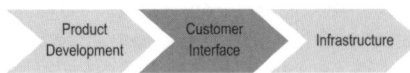

Looking at the increasing competition for clients in general and for the most profitable business areas, i.e. affluent clients or the most profitable businesses from the average client, retail banks will need to use all their wits to be successful at the customer interface. At this interface, like in many markets, there is space for two main types of players: Those catering to the entire market and those selecting specific niches for their business. Among the mass marketers, several distinct types of positioning are imaginable: the price leader, the convenience leader, and the quality leader. In this case, »quality« can take on a number of shapes, for example outstanding service, focus on innovation leadership, or literally the quality of the products. The players addressing the entire market offer a wide range of products and attempt to stand out either through a low price, convenience, or various quality attributes. Niche players, however, are targeting such a narrow customer group that, rather than offering a broad product range, they offer a deep and specialized one. In clothes retailing, consider the differences between the offers of »Woolworth« (price), the clothing section at Tesco or Carrefour (convenience), »Saks Fifth Avenue« (quality and service), or a specialized fur store or hat boutique (niche).

In retail banking, we expect all types of players to develop including price leaders (»Aldi Banks«), convenience leaders (»McDonald's Banks«), quality leaders (»Delicatessen Banks«), and niche players (»Fur-Hats-Are-Us Banks«). In looking at the respective business models, two areas have to be distinguished. On one hand, there is the appearance and positioning at the customer interface itself, which correspond to the four categories we have chosen. On the other hand, each bank within these groups will have its own underlying business system that determines how the company sources its products, brands them, and coordinates its production, i. e. the transactions. In this area, precise predictions as to which group of players will choose which approaches will be difficult to make. A comparison of these »Distributors« to today's food retailers makes the issue clearer. Almost independent of whether you are a Sainsbury, Marks & Spencer, Carrefour, or Mom and Pop shop, you may carry branded products, no-name products, or you might have a house brand. On this level of detail, it is impossible to predict specific choices – there are too many and they are too independent of the positioning at the customer interface. We will therefore limit ourselves to offering generic insights as to whether certain players are likely to outsource or not, but we will not go into the detail. Talking about »McDonald's Banking« will therefore not mean that the players who choose the respective positioning towards the market also will produce their products as McDonald's does – on the premises, in a standardized process, from standardized, purchased components.

All of these various players will need to structure their offers to address their targeted customer groups, and they will need to align their internal processes to deliver the services promised at the costs necessary to be competitive. When designing their offerings, they will need to think about all components: A good (i.e. targeted) offer consists of specific products combined with specific services at a specific price, branded and marketed in a specific way, and distributed through specific channels. Throughout this chapter, the term »offer« will therefore denote this combination of products, services, pricing, branding, marketing, and distribution.

Price Leaders – the »Aldi Banks«

When Aldi's discount supermarkets started to really expand in Germany in the sixties, people were horrified: The concept was disturbingly different from what they were used to. The products were not unpacked from the cartons they came in. Rather, the cartons were stacked in very wide shelves or on the floor and the top row of cartons had been simply cut open so that customers could take out what they needed themselves. Apart from the cashiers, there was no additional personnel in the store who could provide help. The product offering included standard products only, the choice per product area was extremely limited, and most of the brands offered were entirely unknown. The prices, however, were rock bottom. Initially, one had to avoid being seen shopping at Aldi. Only the poor people, it was rumored, went to Aldi. Today, this has changed completely. Shopping at Aldi is hip. There is a special Aldi cookbook using only Aldi ingredients. Today, it is possible to see as many Mercedes or BMWs parked in front of an Aldi as at any other supermarket – often even more.

How can this concept be transferred to the area of retail banking? An »Aldi Bank« would work similar to the Tesco Personal Finance, described at the beginning of Chapter 4, in that it would offer only a limited range of standard products. However, there would also be important differences as Tesco Personal Finance is a convenience leader rather than a price leader, as will be argued in the next section. An »Aldi Bank« attracts its customers via price and price only. Thus, the entire system must be geared towards only this objective. The product offering must be limited and standardized in order to decrease complexity. Advisory services are not given. Deviations from standard processes must not exist, much as Arkadi Kuhlmann, the CEO of ING Direct USA, described earlier in this chapter.

To offer the lowest prices around, an »Aldi Bank« would not only have to outsource product development and infrastructure, it would have to make sure it ends up with the cheapest and therefore often largest provider. To achieve that, product packages might even be auctioned off. No compromise can, however, be made regarding reliability as this is a *sine qua non* of modern retail banking.

Many on-line banks chose an Aldi approach, but deviated from that route when they began offering advice or opening braches, actions not consistent with the original idea of being a low cost provider. However, »Aldi Banks« do not necessarily have to be on-line banks. As there are low cost airlines, the respective model of a bank could exist. Such an »Aldi Bank« could have a regular branch network, but operate with very small branches and very limited service; for example, no advice and no withdrawal of cash or account statements at the counter. Like at ING Direct, deviating behavior would not lead to additional charges but, instead, to a request to close the account. As long as an »Aldi Bank« succeeds in offering the lowest prices for a standard product offering, it will find customers.

Convenience Leaders – the »McDonald's Banks«

Eating at McDonald's is convenient, i. e., fast and easily accessible. It fulfills a basic need for »food« in a standardized, but reliable and expected manner. It is not exactly cheap, but it is certainly not expensive. It is neither gourmet food nor a gourmet brand, but has been very successful.

In banking, the corresponding business model is demonstrated by Tesco Personal Finance in the UK: Fast and convenient, standardized processes and products, and a low price, but not necessarily the lowest around. The business model behind this approach is powerful, as already existing players have shown. The golden rule is to choose channels that are highly convenient for the customer as they combine very good accessibility with the ability to fulfill basic needs in a very satisfactory manner. Good access can mean that the channels or locations fit easily into the clients' daily or weekly routines, that they are combined with other useful offers, or that they simply have long opening hours. Fulfilling basic needs in retail banking can be realized by a standard product range that covers most or all day-to-day requirements, but can leave gaps for specialists to enter. »In a satisfactory manner« signifies not only faultless processes, as that is already a must for today's banks, it also means, at least for some time to come, face-to-face contact and not only contact with a computer terminal or a voice on the telephone.

In order to deliver the comparatively expensive degree of human interaction at the expected low- to medium-range price level, »McDonald's banks«, just like McDonald's itself, will need to compromise both in terms of the breadth of their product range and in how much the products can be adapted to customers' preferences. The products offered will be standardized, allowing for no modifications or additions, and the product range will include only a limited number of standard products. In addition, this kind of retail bank, even more than other banks at the customer interface, will have to outsource its transactions and administration to the »Administrators« in order to be able to offer low prices. This, however, should not be too demanding a requirement for a product range as standardized as the one described above.

In addition, no product development will be undertaken by the »McDonald's Bank«. After all, it is not the »quality« of the products, i. e. better performance or the lowest rates, that attracts customers – it is the convenience of the banking experience and the accessibility of the locations. »McDonald's Banks« are, however, susceptible to potential economic dips in the »underlying« businesses. For example, if Tesco's sales go down, fewer customers may also use the services of Tesco Personal Finance.

The »Real« Banks Behind the Aldi and McDonald's Banks – the »Gray Eminences«

At this point, we need to pause for a moment to discuss the »banks behind the banks«. The business models just described, the Aldi and McDonald's Banks, actually require two players to fulfill the various tasks, rather than just one, even if we do not consider the outsourcing of transactions and product development. One player sits directly at the customer interface and is, in fact, not very specialized in banking: He provides only the brand and possibly even the marketing. The other bank, in the background, is a »real« retail bank and does the »real« banking activities such as managing the accounts, processing transfers, buying and selling shares, whatever is required. Tesco Personal Finance (»TPF«, a joint venture between The Royal Bank of Scotland plc and Tesco plc) uses exactly this system with The Royal Bank of Scotland (RBoS): TPF (the player directly at the customer interface) uses RBoS (the player in the background) to provide the actual banking services (UK Insurance Ltd. and Norwich Union provide the actual insurance products). This second player – RBoS in this example – may, and even probably should, outsource the classic »outsourceable« transactions such as transfers, clearing and settlement, custody, and IT infrastructure. RBoS's value added is to coordinate the various outsourced transactions with those that remain in-house, for example current account management and credit applications, and to provide a seamless interface with the TPF »store front«.

Looking from the point of view of RBoS, the company uses TPF as distribution channel for their own products. Similar to many consumer goods companies, RBoS simply distributes similar products under both their own brand and the partner channel's or a no-name brand. From here on, we will refer to such banks as »Gray Eminences«.

Contrary to the relationships between other »Distributors«, the RBoSs of this world, in their role as »Gray Eminences«, are not in competition with all other »Distributors«. Rather, they have a symbiotic relationship with the »Aldi Banks« and the »McDonald's Banks« we have just spoken about. In addition, however, the »Gray Eminences« usually have business, and a brand, of their own – much like the manufacturers of a no-name or channel-branded sugar who also manufacture sugar under their own brand name. Regarding their own business, the »Gray Eminences« will be competitors to every other player at the customer interface.

With regard to both »Delicatessen Banks« and »Fur-Hats-Are-Us Banks«, these models will not require the services of a »Gray Eminence«. As these two models focus on the service intensive parts of the customer interface, they will need the »real« banking capabilities in-house (see below).

Quality Leaders – the »Delicatessen Banks«

In the same way today's food retailers leave room for delicatessen shops, the future retail banking market will do the same. At the delicatessen food store, they offer around ten varieties of ham at a counter – not even counting the cooked ones – plus five packaged varieties in the self serve aisles. This compares with the only three or so pre-packaged ones at Aldi. You can ask the shop assistant behind the counter to trim off some of the fat, or to cut the slices thinner or thicker. You can buy 100 grams, 120, 140, or 300, if you like. The product will be tailored to your exact wishes, and you pay a certain price for that amount of service. Aldi ham might cost half or two thirds of what you will pay at the deli. However, despite the high prices, the delis are crowded. That is not only because of the overwhelming choice and the personal service, it is also due to the wider product selection that includes specialties such as fresh fish, live lobsters, or ostrich meat.

Delicatessen Banking will be much the same. Whether they will offer more than one or even at a maximum a few varieties of current accounts and money transfers is unlikely – and unimportant. The food deli probably only has one or two types of bananas as well. Like their food counterparts, »Delicatessen Banks« will excel at the high end of the product range. Regarding investments, retirement provisions, insurances, and perhaps mortgages, they will offer not only a large choice of products, but also excellent service and advice. At this point, we are still not talking about private banking, but about retail banking for two main target groups. First, for the mass affluent, the number of which is growing rapidly throughout Europe both due to their own success as well as inheritance. This segment is at the same time below the threshold of traditional private banks and the customers are not being served according to their needs by today's retail banks or the other »Distributors« we have been discussing here. Second, »Delicatessen Banks« will be able to fill the product gaps left by the »Aldi Banks« or »McDonald's Banks« for those clients who prefer standardized, cheap products for their daily requirements but want to complement these with individually tailored products for their more complex needs such as investments.

To distinguish themselves, »Delicatessen Banks« will need to develop and market a brand name that customers will recognize and will be willing to pay for. In the world of financial services, for instance, both American Express Gold Card or Sal. Oppenheim have already managed to do this for credit cards and private banking respectively.

Regarding their internal processes, »Delicatessen Banks«, as most »Distributors«, will outsource whatever they can to the »Administrators« in order to counter the disadvantages of their comparatively small scale. Different from other »Distributors«, however, they will probably have to resort to many different suppliers of products and transactions to be able to deliver their wide product range and still fulfill their high-quality requirements.

Niche Players – the »Fur-Hats-Are-Us Banks«

As food retailing has shown, the existence of delicatessen stores does not at all hamper the development of niche players. Niche players can either focus on a certain product or on a certain customer group. For example, the bakery around the corner selects its niche according to only one product, for which they offer a large variety to a broad range of customers, while the specialty stores for organically grown food or Asian ingredients that only larger cities might offer choose their niche according to a specific customer group to whom they offer a broad range of products. In both cases, the companies have streamlined their offers to fill exactly their chosen niche.

As current competitors have already shown, also in retail banking there are promising business models which focus on a clearly defined niche. Take the French consumer credit company Cetelem, a subsidiary of BNP Paribas: Cetelem uses all sorts of different (and well known) channels to sell its products, for example in France, Carrefour or the furniture chain Conforama.

Active in 21 countries in Europe, Asia, Africa, and Latin America, Cetelem has issued more than 38 million cards, including 13 million of its flagship product »Aurore«, a fixed payments card. The secret behind the surprisingly high financial margins of the Aurore card, 12.1 percent in Belgium, 13.0 percent in France, 14.4 percent in Italy, and 16.9 percent in Spain, according to CEO Labruyère, is an intelligent customer segmentation with tailored payments solutions for each segment[18].

In Germany, MLP is a also good example. MLP was the first to successfully tailor its offer (investment advice and insurances) to a rather limited group of clients that were not selected according to their current, but to their future wealth. Founded in 1971, MLP originally catered to law students only, but one year later included students of medicine and dentistry. In 1985, the business model was widened to cater to business and economics students, engineers, and technical students as well. As the students became professionals, MLP's offers became more sophisticated, and the company grew with its clients. For a long time, however, the acquisition of new customers was limited to the campuses. By now, MLP has widened its approach to serve all academics, students and professionals alike, and offers banking products as well. MLP uses a very specific sales force where, in order to match their clients sophistication, virtually all advisors are university educated and, if possible, have worked in the job their clients currently holds. More precisely, the company uses ex-doctors, ex-lawyers, and ex-engineers to advise the customers and address their specific needs.

Both Cetelem and MPL have focused their entire operations on the chosen product or customer niche, for example their brand, presence, product range, services, employee selection, model of distribution, channels, and so on. The business model looks easy: Optimize your offer precisely towards a chosen product or client niche, thus specializing on the products or services that the respective clients require. The difficult part is to consciously cut out other client segments, products, channels, or services that represent no real value added and which dilute the chosen areas of product or client specialization and unnecessarily increase costs.

Market players who want to focus on a specific niche have to also be careful to define their business well. The market niche chosen must be big enough to warrant the specialization, but it must not be so big as that existing players have already adapted their offers to the needs of the customer group concerned. Moreover, for the chosen clientele, a range of products and services must be put together that offers enough advantages so that the prospective client is willing to either leave an existing banking – or rather financial services – relationship or to add a new one to the existing repertoire. The value proposition must not only be strong enough to attract clients, but must also be defendable, i. e. difficult for competitors to replicate – most notably for the still omnipresent full service retail banks.

In this quest for differentiation, both cost structure and services offer themselves as distinguishing criteria. Concerning costs, new on-line banks like ING direct not only operate without the very costly overhead of most existing players, they also do not need to worry about equally costly and maintenance-intensive legacy systems. For a niche player seeking differentiation through the services offered, the ability to defend his position might be less obvious but is almost equally as strong: Any full service retail bank can try to emulate a specifically targeted offer, but its success in fitting such a service into its existing processes and systems without either creating tremendous costs in the process or compromising on the breadth, depth, or quality of its offer are extremely slim. The resulting offer cannot be sustainable and competitive in the long run.

In order to be efficient despite being small, niche players will have to outsource both product development and transactions as much as possible. There is one obvious limit to outsourcing: For some niche players, it might be precisely the well-designed products or processes that give them their competitive advantage. If they turn to developing all or some of their products in-house, they cross over to the business model of the »Client Specialists«. For everything else that is not a key success factor, however, outsourcing becomes imperative.

The clients that niche players will be able to attract will be those dissatisfied with the current offer they get – potentially nearly everybody. What niches are possible? Given the development of the age structures in Europe, a bank focusing on the needs of the elderly might be successful. For this specific customer group, the bank would need to offer easy access to personal interfaces. In terms of products, the bank could specialize on optimizing investments for retirement needs, giving support with pensions, offering special savings products, giving advice on tax-optimizing the bequeathing of assets to the next generation, etc. As a relatively dense local coverage would be needed, such a bank might also focus geographically, for example on those parts of Europe where elderly people tend to retire like the Cote d'Azur.

Another bank might choose to focus on families with young children, offering not only play areas in their branches, but also advice around the issues of public support or tax breaks for children, life insurance, health insurance, saving for the children's education, opening a child's first account, and providing some education about money or financial planning.

A third, and long term potentially quite profitable niche could be those customers who show high future revenue potential, but are relatively uninteresting to retail banks right now. In the end, that is why MLP started out targeting students and now has many high earning academics as clients.

Looking at the established retail banks, their current full-service orientation, and their associated cost structures, it is unlikely that one of them will specialize enough to develop into a future niche competitor. In order to be profitable despite a narrow customer group, niche players need to be imaginative, adaptable, and lean. Like ING Direct, niche players are therefore much more likely to be independent spin-offs from existing players – if they are given the necessary independence and managerial freedom – or they will develop from scratch. As it is virtually impossible to offer even just fundamental banking services to the clients when a company starts from scratch, these start-ups will need to develop out of an even more specific niche that is likely to make money almost from the beginning. A classical path is entering via advisory services. In this way, the company can make money based on advice until the client base is big enough to warrant offering selected banking services as well. This is also the path that MLP, for instance, took in Germany.

One should not discount the future influence and market power of niche players. Already today, there are many of them who are cherry picking the best customers or the most profitable businesses away from general retail banking. Private banks focusing on affluent customers belong to this segment, as does MLP with its focus on academics, as well as investment specialists which offer hedge funds implicitly only to affluent customers, as the minimum investment excludes virtually everybody else. The more niche players manage to draw the most attractive business segments, the less profitable the remaining market will become.

Customer Targeting via Self-Selection

In talking about these various types of »Distributors«, we have focused very much on the different target groups they may choose to cater to. While this is correct, there is also one other method of selecting one's clients, that is, to select them according to similar behavior as ING Direct has done. In the end, Aldi does not worry whether their clients are poor, greedy, or simply consider it hip to shop there. McDonald's does not care whether they are serving the guy on the road who needs a quick bite before driving for another seven hours, or the mother who promised her kids to take them to

McDonald's if they were good at the grocery store. As long as the customers fit the respective business model, they are welcome. As soon as they do not, they are not. Similarly, different »Distributor« business models will »find« their customers through self-selection as customers decide on their own whether they like or do not like the offers. As a consequence, it is up to the bank to make sure it does not begin »overstretching« its model to accommodate for those clients who originally would not quite fit into the business model. The rule will be to keep the system slim and focused, and let the »others« go.

Franchising as an Alternative to Traditional Distribution Models

One way of keeping the system – and the branches – slim is to use franchising. Abbey National, the 6th largest bank in the UK, has been the first to try franchising its branches on a large scale. According to Mark Melvin, Director of Franchising, Abbey National wants to use the »ownership and empowerment to increase revenues, manage costs, and provide a consistent branded customer experience which will grow the business organically«[19]. In their franchising system, Abbey provides the brand, the branch network, operating systems, policies, procedures, and support from head office functions. The franchise manager then adds the local knowledge, commitment, entrepreneurship, and a limited amount of capital.

Since 2000, the bank has run various pilots to test different franchising schemes. The results of the test phase have been very promising. Sales increases pre- to post-franchising amounted to an average of 28 percent for »internal franchises« and between 36 and 66 percent for »external franchises« (see also p. 45). Customer satisfaction was found to increase by ten percent compared to non-franchised branches. At the same time, overall colleague satisfaction also rose from 64 to 70 percent, with the most significant increase observed for leadership style and management.

Many factors have contributed to this success. Most obviously, a local manager will always be superior to central management when it comes to managing employees, managing the local costs, and spotting sales opportunities. Due to the franchisee's financial involvement, his motivation will also be higher than that of »just« an employee. There are, however, further effects: For most banks, serious careers are only made in the head office, not in the branches. As a consequence, that is where the ambitious and capable managers go. For a franchisee, this is different. With a sizeable earnings upside and a time horizon of at least six years, running branches becomes a career in itself and attracts entrepreneurial managers who are convinced of their capabilities.

Abbey National also experienced other positive impacts on the entire organization. Setting up a franchising program requires a bank to formalize fundamental issues, for example what a branch network is supposed to deliver and what constitutes a good branch manager. As well, processes might need to be formalized and streamlined. In addition, as a franchisee has a direct incentive to make his branch a commercial success, he will instantly challenge the head office where he sees bad quality, be it in inefficient processes or badly designed products, leaflets, or marketing campaigns. Such complaints, often the most efficient form of feedback, should be handled very seriously in order to improve the entire operation. Lastly, Abbey's franchised branches also display an improved sales and credit quality.

However, the bank also faced challenges. The franchise agreement including incentives and disincentives had to be designed very carefully in order to stimulate the aimed-for behaviors. Protection of the brand remains crucial and minimum service standards needed to be set in all franchise contracts. In addition, compliance with tax and supervisory rules had to be assured and approval of the relevant supervisory authorities was necessary.

For Abbey National, the conclusions from the pilots were straightforward: The bank sees franchising as sustainable and scaleable innovation to grow revenues, attract talented employees, and make the bank »a great place to work«[20]. By end of 2002, Abbey had already rolled out the franchising system to roughly half of their branch network[21].

Model 3: ›The Administrators‹ — Companies Focusing on Infrastructure

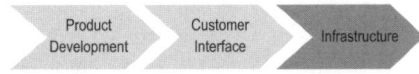

The »Administrator« business models have developed the furthest and already have the greatest presence in today's retail banking world. The »Administrators« will be important components in the networks of specialized companies who will form the future retail banking system. By insourcing processes from the »Distributors«, they will make sure that processes taking place »in the background«, i.e. invisible to customers, offering no added value for clients, and which are competitively irrelevant, will be performed in a cost efficient way with the appropriate scale economies.

When talking about the single value chain steps, we already gave many examples of existing outsourcing relationships. Within the »Administrators«, two specializations should be distinguished. The first are the »Transaction Specialists«, who focus on the production of transactions at a large scale and at low cost (transaction banking). The second are the »IT or Administration Specialists«, who insource the entire IT operations or support functions of financial service institutions. Of these two types of »Administrators«, quite a few players exist already. Especially in IT, large savings are possible: Within a bank's cost of materials, IT costs are by far the largest, and amount to over twelve percent of the total cost base[22]. Unfortunately, due to legislation prohibiting the outsourcing of credit and risk management, the third variety of »Administrators«, the »Risk Managers«, will not exist.

For »Distributors« or others wanting to outsource activities to an »Administrator«, it is essential to assess the future business potential of the possible business partner. It is important to know whether the service provider is likely to be competitive in the long run. Transaction banking especially, is a field where consolidation is ongoing and in which nobody wants to end up with one system, while everyone else in the market migrates to another. The switching costs at such a late stage would simply be too high.

Transaction Specialists – the »Assembly Lines«

The »Assembly Lines« have focused on processing transfers (e. g. ETB), processing checks (e. g. iPSL, UK), clearing and settlement (e. g. Clearstream International), credit card management (e. g. Bayerische Landesbank), and asset servicing and custody (e. g. State Street). So far, there is little evidence of further types of transactions joining this list of »usual suspects« for outsourcing.

Nevertheless, the degree of consolidation in this sector is still much lower than it could and should be. Not only do many players still perform these processes in-house, current consolidation efforts are also largely overshadowed by political issues as well, for example, private retail banks refusing to give their business to competitors. Co-operative or savings banks, too, do not give their business just to anybody, except sometimes – grudgingly – to their own central bodies. A break-through happened in Germany in January 2003. There, the clearing and settlement provider WPS, which is owned by two savings banks associations, and the clearing and settlement provider BWS, which is owned by two co-operative central institutions, agreed to merge »as soon as possible«[23]. Generally, however, vanity creates enormous inefficiencies. These markets should be dominated by between five and 20 players in Europe, so the consolidation of the number of credit institutions in the European Union from around 8 000 to around 7 000 between 1998 and 2001 is a start, but does not help much. In order to really realize the possible scale economies and therefore cost efficiencies, all types of retail banks will have to focus less on political issues and increasingly think about business economics.

Of course, competitive considerations are also important. As we argued already when discussing the value chain step of transaction/administration, competition with one's customers, or the lack thereof, is what determines the chances of success for an insourcer. It must also be completely clear that the company will not in any way breach confidentiality. In this matter, a direct competitor usually is not regarded as trustworthy, and neither is his spun-off subsidiary. An ex-competitor, however, who is specialized in a transaction or process to such a degree that he is no longer a competitor to the regular business, certainly qualifies. As do specialized transaction companies that are either stand-alone – and always were – or that were built and are supervised jointly by several competitors.

This is where the secret of success lies for becoming a successful »Assembly Line«: The company needs to be fully independent and impartial, and it needs to be viewed as such. Only then will the »Distributors« of the future be willing to outsource their transactions to a third party. And only then will the respective transaction specialist be able to gain enough scale to survive the consolidation process, which will have to and will take place around the transaction activities of the »Administrators«.

IT or Administration Specialists

In recent years, outsourcing the entire IT operations has started to take off among financial services institutions. As mentioned before, IBM has been especially active in this field, but also others like EDS, Cap Gemini, Accenture, or CSC are fighting for their share in the market. Outsourcing the entire IT operations has been a recent phenomenon, but in view of both the increased efficiency requirements and the increased focus of the single players on specific value chain steps, the trend is likely to continue to increase.

Regarding classic support functions, the trend towards outsourcing is already much more advanced in other industries. Whether it be payroll, purchasing of office supplies, or facility management, such support processes have already begun to be outsourced years ago and the trend is continuing to grow. Retail banking as well will have to use the cost advantages offered by these third parties.

In this area, there is less necessity for new players to develop than, for example, among the »Distributors« or »Product Developers«. For IT outsourcing, strong and successful players already exist. For other administration functions, there are no fundamental differences compared to other industries, so the established players could also be used to fulfill the needs of the retail banking community. This is not to say that there is no room for new players. However, different from the many other business models developed here, there is less of a need for new entrants as companies are already in existence that follow more or less the models described here.

Model 4: The ›Client Specialists‹ – Retail Banks Focusing on Product Development and the Customer Interface

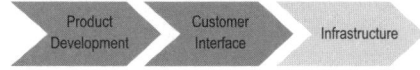

A »Distributor« can buy his products from »Product Developers«, be they standard or specialist products. In some cases, however, there is also a strong argument for combining product development and the customer interface activities in one business model. When the target group of a bank's offer becomes very distinct, at some point only the company at the customer interface itself knows its customers well enough to develop the right, custom-made products and services targeted specifically at its special customer segment. We call such competitors »Client Specialists«, because they aim at fulfilling their (small) customer group's every wish in a comprehensive way, including developing and distributing a differentiated product offer.

This need can arise predominantly for »Fur-Hats-Are-Us Banks« or perhaps also for »Delicatessen Banks«, which might then end up drifting towards the »Client Specialist« business model. However, if an »Aldi Bank« or »McDonald's Bank« were to think about developing own products, it would deviate from its price and convenience focus significantly and thereby jeopardize its entire business model.

These »Client Specialists« can neither compete with full line »Distributors«, nor does their product development compete with the preciously discussed »Product Developers«. On both of these fronts, they would lose against their adversary's larger scale and therefore cost advantages. Most likely, »Client Specialists« will outsource their infrastructure needs to the greatest extent possible because – due to the fact that they serve a niche only

– they are small and want to participate in the insourcers' scale economies. Even as far as the development of standard products is concerned, they might choose to outsource. But as soon as it comes to their differentiated offers, they will want it to be proprietary and will develop it themselves.

By definition, as the »Client Specialists« focus on niches, there will not be very many of them. But, depending on what niche they focus on (for possible target groups, see »niche players« earlier in this chapter) they could be quite successful.

Model 5: ›The Engineers‹ — Companies Focusing on Product Development and Transactions

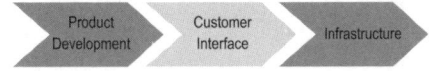

There is one more combination of aggregated value chain steps that offers the opportunity to create additional value: That is, combining product development with the processing of transactions. There are two sources of additional value: First, the example of the product developing reinsurer described earlier can be transferred into retail banking. As illustrated in the first part of this chapter, the company uses their customers' data to obtain a better understanding of the underlying mechanisms and risks than its customers have. Based on this understanding, the reinsurer develops new products for their customers, the primary insurers, to sell to their customers, the mass market. In a similar fashion, transaction banks could use their insight« from processing the transactions of their many »Distributor« clients to get an overview that allows them to develop products with better features or at better conditions. In order to be successful, the »Engineers« must make sure they respect the confidentiality of the data they use. This could mean aggregating it, making it anonymous, or doing whatever the customers demand in order for the company not to compromise its role as an independent, unbiased, and reliable partner for outsourcing. Second, the »Engineers« could use their detailed understanding of their own processing capabilities, costs, and processes to streamline products to their own processing platform. Again, the result would be products with better features or at better conditions.

Like the product developing reinsurer, the »Engineers« would offer their improved products not to the retail banking customers directly but to their clientele of »Distributors«. They would do this so as not to endanger their business model by getting into a competitive situation with their clients as they would then lose their business. In these two ways, the combination of transaction and product development capabilities could be combined to tap into additional value, which would be inaccessible to players operating in only one of the two areas.

Forming the Future Retail Banking Industry

These business models – or similarly focused ones – will make up the future network within the retail banking industry. The question for today's players is not whether to specialize, but when to start. The two most important issues will certainly be which business to specialize in, and how to get there, i.e. how to transform today's »universal retail bank« into a more focused and specialized player.

So far, European retail banks have only begun to adapt to these trends. To evaluate the advance in more detail, we conducted a European survey among 86 leading banks during the end of 2002. The questions covered how active the organizations were in the in- or outsourcing of processes, and whether the banks were already using external distribution channels either under their own brand, or under the distribution channel's brand, to distribute their products (see Exhibit 16: Results of the Survey on Trends in European Retail Banking (I and II)).

The results are hardly surprising. Generally, in both areas of the survey – in- and outsourcing and the use of external distribution channels – the level of activity is low. The outsourcing of processes is, however, clearly the most developed of the four processes covered in the questionnaire. In this area, there were no banks that had not taken one step or the other, whereas almost a quarter of respondents were not active at all in insourcing. About 40 percent had not even thought about external distribution under their own brand, and almost 50 percent were equally as inactive in external distribution under the distribution channel's brand.

It is most instructive to compare the »insourcing« and »outsourcing« lines. Consider »back-office infrastructure«: Many respondents consider outsourcing this activity attractive, but insourcing it »is not an issue« for most of them. Clearly, the demand for outsourcing these backbone activities needs to be met by other players, namely highly specialized IT service providers such as IBM. This is hardly surprising, as these activities do not fall into most banks' core competencies.

For the other activities, interest in both out- and insourcing is roughly equal. This indicates that whatever demand there is for outsourcing a given activity, there are other banking players who deem insourcing that same activity attractive and who could therefore meet the demand. In other words: A functioning market for out- and insourcing seems to be developing *within* the retail banking community.

Regarding the use of external distribution channels, the level of activities is very low. Where external channels are used, they usually originate from within the financial services industry, for example financial intermediaries, mortgage banks, or simply other banks. So far, only very few European retail banks are using or planning to use innovative external channels from outside the banking world.

»How do you feel about outsourcing/insourcing any of these activities?«

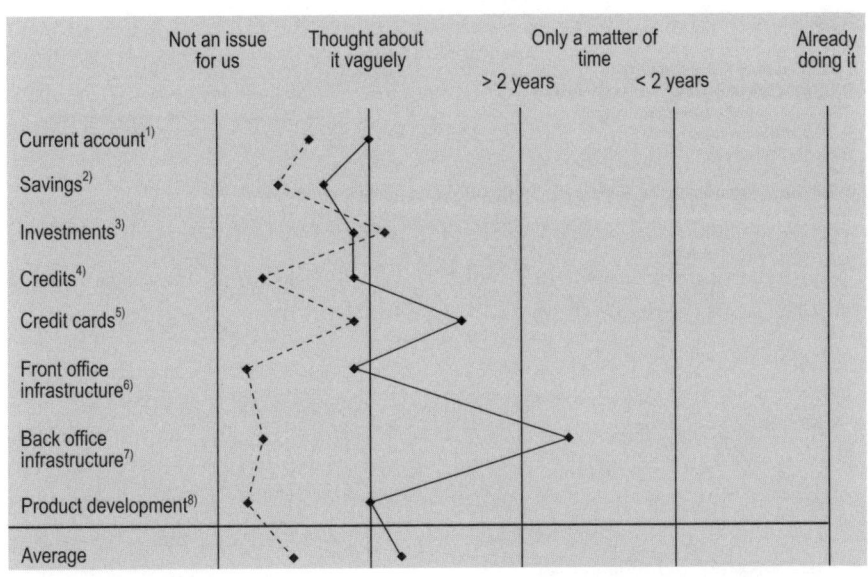

1) Account management, money transfer
2) Account management
3) Account management, clearing and settlement, custody, investment servicing
4) Credit assessment, dunning and collection
5) Account management, settlement
6) Call centers, ATMs, service terminals, Internet, Intranet

7) Software development, sofware maintanance, data processing centers
8) Mutual funds, retirement provisions, tax driven investments

Legend:
——— Average answers for outsourcing
- - - - Average answers for insourcing

Exhibit 16: Results of the Survey on Trends in European Retail Banking (I)

The European
Retail Banking
Landscape in the
Future

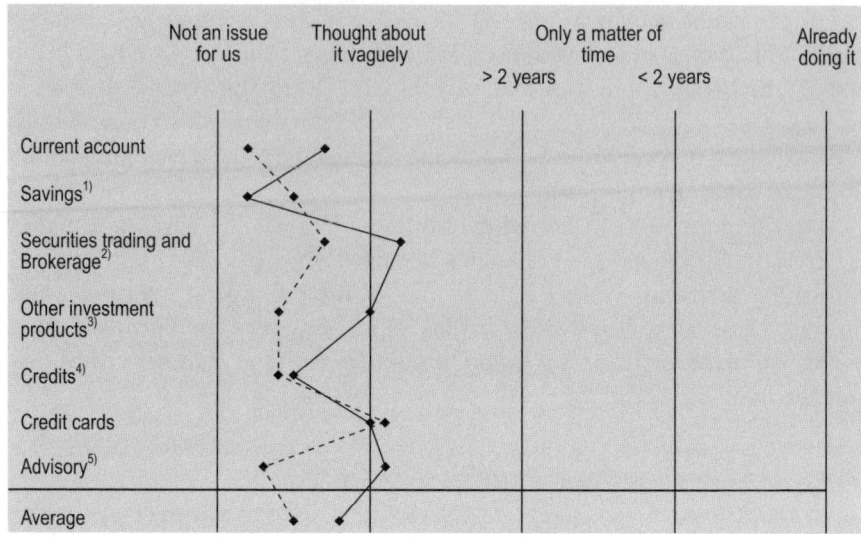

»Do you use any external distribution channels to distribute your products under your own brand / under the distribution channel's brand?«

1) Savings account, fixed term deposits
2) Account, shares, bonds, mutual funds, derivatives
3) Tax driven investments, retirement provisions
4) Overdraft credit, consumer credit
5) Investments, financing

Legend:
——— Average answers for own brand
- - - - - Average answers for distribution channel's brand

Exhibit 16: Results of the Survey on Trends in European Retail Banking (II)

As these figures show, much work remains to be done. How can today's retail banks best refocus themselves on a more promising business model?

5
Transformation Strategies

Throughout the last chapter we argue that, in fact, retail banks will have to make a choice. Either they see product development or transactions as a core competence, in which case they should think about focusing on these activities and getting rid of the part of operations dealing with the customers, or they accept the challenge from the new entrants at the customer interface and focus their efforts there, most often leading to outsourcing of product development and transactions/administration. However, of those future players we described, very few exist already. Today's retail banks will have to decide which direction to move into in order to keep up with the increasing and accelerating tendency towards specialization.

Such a transformation may be difficult, but is not impossible, as State Street has shown. Based in the US, State Street is notable for successfully having shifted its business from being a full-service bank to offering outsourcing services around the investment process. For a detailed description of State Street's services, please refer to Chapter 4.1, Transaction/Administration. Admittedly, the company has been in this business for a long time. In 1924, the then »State Street Bank« was asked to administer the first ever US mutual fund. When ERISA, the Employee Retirement Income Security Act, became a law in 1974, this reconfirmed the business model of asset servicing. By the mid eighties, State Street Bank had grown into a global financial services provider while still pursuing its traditional business of being a regional retail bank. The transition was further refined in 1997, when the bank launched its new brand identity »State Street«, singularly focusing on institutional investors worldwide, and losing the »Bank« from its name. The consequent confirmation of the move for State Street came in 1999, when the company sold its retail and commercial banking arms to focus entirely on investment services.

This change in business focus was not pursued in response to problems in the retail-banking arm. The company has experienced double digit growth for the last 24 consecutive years. Rather, it was the recognition of a niche business that produced a nicely stable flow of fee revenues where State Street could build upon its competitive advantage.

»We are permanently adjusting our portfolio,« says Thomas A. Bergenroth, Senior Vice President and Managing Director of State Street and General Manager of State Street Bank GmbH. In 2001, State Street acquired DST's Portfolio Accounting System in order to complete their accounting capabilities. In response to a growing market in hedge funds, the company acquired IFS in 2002, a leading provider of fund accounting and administration as well as trade support and middle office services for alternative investment portfolios. Around the same time, State Street sold its corporate trust business, again in order to focus even more precisely on the two business lines of asset servicing and asset management. »Over all these years, of course there has been tremendous internal change«, Bergenroth concedes. »Naturally, we bought and sold some of our employees together with the respective businesses; but up to now, our growth has been largely organic and the pace of change self determined.«

In November 2002, State Street entered into an agreement to purchase substantial portions of Deutsche Bank's Global Securities Service Business GSS. As a result of the 1.5 billion US Dollars deal, State Street will acquire Deutsche Bank's global custody business, fund administration services, and other related operations – including approximately 3 200 DB employees worldwide. The days of largely organic growth are over.

State Street's commitment to a clear and focused strategy has clearly paid off. Today, including the newly acquired GSS operations, State Street is the largest global custodian, the sixth-largest investment manager, the number one servicer of US mutual funds and US pension plans, as well as the number one provider of foreign exchange services worldwide.

In Chapter 4, we described a number of generic market opportunities. In the end, each bank will have to select its future position individually, according to its own individual capabilities, current business focus, and possible restrictions. Independent of the selected positioning, however, banks will have to follow similar processes in order to manage such a transition well.

Achieving a viable position for the future hinges on the successful completion of three steps (see Exhibit 17: Three Steps Towards a Successful Future Business Model). In the first step, a realistic and viable business model must be chosen. Secondly, the entire future operations have to be designed around the chosen business model down to the most detailed level. Lastly, the implementation itself, frequently spanning several years, has to be managed carefully. The implementation often consists of one or several external transactions, i. e. mergers, acquisitions, or divestments, and a phase of internal transition, i. e. the internal change of the company. In the long term, the business needs to be streamlined continuously in order to follow the chosen business model as closely as possible.

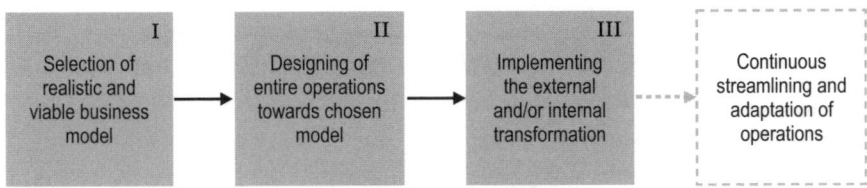

I	II	III	
Selection of realistic and viable business model	Designing of entire operations towards chosen model	Implementing the external and/or internal transformation	Continuous streamlining and adaptation of operations

Exhibit 17: Three Steps Towards a Successful Future Business Model

Step I: Selection of a Realistic and Viable Business Model

What future business model do I want to follow? This is the central question today's banks will have to ask themselves when thinking about the future. Along the chain of analyses, judgments, and decisions that will lead to an answer (see Exhibit 18: Process to Select a Realistic and Viable Business Model), the very first issue is already a difficult one: What am I good at? Why do customers choose me? Why do they buy my products or services? And, finally, what are the key capabilities within my business system which support whatever it is that my customers like? If we take the example of BMW, customers might choose the cars because they feel BMW is a »sporty« brand and offers technically sound cars of »German quality«. But what does that say about the key capabilities within the underlying business systems? Is the success due to superior marketing, superior design, superior engine know-how, a combination of these things, or something else? Retail banks – and companies in general – will have to develop a deep understanding of these issues in order to identify their key capabilities, that is the specific advantages they have over the competition which matter most to the customers. In this context, »customers« can be end-customers as well as specialized players within the future retail banking industry. If no singular customer relevant current key capabilities can be identified, the company will have to assess in which areas it has the know-how to build or acquire significant capabilities within a reasonable time frame.

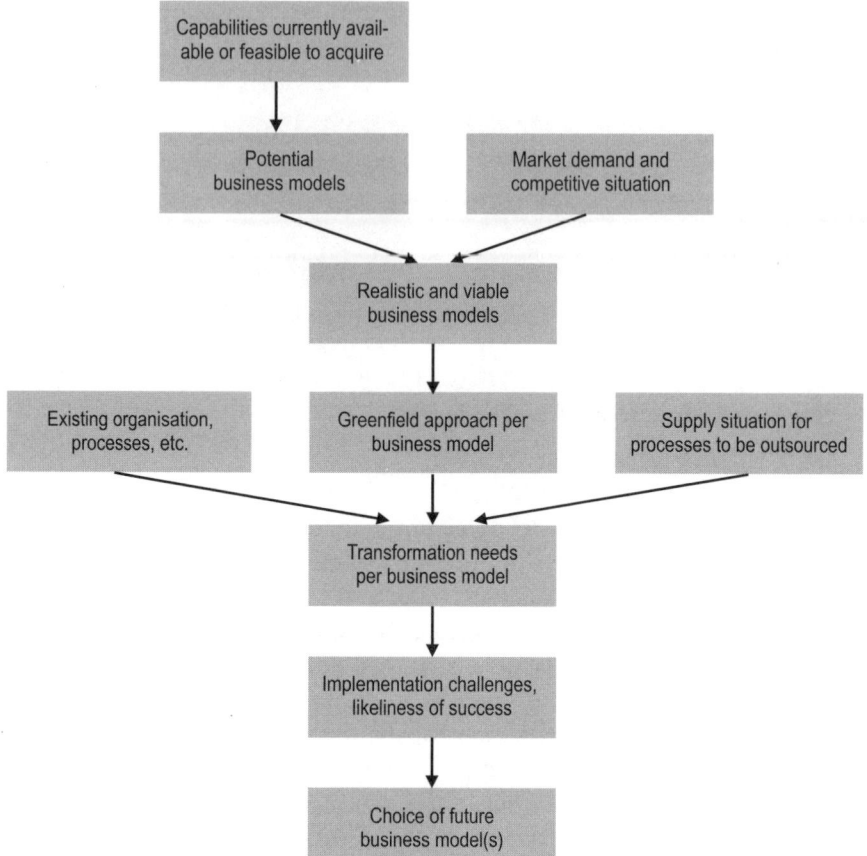

Exhibit 18: Process to Select a Realistic and Viable Business Model

Once the key capabilities are clear, a number of possible business models can be deduced and the viability of each will have to be verified. Is there a demand for the services of the respective business model? Are there enough customers, and are they willing to pay an appropriate price? Are there already too many competitors active in the segment whose offering I will not be able to beat to a sufficient degree that I am able to create an attractive value proposition for my future clients?

For the realistic and viable business models passing this check, a set of deeper analyses has to be performed. If I were to use a green-field approach and design the new entity from scratch, what would it look like? What would I do in-house, what would I outsource? What, roughly, would the organization and processes look like? And, are we talking only about an array of mutually exclusive potential business models, or do I have key capabilities different enough and strong enough to think about transforming myself into several different future players? Of course, they would all have to be separate and specialized in order not to lose the value of focus, but still – may I be transforming into, and spinning off, several future businesses?

Regarding the processes to be outsourced, particularly at the beginning of this industry-wide process of forming specialized players, the existence of outsourcing providers will become an issue. Do providers of these services exist already? Will one of my own new offshoots perhaps become my supplier? If I cannot find an external provider and if at the same time my own capabilities are not strong enough to spin-off a viable entity, will I have to endure a transition period during which I will have to keep the process in-house even though this contradicts my ideal business model? This set of decisions is extremely sensitive and needs to be managed very carefully. It is very easy to spin off an external unit only because its services are needed, despite the fact that I may not be good enough at whatever it is this entity is supposed to do in order to attract external clients. It is equally easy to keep the process in-house and to continue devoting a lot of managerial effort into the process, thus »forgetting« to focus on the actual chosen business model. Alternatively, I might »forget« to look for alternative external options later in time. In this matter of how to provide for those business processes I do not want to do myself, but where no external service provider is currently available, only extreme honesty regarding one's own capabilities and continuous focus on the big picture can prevent making the wrong decisions.

Now that I know how the future business systems underlying my future business model(s) could look like, how do they match up with my existing organization? What transformation needs exist? What are the challenges during a possible implementation, and – ultimately – how likely am I to succeed? The decision about which future business model or models to transform into can only be made after these questions in the chain of necessary analyses have been answered.

Step II: Designing the Entire Operations Towards the Chosen Business Model

Whichever business model is chosen, what matters most is the focus and the single-mindedness with which the supporting operations, or the »business system«, are thought through and implemented.

Let us look to the example of the German discounter chain Aldi again[1]. In Chapter 4, we highlighted Aldi's positioning as a low cost (»discount«) provider and named the business model of the price leader after the company. »Aldi Banking« was meant to be synonymous with a focus on price. Let us now take a look at how the Albrecht brothers, the owners of the chain who lent their name to the »ALbrecht DIscount« markets over 50 years ago, streamlined the operations to deliver their value proposition of low prices. We do not want to suggest that this is in any way directly comparable to how the future price leaders in retail banking, the so called »Aldi Banks«, should run their business. What we do want to point out is how much attention to the details is required in order for a business to be sustainable and successful in the long-term.

From the beginning, Aldi's idea was simple: Be cheaper than the competition. After the Second World War, Germany's food retailing was dominated by union-owned shops. At the end of the year, customers could claim a three percent rebate on all shopping bills presented. The Albrecht brothers' idea was simple: Why not grant this three percent savings right away, thereby beating the union shops' prices? This idea proved to be hugely successful, and the focus on low prices was born.

Since then, the system has been refined almost beyond recognition. What has remained untouched is the focus on price. Today, in the food section, Aldi offers a selection of fresh fruit and vegetables as well as frozen food and refrigerated goods. Non-food items include cleansing agents, personal hygiene products, and household supplies. In addition, there are always special offers ranging from clothing or CDs to microwave ovens and sometimes even personal computers. This has not always been the case. For years, Aldi had no frozen food at all and only an extremely limited supply of fresh produce. The logistics system was not geared to handle these perishable goods and therefore – sensibly – they were excluded from the shops. As Aldi's logistics capabilities grew, the model could be expanded to include such sensitive items. When a deposit on one-way cans and bottles was introduced in Germany in January 2003, Aldi sold off all their stock of the affected products before year-end 2002 at vastly reduced prices because it was unwilling to build the costly capability of handling returns right away. Whether these products will be readmitted to the shops – and returns made possible – is still an open question. A good business model rests on the knowledge not only of what you can do, but also, and equally importantly, of what you cannot do.

In line with their cost consciousness, Aldi has no press office, no public relations unit, and no advertising department. No advertising agency has ever had an assignment from Aldi. The weekly newspaper ads advertising the special offers of the week come with the rather matter-of-fact header »Aldi informs«. This sober wording reinforces the image of cost consciousness and subsequent low prices.

Up to today, the system continues to be constantly challenged and streamlined. Introducing those new scanner checkouts would have unnecessarily slowed down the (extremely fast and efficient) checkout process as it takes too much time to turn the products around and search for the bar code. Aldi used its market power to »convince« the manufacturers to place several bar codes on each product – in the front, in the back, and, if possible, also on the sides, top and bottom – and is introducing scanner checkouts as well. For fear of a negative brand impact, brand manufacturers refused to give Aldi the cheap prices the discounter needed for its business model to work? For Aldi, they agreed to produce under new, unknown brands, which could not be connected to the original manufacturers and which are not marketed anywhere else. Available forklifts did not fit Aldi's requirements of a just-in-time distribution process? Different from the processes at many other supermarkets' central warehouses, at Aldi, the goods are not really stored but just redistributed from the suppliers' incoming trucks to Aldi's waiting outgoing trucks. Forklifts therefore are not required to lift pallets, but rather move them from one side of the hall to the other. To be able to quicken the process, Aldi nagged forklift manufacturers for long enough to have a specific model developed for them. This model is able to push three pallets at the same time rather than moving and lifting only one. Many of the (often female) staff developed back problems, because, on average, each of them had to stack goods worth over 100 000 Euros a month due to the high turnover? Aldi got the manufacturers to develop a hand pallet transporter that in addition to moving the pallets through the shop also lifts them up to 70 centimeters so that the personnel can stand upright while unloading. Due to less sick leaves, everybody benefits.

Throughout the entire company, the structure, processes, and efficiencies are optimized to the smallest detail such that less financial and personnel resources are required. Again, everything is geared towards the value proposition of low prices.

The success of the concept is enormous. New stores are opened by the week, over 70 within the last six months. Today, the Albrecht brothers run more than 3 700 markets in Germany and over 2 600 abroad.

What retail banks – like every other company – can learn from this is how to successfully streamline operations towards one overarching goal. The impression one gets from the Aldi system is somewhere between »single-minded« and »obsessed« – but it is precisely this single-mindedness or obsession that made and continues to make the company successful. One other fact becomes also clear: Business systems develop over time as new technologies become available and customer preferences or competitive situations change. Sometimes, an entire business model might have to be abandoned, but most often, adaptations to the supporting operations within the existing framework are sufficient. That is not to say that in order to build a new business model, sub-optimal operations are sufficient, which can later be improved. Rather, at any given time, the company's operations have to support the given model in an optimal way; just what that »optimal way« looks like can change. If there is one central message to be learned from the Albrecht brothers, it is certainly to »be obsessed«.

Admittedly, it is often quite difficult to design the business system (step II) without being influenced by step III (the realities of how to get there). Nevertheless, clarifying the business system without thinking about the constraints of the existing operations can be a very enlightening and liberating process. To a certain degree, this is the same as using the green-field approach during step I, the decision process about what business model(s) to adopt in the future. During step I, however, it was sufficient to roughly design the respective underlying business systems for many different models. In step II, the entire new company must be redesigned down to the most minute detail. Design the optimal system, question everything you do today, and do so by not using your current operations as a basis for your considerations. You can worry about those »holy cows« that may need to be slaughtered later.

Step III: Implementing the Transformation

Once both the future business model and the supporting business systems are clear, the implementation process begins. First, the path of how to reach the desired end-state will have to be designed. The radical changes we are proposing here – focusing on a few activities and outsourcing the others – can most likely not be implemented without some M&A activities. Which parts of the existing operations are not required anymore? Which parts will need to remain to form the optimal future business system? If two or more business models are to be sculpted out of one company, how can the existing operation be split into several separate and focused entities? Does an existing player need to be acquired in order to support (one of) the future business model(s)? Does the bank need to form a joint venture – and with whom – in order to reach its objectives?

Equally importantly, internal changes will have to be planned. In preparation for M&A activities as well as spin-offs, the bank will have to answer many questions: Which parts have to be disentangled from the rest of the operations? Which of the remaining operations might have to be consolidated? How does the remaining part of the business need to be transformed into the new business model? What will the new organization and processes look like? How do responsibilities need to be reallocated, how do interfaces to external suppliers have to be designed and the respective processes adapted? How are external suppliers identified and selected to begin with?

Quite rightfully, a transformation like this appears to be a daunting task, and it is. There are, however, some key considerations which can increase the likeliness of success for both internal and external transformations.

Key Success Factors for External Transformation

External Transformations can take many shapes, i. e. mergers, acquisitions, joint ventures, or divestments. When it comes to M&A, three general issues matter the most. To begin, the target needs to be chosen well, so that the transaction has the potential to lead to the intended results. In addition, the price paid for the target must be lower than the possible gains, i. e. possible cost and revenues synergies have to be evaluated realistically, and the offer price aligned accordingly. Lastly, the transaction and the following integration into the existing business systems have to be managed such that the intended results are reached. More specifically, eight crucial tasks can be distinguished (see Exhibit 19: Eight Key Success Factors for External Transformation).

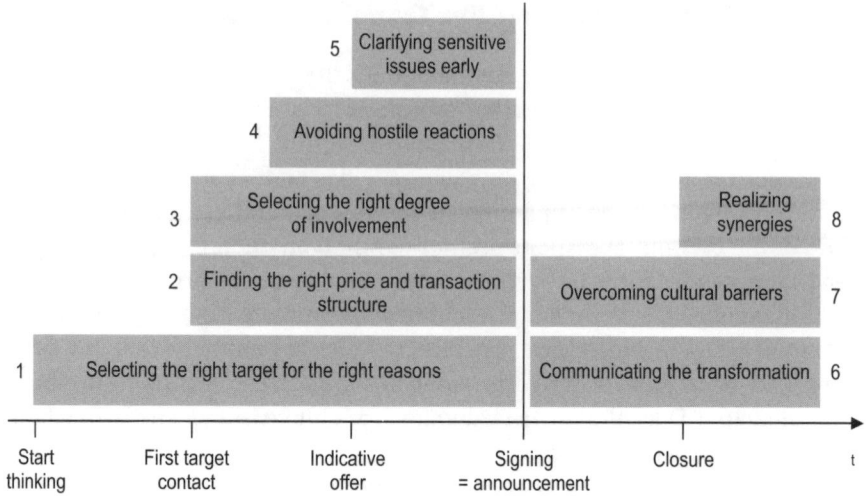

Exhibit 19: Eight Key Success Factors for External Transformation

1. Selecting the Right Target for the Right Reasons

The first and key issue to be considered is the selection of the target company. When it comes to boosting revenues or entering new markets via acquisitions, there is no limit to an executive's ambition. Here, a »vision«, for example Edzard Reuter's idea of turning Daimler Benz into an »integrated technology group«, can take on a life of its own and lose all contact with reality, with the result that painful truths may cease to be acknowledged and the chosen path followed blindly. This can apply for mergers just as much as for strategic changes. In those circumstances, the players sometimes seem to want to raise a monument for themselves or to be driven by the enlargement of their power base rather than by the value they must create for the shareholders. When an M&A project takes on a life of its own, it can be difficult to back down, particularly if negotiations have already been made public. Some transactions may even take place for their own sake without the key players being convinced of their advantages anymore. Therefore, one should use great care at the onset in selecting the right company for a takeover.

Before the question of the target can be solved, which strategy the retail bank wants to pursue and the objectives of the transaction must be clear. Personal ambitions or the simple availability of a target must not compromise the overall transformation processes described here from a »universal retail bank« into a focused player. To make it simple, the transaction in question must make sense in the framework of the targeted business model.

What advantages can a transaction bring? For divestments, two spring to mind: First, the divestments of certain activities or business areas may be necessary in order to (re)focus the business. Second, when a certain market sector is valued very highly (like telecoms in early 2000) and selling the business is likely to generate higher returns than continuation, the sale of the entire operations should be considered. When thinking about mergers and acquisitions, synergies are most often cited as a reason for a transaction. This is true for retail banking as well, but in the future world of specialized players, the answer will have to be more precise; in its general form, »synergies« will not be true anymore in all cases. Between revenue and cost synergies, cost synergies are easier to plan, easier to measure, and easier to implement, which is why, as we will discuss in more detail later, they are the most important synergies to be aimed for in a merger. Cost synergies most frequently are reaped from the middle- and back-office, in the areas of product development, transaction, and administration. In the front office, cost synergies can only be realized if the two merging banks have a local presence, i. e. branches, in the same geography.

However, in the future retail banking industry, the »Distributors« at the customer interface will source out virtually all product development, transaction, and administration that display economies of scale (a prerequisite for making synergies possible) to the »Rocket Scientists«, the »Assembly Lines«, the »IT or Administration Specialists«, or the »Engineers« (see Exhibit 15: Realistic Future Business Models in Retail Banking, p. 87). For the future »Distributors«, there are therefore only very few efficiencies left to gain in the middle- and back-office. Unless a geographical overlap makes it possible to cut costs in the branch network – why should these players take over other »Distributors« at all? Why should they expand cross border? Some niche players might focus on an international clientele. For all others, the one remaining reason is a very powerful one: In order to transport one's own business model with the corresponding unique capabilities to another, less focused, less successful, player. A »Distributor« or »Client Specialist«, for example, who has figured out how to change his branding, marketing, sales, and client-management processes so that he can significantly improve cross-selling rates, customer acquisition, or customer retention, can and should successfully expand his business model internationally via M&A.

For the »Rocket Scientists«, the »Assembly Lines«, the »IT or Administration Specialists«, or the »Engineers«, merging is straightforward. By definition, their businesses display the necessary economies of scale or scope to make a merger successful as long as it is strategically sensible and well executed.

2. Finding the Right Price and Transaction Structure

When planning an acquisition, the buyer possesses only very little, publicly available, information about the target's internal structure, strengths, weaknesses, customer base, and so on. This is especially true for non-listed companies. The buyer must therefore use the time before the final negotiations to get to know as much as possible of the target so as to offer an appropriate price and face less future uncertainties when making the bid. The seller, too, has a strong interest in reducing the information asymmetry, as high uncertainty will make the buyer use a high risk discount and make a correspondingly lower offer.

The approach to overcoming this information asymmetry without disclosing too sensitive details is to offer information step by step. First of all, a good and detailed information memorandum should contain all necessary information required for the potential acquirer to make an indicative bid. Next, an initial due diligence process and management interviews enable interested players to gather detailed, non-public information about the target. During this due diligence, potential bidders gain access to a broad range of the target company's documents, which are set up in the »data room«. The documents give insight into the financial, legal, tax, environmental, and strategic situation of the target. This process usually starts only after a preselection is made based on the indicative offers. Thus, the target can exclude less serious bidders and reduce the number of companies – often competitors – who gain insight into confidential and highly sensitive data. Based on the gathered information as well as additional discussions with the target management, the bidding companies produce a due diligence report, which is the basis for the binding offer, including the price and further conditions. After the acquisition agreement, a confirmatory due diligence may be carried out in order to clarify the final details. These are usually agreed upon before the signing and are directly linked to the amount paid in the transaction.

If, after this elaborate process, the potential buyer still feels uncertain about the future business potential of the target or of the future combined entity and perceives the transaction as too risky, the downside of a transaction can be limited by structuring the deal accordingly. The most frequently used methods are earn-out structures, and put and call options.

An earn-out means that the final price paid for an acquisition is linked to achieving certain milestones after the transaction has taken place. By thus linking the purchase price to future success, the buyer can overcome the remaining uncertainties and reduce his risk. In transaction banking, for example, the future volumes, and therefore the company's performance, strongly depends on the future stock market performance. The risks for the buyer are evident, especially as many business plans contain »hockey stick« developments, in which the target expects a drastic increase in business volume and net income after a historically mediocre performance. Most buyers will doubt such a plan. In order not to derail the entire negotiation, the buyer can opt for an earn-out structure, and both parties will agree that the purchase price depends on the post-transaction performance of the target. If, for instance, a certain earnings level is not reached within a certain time frame, the price would be reduced by an agreed upon amount.

Alternatively, a buyer may make use of options to reduce his risk, be it due to information asymmetry or to a general uncertainty about the future development of the market. He may agree to buy 60 percent of the shares now plus a call option to purchase the remaining 40 percent at the same price in two years. In two years, if the value of the target proves to be equal to or above the value assured by the seller and agreed upon in the transaction, the buyer will exercise his call option. If it is not, he will not increase his share and might even, if a corresponding put option has been included originally, put his 60 percent back to the seller.

A good example of a transaction involving such options was BSkyB's acquisition of Kirch PayTV. In late 1999, British Sky Broadcasting Group (BSkyB), which was 40 percent-owned by Rupert Murdoch, acquired 24 percent of Kirch PayTV for 1.53 billion Euros (paid roughly one third in cash and the rest in BSkyB shares). As the concept of PayTV was new in Germany, the contract included a put option in order to reduce the risk. If Kirch Pay TV missed the targets specified in the business plan in the years to come, for example the number of subscribers, Kirch would have to buy back the 24 percent stake at the original selling price. Should Kirch not be able to do this, Murdoch would have the right to acquire a majority stake in Kirch Pay TV. As Kirch Pay TV missed its targets, Murdoch chose to exercise the put option in 2002. By that time, the Kirch media empire was already facing bankruptcy, however, and BSkyB had to write off its whole stake.

In the end, information asymmetries can never be overcome completely in time to make a fully informed offer. Due to legal restraints, certain pieces of information cannot even be exchanged before the closure of the deal. In addition, the future development of the market will always remain uncertain. It will be up to the good judgment of the buyer, his confidence in his capabilities to realize the value of an acquisition, the cooperation of the target both pre- and post-closure, and to the actual structuring of the deal, whether a justified and adequate price can be established.

3. Selecting the Right Degree of Involvement

When thinking about acquiring, merging, investing in, or joining forces with another company, the buyer has to evaluate carefully to what degree he would like to get involved. Two questions need to be answered: To what degree does the buyer want to control the resulting entity (financial involvement), and how deeply does he want the two entities to be integrated in order to (usually) reap synergies (operational involvement, see Exhibit 20: Framework for Choosing Integration Depth and Financial Involvement).

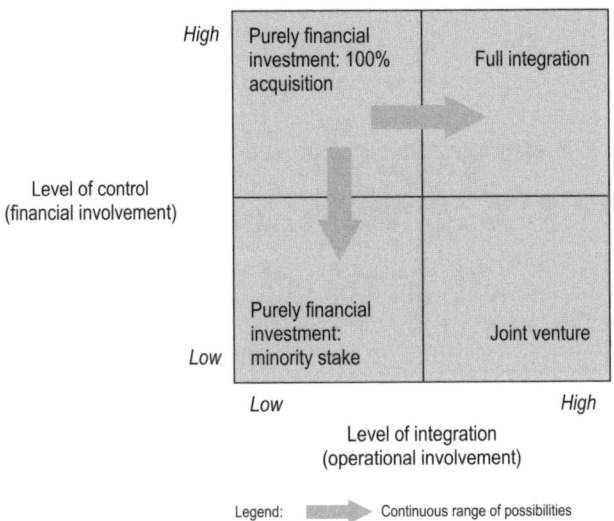

Exhibit 20: Framework for Choosing Integration Depth and Financial Involvement

The first answer usually depends on whether the core business or a more peripheral activity is concerned. In the core business, 100 percent control of the resulting entity is essential, so that a full acquisition or merger is necessary. Even in the so-called »mergers of equals«, there is invariably one party who will ultimately have the say, and both parties usually know who that is before the deal is closed. For a less vital part of the business, acquiring less

Transformation
Strategies

than 100 percent, i.e. a majority or even only a minority stake, or forming a joint venture (thereby splitting the control with the other venture partner(s)) is an option.

The second answer depends on to what degree synergies are supposed to be reaped from the transaction. Using examples from other industries, is the transaction intended to give the purchaser future access to a promising technology (for example, a small biotech company acquired by pharma giant), sales channel (Internet company acquired by media conglomerate) or the like? In those cases, meddling with the acquired company's structure or processes could destroy its competitive advantage, which is often based on (among other things) being much smaller and less bureaucratic than the acquirer. In these cases, the acquired company will be kept at arm's length and a pure acquisition will take place, without merging the two entities afterwards. The only issues that have to be considered here are possible knowledge transfer and the amount and type of control (if any) the new parent wants to exercise. Is the transition meant to shift the strategic focus of the acquiring company to new, more promising businesses – like German Mannesmann transforming from a steel company into a telecommunication company or Preussag turning from yet another steel and industrial goods company into a tourism conglomerate. Or, is it meant to diversify the company due to the cyclical exposure or risk of the existing portfolio – like Philip Morris' acquisition of General Foods in the mid eighties, using up the cash generated by the tobacco business in the process? Again, integration is needed only insofar as reporting, control, and the appropriate flow of funds is to be secured. Things are different, however, once the transaction is meant to bring together two sets of know-how, experience, businesses, or customer groups in order to form an entirely new business or explore a new market. Here, a full integration of the two businesses will be necessary in order to reap intended benefits along all of the affected steps of the value chain. Depending on the level of control, full integration can either mean a full-fledged merger or the establishment of a (by nature) fully integrated joint venture. In financial services as well, the degree of synergies to be reaped determines how closely the two entities in question need to be joined or merged.

Joint Ventures, Acquisitions, Mergers, Merging onto a New Entity (»NewCo«), and »Mergers of Equals«

In a *joint venture*, certain activities are brought into a new entity, the ownership of which is usually divided equally between the joint venture partners. Depending on the relative value of the parts brought into the joint venture, compensation payments may be made. In another less common form of a joint venture, the respective activities are spun off into separate entities, which are then hung beneath a newly created holding company. The joint venture partners in turn become the joint owners of the holding company, which then owns 100 percent of the spun-off entities. Sometimes, joint ventures are planned to be temporary arrangements from the very outset. They combine the strengths of two companies in order to serve a special purpose, and may be dissolved when the goal is achieved. By their nature, however, joint ventures only combine a subset of their parents' organizations and capabilities. They can therefore only be used to create a business that is comparatively narrow in scope in comparison with their parents' activities.

In the classical *acquisition*, one company makes a friendly or hostile bid to take over another company. Large, listed companies can also make use of their shares as take-over currency without risking too much influence of the target's shareholders after the transaction. Usually, the bigger company acquires the smaller one. However, this is only a rough rule. Royal Bank of Scotland, for instance, acquired NatWest in 2000, although it was only half the size of the target.

After an acquisition, the target company can remain a separate legal entity, which is fully or partly owned by the acquiring company, or it can be *merged* into the acquiring company. Citibank, who buys banks all over the world, for instance, follows a middle road by integrating their acquisitions into other subsidiaries or into the parent corporation often only after some time has passed.

As an alternative to merging the target into the acquirer, a *new entity* (NewCo = new company) can be created into which both parties are brought in. One of the largest examples for this approach has been the merger of Daimler-Benz and Chrysler into DaimlerChrysler in 1998. There are two main reasons to use this approach. Firstly, especially in cross-border mergers, political reasons often make it necessary to present a merger as »merger of equals« when it is not. Merging the two companies onto a »NewCo« is a particularly suitable instrument to give the impression of equality. In this way, the takeover of Chrysler by Daimler-Benz could be presented as a merger of equals. Second, when merging onto a NewCo, legal and tax issues often play a role. In the DaimlerChrysler example, a NewCo made it possible to transfer hidden reserves into the new entity, which would have had to be lifted otherwise.

A word of caution is needed, however, about the famous »*merger of equals*«. It is often talked about, and the concept sounds nice, but it does not work. In the truest sense of the word, »merger of equals« means using a leadership-duo from the merging companies (for example, two CEOs) and a basic-democratic process to run the integration down to the lowest level. There is no better recipe for disaster than using this set-up, i.e. a set-up lacking firm and unambiguous leadership. The only way something like a »merger of equals« can work, is using a »best-of-both-worlds« approach steered by a clear set of decision rules and one strong leader. Experience shows that no more than one CEO must be appointed except for a very brief transition time. A CEO team will not be able to exercise the leadership degree required.

Choosing the appropriate integration depth is critical for the success of any transaction. In the case of bancassurance, the combination of banking and insurance activities for instance, the complete merger of a retail bank and an insurance company shows far better results than forming a joint-venture[2].

Both decisions, whether fully integrated operations are necessary to reap the benefits aimed for in the transaction, and how much control of the final entity is required, will determine what the transaction will look like. Nothing but business logic and strategic thinking should be used to find the appropriate solutions. Ultimately, these two decisions will form the basis for future success or failure of the transaction.

Deciding on the Appropriate Brand Architecture

As banks grow in their global reach, the concepts of brand architecture become ever more important. At the very latest when deciding on possible re-branding after an acquisition, the overall brand architecture must be clear. Possible approaches span a spectrum from the establishment of several unambiguous individual brands, each focused on a specific business or customer group, to the development of a strong corporate brand to span all customer groups and businesses (see Exhibit 21: The Brand Architecture Continuum). Maintaining unambiguous individual brands opens the option to maintain the strength and brand equity of acquired brands, limits the danger of brand overstretch, and enables unambiguous positioning and targeting of specific customer groups. Establishing one dominant corporate brand, on the other hand, provides the option to build a strong, international brand with a global positioning and a correspondingly high brand equity, and to reap brand synergies.

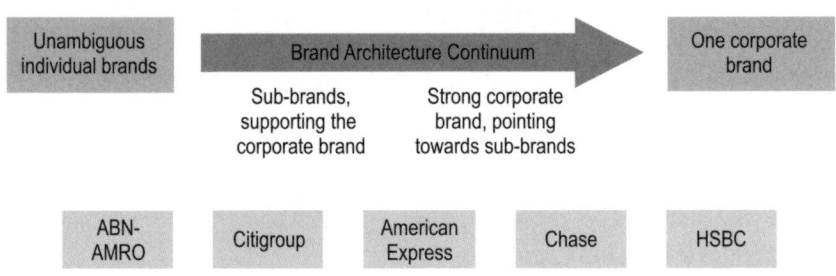

Exhibit 21: The Brand Architecture Continuum

Despite the fact that in our new world of retail banking only a network of specialized players will exist, the question of whether or not to have a dominant corporate brand spanning customer groups or businesses remains an issue. Even in a future market, a Citibank, for example, could still provide services to corporate and retail customers – but more likely with two different subsidiaries. Even considering only one customer group – retail customers – several businesses could be offered by several focused subsidiaries. Perhaps there would be a Citi convenience retail bank, some Citi niche players, a Citi mortgage bank, Citi insurances, a Citi building society, or Citi asset management.

In addition, there is the issue of whether or not to rebrand the acquisition of a similar player, be it in a new country or where the acquirer is present already. Targeted positioning or brand overstretch are no issues in this case. But both brand equity – the loss of the target's existing brand equity and the acquirers' potential to build a global brand equity – and possible brand synergies need to be evaluated.

HSBC has probably displayed the most radical focus on the one-brand concept. In 1998, HSBC decided to create a unified brand for the HSBC Group, using HSBC and the company's hexagon symbol as its identity in all markets where it operates. HongkongBank of Australia, Midland Bank, HongkongBank, Hongkong Bank Malaysia, Marine Midland Bank, Hongkong Bank of Canada, Banco HSBC Bamerindus, HSBC Banco Roberts, and The British Bank of the Middle East all adopted the HSBC branding, regardless of potential losses of existing brand equity. CCF (France), during whose acquisition the continued use of the CCF brand name had to be guaranteed, at least soon displayed the familiar HSBC logo next to its name and adapted its color to HSBC's red.

In the company's on-line press room, HSBC Group Chairman John Bond is quoted as saying: »...we are placing increased emphasis in many countries on the development of banking and other financial services for personal customers. Our strategy calls for the development of a strong consumer brand ... We want the HSBC brand to be known in every country and in every sector in which we operate as synonymous with integrity, trust and excellent customer service.«

HSBC's intended positioning is at the same time a good example for the constraints of establishing a corporate brand across many businesses and customer groups: The wider the brand stretches, the less technical and the more emotional it must be. A large variety of customer groups can only relate to a single brand (message) when it is an emotional (and not a technical) one like HSBC's. However, this limit is not a disadvantage; compared to other industries, emotional brands are precisely what is lacking in retail banking

4. Avoiding Hostile Reactions

A company has a variety of options to protect itself from a takeover it regards as unattractive be it due to business considerations, like differences in strategy, or due to managers' own interests, for example, their fear of being made redundant after the transaction. The aim of these strategies is to make the target less attractive, for instance by selling key assets, or to make the transaction more costly for the acquirer, for example by entering long lasting contracts that are not desired by the buyer, and which might include significant penalties if dissolved early. In some cases, the management may even ask another company to make a more suitable bid (a »White Knight«).

Possible Hostile Reactions

Poison Pills are provisions that aim at making unfriendly takeovers too expensive. A poison pill is triggered when the potential acquirer buys a certain percentage of the shares. When a certain threshold is reached, the target can then issue additional shares with original shareholders having the chance to purchase them at very low prices, thus diluting the acquirer's position. Poison pills are particularly favored by technology companies and were used, for example, by both WorldCom and Commerce One.

Golden Parachutes are clauses in the contracts of executive management specifying that they will receive large benefits in case of the termination of the executive's employment (which is usually one of the consequences of a takeover). These benefits may consist of severance pay, a bonus, stock options, or a combination thereof. If a large payment is made when the employment is terminated, this is also called a Golden Handshake.

If a target does not want to be acquired by a certain bidder (threat of hostile takeover), it might look for a *White Knight*. A White Knight is a third company who is willing to make a competing bid for the target and whom the target's management would prefer as future owner, no matter what the reasons are.

The *Sale of the Crown Jewels* denotes the sale of the target's best assets or entities in order to make the company unattractive and prevent the acquirer from submitting a bid. A transaction bank, for instance, could sell its IT system to an IT service provider in combination with an outsourcing contract.

Note that not all of these reactions can be used in all European countries due to legal restrictions.

To defend itself against the hostile takeover bids from its then-rivals Royal Bank of Scotland and Bank of Scotland in 1999, NatWest put its Ulster Bank up for sale to make a takeover less attractive. Potential buyers for Ulster Bank were Allied Irish Banks (AIB) and Bank of Ireland. However, the move failed and the Royal Bank of Scotland acquired NatWest – including Ulster Bank – in March 2000.

To avoid bad surprises during the transaction, the absence of such strategies should be ensured from the beginning. As mentioned before, the best method to achieve this is to involve the target's management as well as other share- and stakeholders as much and as early as possible. If, for instance, the key supplier or customer of a target threatens to end all business, the deal is unlikely to succeed.

One other last resort a target may utilize is to intentionally misinterpret the law and deny interested buyers access to detailed information. In these cases, the target's management literally locks the door to the data room and justifies this behavior with corporate law. In Germany, for example, members of the board are obliged not to disclose any confidential information according to § 93 AktG. The term »confidential information«, however, is not defined precisely, and this loophole can be exploited as described. In court, the target will usually lose such a case, but the delay is often enough for a potential transaction to not be carried out. Only an inclusion of a mandatory due diligence into the legal sales process would eliminate this threat to takeovers.

5. Clarifying Sensitive Issues Early

Again and again, mergers fail after their announcement – for example the takeover of Honeywell by GE, which was rejected by the European Commission in July 2001. But not all failures can be attributed to external sources: In April 2000, the German Deutsche Bank and Dresdner Bank had to renounce their merger plans (which had been public for almost one month), because it had become clear during the later-stage negotiations that no agreement could be found over the fate of Dresdner's investment bank subsidiary Dresdner Kleinwort Benson.

Accidents like this can happen both before and after the main contract has been signed. Even if the transaction takes place as planned, the internal cooperation between the merger or joint venture partners can still be jeopardized when emotional discussions crop up late in the process. The chances for such difficulties and internal collapses can be reduced sharply, however, by clarifying the most controversial and emotional topics – predominantly corporate governance issues – early on in the negotiation phase before publicizing the deal. Who will be appointed CEO, how many members (and even more importantly, from what firm) of the managing boards will be on the board of the new entity? How is the supervisory board constructed? How will the voting rights be divided? In addition to these corporate government issues, and especially for a joint venture or a »merger of equals« where no natural leader exists, some operational details need to be clarified beforehand as well. For example, what will the top-level organization look like? What is the future strategy and positioning of the combined entity? What is the scope and speed of the integration? What is the future name of the company and the headquarters location? Especially when integrating two transaction banks, the »system issues« also need to be clarified: Which system will be shut down (most often implying, which site will be closed)?

Even in a regular takeover, where the acquiring bank usually has the power to decide on these issues single-handedly, each of these considerations should be addressed carefully. In particular the involvement of the target's management is critical in order to avoid desperate reactions, such as those described above, or just plain resistance, which can be equally effective in compromising the success of the transaction – albeit only after the takeover has taken place.

6. Communicating the Transformation

Usually beginning with the public announcement of a transaction, communication both within the acquiring and, sometimes even more importantly, the target company is essential. Employees are afraid of change, of losing their responsibilities, their position, their familiar environment, and – most importantly – their jobs in the process of the transaction. If those fears are not addressed, the corporate climate can decline drastically, leading to bad performance, making any integration even more difficult, and ultimately significantly lowering the chances for success.

In particular, key personnel should be catered to during the process: Their future within the new entity must be assured and their new position be decided upon as soon as possible. Otherwise, highly capable individuals are likely to leave the company, making the acquisition less attractive. The retention of key managers must, therefore, be an important point on the agenda of the acquirer. This is less important if the two companies' businesses are rather complementary, but is especially urgent if the dismissal of some of the management is to be expected due to overlapping businesses.

In addition to addressing more personal fears and uncertainties, both employees and shareholders have to be united behind the new company. To achieve this alignment, the overall strategy, aspired positioning, merger logic, and planned benefits for all stakeholders must be communicated early, clearly, and in detail.

Despite being such a »soft factor«, efforts in communication have proven to pay off: In their 1999 study about success and failures of cross-border

M&A[3], KPMG found that companies who prioritize communication during the merger process were 13 percent more likely to be successful than the average.

7. Overcoming Cultural Barriers

Another often neglected aspect of creating alliances is the cultural compatibility of the different banks or the different companies in general. Even in Western Europe, there are considerable differences in language, behavior, and value systems – the way things are perceived and done – across different geographies. During the transaction as well as the post merger integration (PMI), these differences can lead to the ultimate failure of the deal. While top- and middle-management are often accustomed to working in an international setting, particularly lower management and employees may have difficulties bridging cultural barriers. When it comes to different attitudes and corporate cultures, or the existence of informal structures, information paths, or processes that outsiders may not know and follow, employees across all ranks will have difficulties cooperating openly and constructively with their new colleagues. In banks as in other companies, these issues – together with a certain unwillingness or laziness to leave the trodden paths – can lead to the establishment of »old boys' networks«, i. e. the workforces of both players stick to themselves and often disregard explicit new processes or organizational structures. Both Siemens Nixdorf and Daimler-Chrysler, for example, were rumored to have faced this problem for a long time. Whatever the reasons for such behavior, once it is there it is difficult to eliminate, and a proper integration is even harder to achieve.

Here as well, KPMG has found clear evidence that cultural issues are important[4]. First, those companies focusing on identifying and resolving cultural issues were an astonishing 26 percent more likely to be successful than on average. Secondly, the success of international mergers clearly depended on the origin of the two (or more) companies: US/UK deals were 45 percent and UK/Rest of Europe deals still 19 percent more likely to be successful than on average, whereas for US/Rest of Europe deal success was eleven percent *less* likely than on average. These results clearly show how cultural proximity, or the lack thereof, can influence merger results and how actively addressing cultural issues can greatly increase the likeliness of success.

8. Realizing Synergies

Synergies, whether on the cost or revenue side, are the main reasons for why transactions take place. As argued before, most synergies can only be reaped if the two entities are merged; synergy capture is much more difficult in a pure acquisition. Joint ventures, too, are very successful in reaping synergies, but in this case the synergies are clearly limited to the comparatively narrow range of joint activities.

As most banks still show a potential for cost reductions, cost synergies are the most frequent key factors for a merger. Not only can scale efficiencies be reaped, mergers also always provide a good opportunity to overhaul the cost base and make required changes to the organization and processes. Different from revenue synergies, cost synergies can be planned and measured quite easily. Past transactions in the banking sector show that the average planned annual cost savings amount to around 20 to 30 percent of the smaller company's cost base. In its 2001 acquisition of Halifax, the Bank of Scotland forecasted cost savings amounting to 22 percent of Halifax's cost base. However, the actual realization of these synergies is another issue. Some banks, as the Royal Bank of Scotland has shown in integrating NatWest after the takeover in 2000, are able to realize cost synergies on schedule or even ahead of schedule, while others face enormous difficulties achieving any synergies at all. In the case of failures to reach the planned synergies, sub-optimal post-merger integration or simply a false estimation of the real synergy potential are the most frequent reasons. Sometimes, the likeliness of reaching the planned synergies can already be roughly judged on the day of announcement: If the buyer is a publicly traded company, the general opinion regarding the likelihood of success can easily be inferred from the directional movement of the buyer's stock price.

Of the possible mergers in the retail banking industry, merging transaction banks can be an especially rewarding task. Usually, one of the two IT systems will be eliminated, leaving one system to handle the combined volumes. As personnel expenses are a minor factor in transaction banking compared to IT costs, the overall cost base will increase only slightly, resulting in dramatically lower per-unit costs. Often, the increase in volume will not only be the result of processing the other partner's business. In a domino effect, such a strengthened company will attract additional business as the chances of becoming one of the »final« players have increased significantly through the merger.

Regarding revenue synergies, often based on the assumption of introducing one partner's products into the other partner's sales channels, the realization of the original plan is often very difficult. Both for very similar and very dissimilar merger partners, little potential for revenue synergies exists. In its planned merger with Dresdner Bank, Deutsche Bank calculated cost synergies of 44 percent of Dresdner's cost base, but no revenue synergies[5]. During other mergers, however, such as the Bank of Scotland's acquisition of Halifax or Banca Intesa's purchase of BCI, managers announced that income from increased sales would account for more value than cost synergies. Allianz's takeover of Dresdner Bank, too, was based largely on revenue synergies. Between 2002 and 2005, total net revenue synergies, i. e. positive minus negative revenue synergies, were estimated to be about as large as total cost synergies, excluding the necessary restructuring costs. After that, future synergies were 70 percent revenue based and 30 percent cost based[6]. However, the realization of the revenue synergies has proved to be extremely difficult. By now, Allianz has sharply increased its focus on cost cutting. Ultimately, revenue synergies are hard to assess as they are based on intangible assumptions such as improved reach of customers or increased marketing success.

Whether cost or revenue synergies are concerned, their realization depends on a rigorously planned and executed PMI process. Among other tasks, merger teams have to be set up to plan the new organization and processes. The staffing of these merger teams has to be chosen carefully, so that the future management is involved and buy-in is generated; a steering committee must review the proposals regularly; processes and manpower must be established to detect overlaps and gaps; to realize the planned synergies, a structured target-setting and planning process must be set up; from this process, a »business plan« has to be written by each merger team, containing the future action plan, objectives, responsibilities, and timetables; and finally, the implementation of these plans must be monitored frequently and in detail.

As in any transformation, the soft factors have to be addressed with as much attention as the hard factors. In this, both communication and the integration of the workforce across possible cultural barriers between the two companies are essential.

External transformations are only one part of changing an organization. Sometimes, they might not even be necessary in order to reach the chosen business model. However, whether the retail bank undergoes an external transition or not, wherever it is coming from today, and wherever it aims to be heading in the future, an internal transformation will always be necessary. Not only will processes and organizations need to be adapted; most

123

importantly, the mind-set of both management and employees will have to be changed in order to fully embrace and live the new concept.

Key Success Factors for Internal Transformation

Many of the issues important here (see Exhibit 22: Key Success Factors for Internal Transformation) were already mentioned when describing post merger integration above. This should be no surprise, as both a purely internal transformation and a PMI process require a significant amount of vision and leadership, project management, and change management.

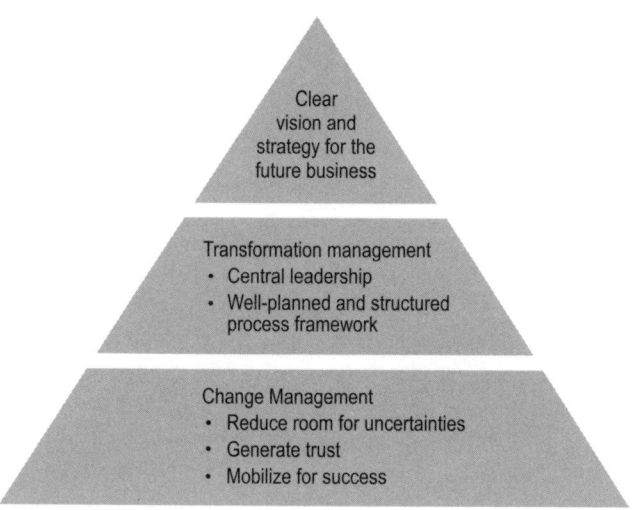

Clear vision and strategy for the future business

Transformation management
- Central leadership
- Well-planned and structured process framework

Change Management
- Reduce room for uncertainties
- Generate trust
- Mobilize for success

Exhibit 22: Key Success Factors for Internal Transformation

Transformations can be traumatic for employees unless they are handled well. The starting point of any transformation must be a clear vision and strategy for the future business. Communicated well, and throughout all levels of the company, the strategy and vision serve as a basis for the reorganization process, as a guide for all decisions, and as a focal point for the employees.

The transformation itself needs to be handled like any major reorganization. Strong central leadership is required to set the pace of change and coordinate the various activities. This is enabled and supported by a well-structured framework for all transformation activities, including the task of communication. Sufficient capacity is needed, and senior managers have to be made available to coordinate and realize this complex task. To reduce uncertainty, new management structures must be announced rapidly.

Last but most certainly not least, change management is needed to form the basis for the future company. As long as the employees do not understand the objective or the process of the transformation, or do not feel understood and taken care of during the change process, the resulting company will be inoperable, as many employees will be distracted, frustrated, and less productive. Change management needs to prepare and accompany the workforce during this period of uncertainty. It needs to give adequate and timely information, address the uncertainties and needs of the individuals, and prepare them for their new responsibilities through training and dissemination of information. Successful change management reduces the room for uncertainties, generates trust, and mobilizes the organization for success. A »can-do-attitude« can be created, the opportunities of the transformation can be pointed out without belittling valid concerns, and the momentum and energy generated by the project can be channeled and focused on positive objectives.

Such a transformation, from today's generalist retail bank to tomorrow's focused player, is certainly not an easy task from strategic, management, and organizational points of view. In this process, top management has two of the most crucial tasks. First, they must be especially candid and honest in assessing the current position, capabilities, strengths, and weaknesses of their own organization. Only by taking an outsider's view, can the status quo be analyzed truthfully and then a viable area of specialization be chosen. Second, once this decision is taken, top management must have a clear picture and a common understanding of the future company, of the »end state« to be reached. During the transformation, there are so many decisions to take (companies to buy, activities to sell or outsource, employees to hire or make redundant, organizational redesigns to be accepted or rejected) and there are so many stakeholders to motivate and convince of the objective and the path to get there, that consistency – and therefore success – is only possible when all the key decision makers follow the same compass to guide their actions and decisions. To which degree deviations from this general direction can be tolerated must be determined on a case-by-case basis. The default, however, should be none. Otherwise, the concept may get lost before it has even had the chance to be implemented. Only with a strong and united leadership team can such a task be mastered.

An overall transformation process as described here may take several years. Compared to the other steps, step I, the choice of which future business model to pursue might even be the easiest decision to make. Even though the decision itself is difficult, because the future of the entire bank hinges upon it, both the process and the result are clear. Regarding step II, the design of the future business model, however, things are more complex. The single largest danger is to underestimate this task. Banks cannot only err in how detailed they do their redesign, more fundamentally, they might not be willing or able to apply the required amount of rigor. Thinking back to the Albrecht brothers' design of the Aldi discounters, a certain obsession is necessary to successfully streamline the underlying business system so that the unique network of activities supports the chosen business model in every way. The final step, the actual transformation of the business, usually takes the longest – often up to many years. Throughout this time, two issues are crucial: First, the final objective must not be let out of sight. Second, all stakeholders, and especially the employees, must be convinced of the benefits of the new concept. Otherwise, the new entity is very likely to fail.

6
Outlook Into The Future

Why should all of this transformation happen? More specifically, why should banks start to specialize, letting go of some of their capabilities and focusing on others, and having other companies do what they will not do themselves anymore? Why should the retail banking industry move to this network of specialists linked by insourcing/outsourcing contracts? Why should the competitors adopt the business models we have described?

Something will have to happen, for three reasons. First, it is happening already in virtually every other industry. Second, the process has already started to happen in banking (although often on a small scale, often only locally, and thus perhaps often going unnoticed by many retail banks). Third, many of the new and focused players will increase their success, great success in some cases, and will begin extending this success thus forcing the established players to make a move.

If that is the case, if the established players do indeed make their moves, why should they move in the directions we have put forward? Would the future retail market necessarily have to look the way we have described? Here, the answer is more mixed: partly yes and partly no. What is certain is the breaking up of the value chain into more specialized players. It has already started and is increasing in speed, and every trend in banking (as for other industries) indicates that it will continue. In order to be operationally effective, these more specialized players will have to subcontract each other, call it outsourcing or not, to focus on the other parts of the value chain. That does not mean, however, that each and every business model will exist exactly as we described.

It is possible that some models will not turn out to be viable or outright successful. Perhaps, there will be no independent product developers whatsoever, and »Client Specialists« and »Engineers« will take their place, combining product development with customer interface activities or transactions. Perhaps there will never be an »Aldi Bank«, because in the end customers dislike the idea of an absolute no-frills bank. Or, customers may demand so many »little extras« that the business model cannot cope and

127

will ultimately collapse or need to be abandoned. On the other side, no-frills airlines have managed to secure a significant market share; 20 years ago people might have felt quite uncomfortable about this idea as well.

The market as a whole will certainly undergo a gradual change as business models are tested, adopted, or discarded, and as customer groups are singled out and targeted, or left again to the mainstream players. Ultimately, market forces will produce the structure and the business models that benefit customers most. But most likely, no single big step or market rupture will occur along the way.

For each player, the transformation process will have to be a very conscious and active one. Each retail bank will have to actively decide where it wants to position itself, which capabilities it wants to nurture, and which it wants to get rid of. If companies avoid active decision making and try to »let the market decide« for them, which it will, they will find themselves falling through the cracks, left behind, and doomed to failure.

And then, there is an entirely different model of the future, one in which most of our players would be irrelevant. Do you remember the »electronic butler«? The portable system that understands your spoken orders and knows enough about you, your preferences, and your banking details to actually do whatever you tell it to do? Ten years might not be enough time for this to happen, but 15, 20, or 30 years might. In such a world, many things would be different, not just banking. Most likely, the industry would be split into those companies who »own« the customer, i. e. who know his preferences and have the necessary databases, and those who provide the hardware for this to happen and the services the customer can purchase. With their current level of customer understanding and proximity, retail banks would probably find themselves among the hardware and service providers – unless they reinvent themselves completely between now and then, learn how to understand their customers, how to cater for their needs, and learn how to address their customers as individuals. Toward such a model, our predictions would merely be a stepping-stone, an intermediary phase along the path to this end-state.

Nevertheless, until this futuristic world becomes reality, we are safe in assuming that the future of retail banking will roughly look as we described: A network of more specialized players. On the whole, the species of retail banks is not endangered, as its services will always be needed. Those players, however, who are incapable or too slow to adapt to the impending changes, may well have the meteor coming right at them.

Appendix: Main Products in Retail Banking

Retail products basically comprise current accounts, savings and credits, credit cards, and brokerage services. Overall, products do not vary much across the European countries.

Current Accounts

Current accounts are very widespread among bank customers. Offering no or very modest interest rates, they are frequently combined with debit cards. The most common card is the EC card, already introduced in most European countries. It enables customers to withdraw cash from teller machines as well as make point-of-sale transactions.

Current accounts address the customers' need for liquidity rather than investment. Since the introduction of the Internet, most activities such as transfers can be conducted on-line.

Savings

Besides credit, savings accounts are probably the most typical retail banking products. Savings products come in many versions, for example fixed term deposits, and offer varying interest rates, usually depending on the amount invested and the flexibility with which the money can be withdrawn.

The importance of savings accounts differs across Europe. While in some countries like the UK there is a high awareness of other investment alternatives with higher returns, people in other countries like Germany still hold a large extent of their wealth in cash or savings accounts.

Credits

Similar to savings products, banks offer a huge variety of credits. Based on an assessment of the potential creditor's financial situation and collateral, interest rate, duration, and amortization are determined. Apart from these traditional credits, the banks' product ranges also comprise drafts, discount and acceptance credit, or leasing agreements. Due to the usually limited credit amount in retail banking, products are typically standardized and the sale therefore follows rather simple procedures.

Credit Cards

While EC cards are widely used throughout the EU, credit cards are more popular in some countries than in others. In the UK for instance, citizens exhibit a high willingness to pay on credit for daily products. In Germany, on the other hand, customers mostly use credit cards for the purchase of rather expensive goods and prefer EC cards or cash for daily transactions.

Securities Trading and Brokerage

Brokerage services enable customers to trade in securities, funds, and derivatives. These products became especially popular during the stock market boom of 1999 and 2000. Coinciding with the increasing acceptance of the Internet, on-line-brokerage accounts were offered with huge success. Investments are mainly in mutual funds and equities, rather than bonds or derivatives. The use of brokerage accounts is cyclical and follows the development of the stock market. In this respect, savings accounts can be seen as complementary products that are now mainly used when stock markets are weak. Accordingly, in the current market situation, on-line-brokers, mostly subsidiaries of commercial banks, face considerable problems as turnover is generally low and costs remain high.

Other Investments, Particularly Tax-Driven Products

In the recent past, tax-driven products have experienced increasing popularity. It has become clear that public retirement schemes will not be able to sufficiently cater for people's retirement needs due to the demographic changes in Europe, i. e. the increasingly aging population. Therefore, private savings schemes are encouraged and supported by many national governments. Again, the impact has already been observed in some countries, while others lag behind, like Germany, where the so-called Riester retirement products have not yet taken off as predicted.

Services, Especially Personal Advice

Apart from the above products, retail banks offer a range of services through their branch network. These include personal advice and investment support as well as project finance. Furthermore, several banking products often are combined, sometimes with modified conditions, to attract different customer groups. For instance, current accounts and EC cards are often free of charge for students.

References

Chapter 2

1 Monitor Group/JPMorgan, *Combining Strengths – Bancassurance*, 2002
2 Leichtfuß, Merkle, Mihov, »Retail Banking: Erfolgsformeln für Aufsteiger«, in: *Die Bank*, October 2002

Chapter 3

1 European Central Bank, *Structural analysis of the EU banking sector 2001*, November 2002
2 Bundesverband deutscher Banken (BdB), *Übersicht über das Bankgewerbe im Euro-Währungsgebiet*, 2002
3 Ibidem
4 European Central Bank, *Structural analysis of the EU banking sector 2001*, November 2002
5 BNP Paribas, interim report 2002
6 BNP Paribas, *European Banks*, broker report, July 2002

Chapter 4

1 Verband der Automobilindustrie (VDA)
2 Monitor survey 2003
3 *Zdnet news*, April 2001
4 *Computerwelt*, November 2002
5 Monitor survey 2003
6 *Bank Marketing International*, July 31, 2000
7 *SDA*, May 11, 2000
8 Reuters, May 10, 2001
9 Euromonitor, *Market Direction, Global Retailing*, February 2002
10 IPA report *Digital Interactive Television – Loved or Abandoned?*, January 2002
11 Presentation by Mark Melvin, Director of Franchising, Abbey National, at the IFS Financial World Seminar »*Future of the Branch*«, April 30, 2002

12 Abbey National press release, September 24, 2001
13 Monitor research
14 money.telegraph.co.uk, January 22, 2003
15 BAI and The Cambridge Group, *Demand Strategy on Consumer Financial Services*, December 2000
16 Respective interim reports for Q3/2002
17 *Berliner Zeitung*, September 19, 1996
18 Lafferty, *Cards International*, July 17, 2002
19 Presentation at the IFS Financial World Seminar »*Future of the Branch*«, April 30, 2002
20 Presentation by Mark Melvin, Director of Franchising, Abbey National, at the IFS Financial World Seminar »*Future of the Branch*«, April 30, 2002
21 Abbey National

22 *Börsenzeitung*, November 23, 2002
23 *Handelsblatt*, January 24, 2003

Chapter 5

1 *Der Spiegel*, November 28, 2002; Monitor research
2 Monitor Group/JPMorgan, *Combining Strengths – Bancassurance*, 2002
3 KPMG, *Unlocking shareholder value: the keys to success*, 1999
4 Ibidem
5 Deutsche and Dresdner Bank, Press conference presentation, March 9, 2000
6 Allianz Group, Analysts' Conference, Munich, June 1, 2001

List of Exhibits

List of Case Studies and Examples

Acknowledgements

Our greatest debt is to the many clients of both Rothschild and Monitor Group. The numerous high level discussions we have led with them allowed us to develop our understanding of this fascinating industry and were the basis for many of the ideas expressed in this book. Client confidentiality prevents us from expressing our gratitude in more detail.

Many individuals from inside and outside of our firms contributed to this effort. Sibylle Pollehn from Monitor Group held the project together, did not tire in challenging our thoughts, and persistently steered us through all the deadlines such a project involves. Philipp Gossow and Joachim Häcker from Rothschild shared with us their varied experience and insights into the industry, and Hendrik Becker supported them with the necessary market research and analyses. Silke Bonarius, Heiko Stutzinger, and Masina Malepeai from Monitor Group read the manuscript in its entirety, often on top of normal client obligations, and gave us valuable comments regarding content, architecture, and style. Silke Möck from Monitor Group did the basic research upon which large parts of this book rest. Jay Ogilvy from Global Business Networks (GBN), a Monitor Group company, and Marc Beylier from BNP Paribas provided us with valuable insights into their respective areas of expertise. We would especially like to thank the participants of our survey who took the time not only to complete the questionnaire but also to answer our detailed follow-up questions.

Lastly, we would like to thank all colleagues at Monitor Group and Rothschild. Frequent debates and the culture of constantly challenging one another's thoughts allowed us to develop the constant feedback way of thinking expressed in this book. Without their schooling, this work would not have been possible

About Monitor Group

Founded in 1983 by Professor Michael Porter and colleagues at Harvard Business School, Monitor Group is a leading global strategy consulting firm with more than 1000 consultants in 29 offices around the world. Since its founding, Monitor Group has remained focused on a core mission: Applying leading-edge analysis to help its clients define robust strategies as well as actions to transform these strategies into sustainable advantage. Monitor's clients come primarily from the financial services, chemical, pharmaceuticals, telecommunication, automotive, consumer goods, retail, and media industries.

While primarily focused on strategy consulting, over time, Monitor Group has developed a broader portfolio of professional services. Building on a strong foundation in corporate and competitive strategy, Monitor Group has developed leading edge skills in marketing strategy, organizational analysis, corporate finance, and private equity.

About Rothschild

Rothschild is a leading worldwide player in investment banking with 32 offices and over 700 investment bankers on five continents. Its specialization on mergers and acquisitions advice allows Rothschild to give recommendations free of conflicts of interest. The trust in its independent advisory work has led Rothschild to be ranked consistently among the top five M&A investment banks in Europe. Around two thirds of Rothschild's investement banking revenues are from repeat business, evidencing the strength of Rothschild's relationship driven approach. In 2002, Rothschild ranked number 1 in European M&A with 125 announced deals representing a value of 101.9 billion US Dollars.

About the Authors

Dr. Holger J. Kern, Vice President of Monitor Group, Munich, is responsible for the Financial Institutions Group in Europe. His consulting work is primarily focused on distribution strategies, segmentation, and branding. Before joining Monitor Group, he was responsible for the Financial Services Practice Group at Roland Berger.

Andreas R. Dombret, Managing Director in the Financial Institutions Group of Rothschild and Co-Head of Rothschild Germany, focuses on financial advice to European financial services companies. Before joining Rothschild he was Managing Director at JPMorgan responsible for German Financial Institutions.

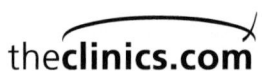

ORAL AND MAXILLOFACIAL SURGERY CLINICS
of North America

Perioperative Management of the Oral and Maxillofacial Surgery Patient, Part II

HARRY DYM, DDS
Guest Editor

RICHARD H. HAUG, DDS
Consulting Editor

May 2006 • Volume 18 • Number 2

SAUNDERS

An Imprint of Elsevier, Inc.
PHILADELPHIA   LONDON   TORONTO   MONTREAL   SYDNEY   TOKYO

W.B. SAUNDERS COMPANY
A Division of Elsevier Inc.

1600 John F. Kennedy Blvd., Suite 1800, Philadelphia, PA 19103-2899

http://www.oralmaxsurgery.theclinics.com

**ORAL AND MAXILLOFACIAL SURGERY
CLINICS OF NORTH AMERICA**
May 2006
Editor: John Vassallo

Volume 18, Number 2
ISSN 1042-3699
ISBN 1-4160-3570-2

Reprints. For copies of 100 or more, of articles in this publication, please contact the Commercial Reprints Department, Elsevier Inc., 360 Park Avenue South, New York, New York 10010-1710. Tel. (212) 633-3813 Fax: (212) 462-1935 email: reprints@elsevier.com

The ideas and opinions expressed in *Oral and Maxillofacial Surgery Clinics of North America* do not necessarily reflect those of the Publisher. The Publisher does not assume any responsibility for any injury and/or damage to persons or property arising out of or related to any use of the material contained in this periodical. The reader is advised to check the appropriate medical literature and the product information currently provided by the manufacturer of each drug to be administered to verify the dosage, the method and duration of administration, or contraindications. It is the responsibility of the treating physician or other health care professional, relying on independent experience and knowledge of the patient, to determine drug dosages and the best treatment for the patient. Mention of any product in this issue should not be construed as endorsement by the contributors, editors, or the Publisher of the product or manufacturers' claims.

Oral and Maxillofacial Surgery Clinics of North America (ISSN 1042-3699) is published quarterly by W.B. Saunders, 360 Park Avenue South, New York, NY 10010-1710. Months of publication are February, May, August, and November. Business and Editorial Offices: 1600 John F. Kennedy Blvd., Suite 1800, Philadelphia, PA 19103-2899. Accounting and Circulation Offices: 6277 Sea Harbor Drive, Orlando, FL 32887-4800. Periodicals postage paid at New York, NY and additional mailing offices. Subscription prices are $195.00 per year for US individuals, $295.00 per year for US institutions, $90.00 per year for US students and residents, $225.00 per year for Canadian individuals, $345.00 per year for Canadian institutions, $245.00 per year for international individuals, $345.00 per year for international institutions and $115.00 per year for Canadian and foreign students/residents. To receive student/resident rate, orders must be accompanied by name or affiliated institution, date of term, and the *signature* of program/residency coordinator on institution letterhead. Orders will be billed at individual rate until proof of status is received. Foreign air speed delivery is included in all *Clinics* subscription prices. All prices are subject to change without notice. **POSTMASTER:** Send address changes to *Oral and Maxillofacial Surgery Clinics of North America*, Elsevier Periodicals Customer Service, 6277 Sea Harbor Drive, Orlando, FL 32887-4800. **Customer Service: 1-800-654-2452 (US). From outside of the US, call 1-407-345-4000.**

Printed in the United States of America.

GUEST EDITOR

HARRY DYM, DDS, Chairman, Department of Oral and Maxillofacial Surgery, The Brooklyn Hospital Center, Brooklyn, New York; Clinical Professor, Columbia University, School of Dental and Oral Surgery, New York, New York; Senior Attending, Woodhull Medical and Mental Health Center, Brooklyn, New York

CONTRIBUTORS

LEON A. ASSAEL, DMD, Professor, Department of Oral and Maxillofacial Surgery, Oregon Health and Sciences University, Portland, Oregon

ERON ALDRIDGE, MD, Department of Oral and Maxillofacial Surgery, University of Kentucky, Lexington, Kentucky

SANJEEV RAJ BHATIA, MDS, FDS RCS (Eng), DDS, Resident, Oral & Maxillofacial Surgery, The Brooklyn Hospital Center, Brooklyn, New York

REMY H. BLANCHAERT, Jr, MD, DDS, Oral & Maxillofacial Surgery Associates, Wichita, Kansas

M. TODD BRANDT, DDS, MD, Department of Oral and Maxillofacial Surgery, University of Kentucky, Lexington, Kentucky

LEE R. CARRASCO, DDS, MD, Assistant Professor of Oral and Maxillofacial Surgery, University of Pennsylvania School of Dental Medicine; Department of Oral and Maxillofacial Surgery, Hospital of University of Pennsylvania, Philadelphia, Pennsylvania

GUILLERMO E. CHACON, DDS, Assistant Professor, Interim Section Head, Residency Program Director, Oral and Maxillofacial Surgery, Section of Oral and Maxillofacial Surgery, Anesthesiology, and Oral and Maxillofacial Pathology, The Ohio State University Medical Center, Columbus, Ohio

JOLI C. CHOU, DMD, MD, Resident, Department of Oral and Maxillofacial Surgery, University of Pennsylvania School of Dental Medicine; Department of Oral and Maxillofacial Surgery, Hospital of University of Pennsylvania, Philadelphia, Pennsylvania

EARL CLARKSON, DDS, Director, Oral & Maxillofacial Surgery, The Brooklyn Hospital Center, Brooklyn, New York

LARRY L. CUNNINGHAM, Jr, DDS, MD, Assistant Professor and Residency Director, Department of Oral and Maxillofacial Surgery, University of Kentucky, Lexington, Kentucky

LADI DOONQUAH, MD, DDS, Consultant Maxillofacial Surgeon, University Hospital of the West Indies; Associate Lecturer, Faculty of Medicine, University of the West Indies, Kingston, Jamaica; Private Practice, Decatur, Georgia

LELEKA DOONQUAH, MD, Consultant in Infectious Diseases, Providence Hospital; Infectious Diseases Specialist, Family and Medical Counseling Services, Washington, District of Columbia

CHRISTOPHER M. HARRIS, MD, DMD, Chief Resident, Department of Oral and Maxillofacial Surgery, University of Missouri—Kansas City, Truman Medical Center, Kansas City, Missouri

BARTLOMIEJ L. NIERZWICKI, MD, DMD, PhD, Resident, Department of Oral and Maxillofacial Surgery, University of Missouri—Kansas City, Truman Medical Center, Kansas City, Missouri

ORRETT E. OGLE, DDS, Chief and Residency Program Director, Division of Oral and Maxillofacial Surgery, Department of Dentistry, Woodhull Medical and Mental Health Center, Brooklyn, New York; Associate Clinical Professor, School of Dentistry and Oral Surgery, Columbia University, New York, New York

ORVILLE D. PALMER, MD, MPH, FRCSC, Division of Otolaryngology, Head and Neck Surgery, Department of Surgery, Harlem Hospital Center; Department of Otolaryngology, Columbia College of Physicians and Surgeons, New York, New York

CAROLYN PINNOCK, MBBS, DM, Bustamante Hospital for Children; Department of Surgery, University of the West Indies, Kingston, Jamaica

MANAF SAKER, DMD, Private Practice, Ridgewood, New Jersey

STEVEN R. SCHWARTZ, DDS, Private Practice; Attending, Woodhull Medical and Mental Health Center, The Brooklyn Hospital Center, Brooklyn, New York

BETHANY L. SERAFIN, DMD, Chief Resident, Department of Oral and Maxillofacial Surgery, Woodhull Medical and Mental Health Center, Brooklyn, New York

BRETT A. UEECK, DMD, MD, Assistant Professor, Department of Oral and Maxillofacial Surgery, Oregon Health and Sciences University, Portland, Oregon

CARLOS M. UGALDE, DDS, Resident, Oral and Maxillofacial Surgery, Section of Oral and Maxillofacial Surgery, Anesthesiology, and Oral and Maxillofacial Pathology, The Ohio State University Medical Center, Columbus, Ohio

VAUGHN WHITTAKER, MD, Department of Surgery, Harlem Hospital Center, New York, New York

HYON K. YOO, DDS, Affiliates in Oral and Maxillofacial Surgery, Cranston, Rhode Island

CONTENTS

Perioperative pain management requires a multifaceted approach. The local inflammatory injury and the local and centrally mediated responses must be understood and evaluated to be treated appropriately. This article reviews the different classes of medications and where each one fits into a pain management plan. The implementation of multimodal therapy, which combines different techniques, routes of administration, and different drugs, must be managed. Our ultimate goals are to provide safe and effective pain management, reduce adverse outcomes, preserve patients' physical and psychological well-being, and improve the quality of life for patients with acute pain during the perioperative period.

Various pharmacologic methods can be used to treat or prevent complications, such as deep venous thrombosis, or other sequelae related to a hypercoagulable state. Patients who take anticoagulation medications may be seen by oral and maxillofacial surgeons for evaluation and surgery in elective, urgent, and emergent situations. The purpose of this article is to familiarize readers with commonly encountered medications and recently published findings regarding their use by patients at risk of thromboembolic events.

Bleeding at the time of surgery has the potential to become a serious complication. Careful patient assessment and review of history are of the utmost importance if this situation is to be avoided on the operating table. Unfortunately, many patients, particularly younger individuals with little to no previous exposure to surgery, are unaware of underlying bleeding disorders that they may have. Understanding the basic pathophysiology and management of these conditions becomes critical for the treating surgeon. For patients who have known conditions, close interconsultation with the treating hematologists and careful observation of preoperative, intraoperative, and postoperative established protocols reduces the risk of complications for patients and makes the possibility of success a reality for these individuals.

believed to be at increased risk for perioperative morbidity and mortality. Appropriate preoperative evaluation is the cornerstone of successful intra- and postoperative management of the effects of anesthesia and surgery and is necessary for combating complications that may result from preexisting liver disease.

FORTHCOMING ISSUES

PREVIOUS ISSUES

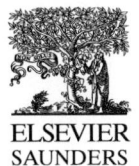

ELSEVIER
SAUNDERS

Oral Maxillofacial Surg Clin N Am 18 (2006) ix – x

**ORAL AND
MAXILLOFACIAL
SURGERY CLINICS
of North America**

Preface

Perioperative Management of the Oral and Maxillofacial Surgery Patient, Part II

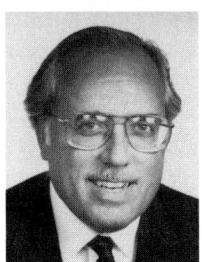

Harry Dym, DDS
Guest Editor

"I have learned much from my teachers and from my colleagues more than from my teachers, but from my students more than from them all." — Rabbi Chanina as related from the Talmud

Perioperative Management of the Oral and Maxillofacial Surgical Patient, Part II marks the completion of my two-volume planned series. The articles selected for this series were meant to assist practicing clinicians and oral and maxillofacial surgery residents in the everyday management of both the complex hospitalized oral and maxillofacial surgery patient admitted with medical issues and/or traumatic injuries, and the outpatient surgical patient who has concomitant significant medical problems.

I sincerely thank all my able contributors, who I feel met and exceeded my expectations by having submitted well-written, lucid, and comprehensive articles. They have succeeded in fulfilling my original vision and goals for this two-volume series, and I hope the readership will agree with my assessment and find this series to be a valuable ongoing reference guide.

As a profession whose scope of practice has grown enormously these past few decades, we must always remember that our roots were grounded in our active presence in hospitals and emergency departments. As such, we must always strive to maintain a vibrant hospital presence, although it may prove difficult and costly at times.

On a personal note, I must once again thank Mr. John Vassallo, the capable editor of *Oral and Maxillofacial Surgery Clinics of North America* for his assistance and patience, and offer special thanks to Corinne Acevedo, my Executive Assistant, for all her help in coordinating this two-volume project. These two volumes could not have been completed without the support of my colleagues and friends, Drs. Earl Clarkson, Orrett Ogle, and Peter Sherman, and my wife Freidy.

I must also acknowledge the Brooklyn Hospital Board of Trustees, Mr. Jonathan Weld, Chairman of the Board, and Mr. Carlos Naudon, Vice Chairman, for their continued confidence in me, and my entire department of Dentistry and Oral and Maxillofacial Surgery and its staff of dedicated employees. My deepest thanks go to Mr. George Harris, a Brooklyn Hospital Trustee, for his friendship and for his generous contributions to our Dental/OMS program

1042-3699/06/$ – see front matter © 2006 Elsevier Inc. All rights reserved.
doi:10.1016/j.coms.2006.03.001

oralmaxsurgery.theclinics.com

on behalf of the Littauer Foundation. Finally, this
year marks my 18th year as an active Oral and Maxillofacial Surgery Residency Program Director at The
Brooklyn Hospital Center, and I wish to dedicate
this current volume to my past, present, and future
OMS residents. They have been and continue to be
my greatest teachers.

Harry Dym, DDS
The Brooklyn Hospital Center
Department of Oral and Maxillofacial Surgery
121 DeKalb Avenue
Brooklyn, NY 11201, USA
E-mail address: hdymdds@yahoo.com

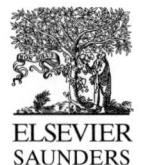

ELSEVIER SAUNDERS

Oral Maxillofacial Surg Clin N Am 18 (2006) 139 – 150

ORAL AND MAXILLOFACIAL SURGERY CLINICS of North America

Perioperative Pain Management

Steven R. Schwartz, DDS[a,b,]*

[a]*Private Practice, 2844 Ocean Parkway, Suite B-2, Brooklyn, NY 11235, USA*
[b]*Department of Oral and Maxillofacial Surgery, Woodhull Medical and Mental Health Center, The Brooklyn Hospital Center, Brooklyn, NY, USA*

Pain management is probably one of the most common problems dealt with in dentistry, especially by oral and maxillofacial surgeons. Patients are often referred to us to deal with painful problems, and the treatment we render in itself can cause pain postoperatively. We must be equipped to deal with pre-, intra-, and postoperative pain and its management. To do this effectively we must understand the biology of pain and the current theories and practices for its management.

Pain is a sensory and emotional experience evoked by stimuli that injure or threaten to destroy tissue. It is often associated with anxiety and increased activity of the sympathetic nervous system. For the purposes of this article we limit ourselves to the discussion and management of acute pain, pain that lasts, or pain that is anticipated to last less than 1 month.

Neuroanatomy of pain

An unpleasant noxious stimulus that injures or destroys tissue is the instigator of pain. It can be thermal, mechanical, chemical, or any combination thereof. At weaker levels these various stimuli may be perceived as only warmth, cold, or pressure.

For an individual to perceive a noxious stimulus as pain it must be transmitted as an electrical event from the site of injury to the higher brain centers. This process is termed nociception. The parts of the

nervous system that are involved in this transmission of painful impulses in sequential order are as follows: (1) nociceptive afferent pain receptors, (2) primary afferent nerve fibers, (3) dorsal horn of spinal cord via the dorsal root ganglia, (4) ascending spinothalamic tract and collateral fibers, (5) thalamus, (6) higher brain centers, and (7) descending (pain modifying) pathways [1].

The two different types of primary afferent neuronal fibers generally associated with pain transmission are A-delta and C-polymodal. There are certain distinct differences between these two classes of fibers based on their diameter and speed of impulse conduction. These disparities account for their functional differences. The A-fibers are of larger diameter and faster conducting (6 – 30 m/s), have a thin myelin sheath, are principally stimulated by mechanical means, and are thought to account for sharp, stabbing, and electrical-type pain. Some A-delta fibers in skin have been found to respond to thermal and chemical stimuli, however. C-polymodal fibers are classified as such because they are capable of responding to multiple different stimuli—thermal, chemical, and mechanical. C-polymodal fibers have a smaller diameter, are slower conducting (0.5 – 2 m/s), are unmyelinated, and are associated with duller, achy, more lingering pain. This prolonged pain is linked with emotional behavior and autonomic and somatic reflexes, predominantly sympathetic in nature (ie, tachycardia, peripheral vasoconstriction, and mydriasis) [2].

The peripheral afferent neurons enter the spinal cord at multiple levels at the dorsal root zone and, through multiple synapses, cross to the contralateral ascending spinothalamic tract. The impulses then course through the brain stem to many regions of the

* 2844 Ocean Parkway, Suite B-2, Brooklyn, NY 11235.
E-mail address: nyoms@hotmail.com

1042-3699/06/$ – see front matter © 2006 Elsevier Inc. All rights reserved.
doi:10.1016/j.coms.2006.02.002

brain and supply inputs to the reticular formation, limbic system, thalamus, and somatosensory cortex. Pain fibers from the oral cavity, sinuses, face, and corneas are carried in the trigeminal nerve (V^{th} CN) and the trigeminal ganglion. They enter the brain stem in the pontine region and ultimately synapse and cross to the opposite side, where they ascend as the anterior (ventral) trigeminothalamic tract to the thalamus and somatosensory cortex. Descending inhibitory pathways from the cerebral cortex synapse in the dorsal horn and modify the pain sensations [3], which could explain the "gate control theory" of pain by Melzack and Wall, in which emotional behavior and other sensory modalities can influence pain. A "target" cell in the dorsal horn is stimulated by large mechanofibers and smaller pain-conducting fibers. When the large mechanofibers are stimulated (eg, cold, pressure, rubbing the area, transcutaneous electrical nerve stimulation), pain perception is reduced. The response of the limbic system may determine how an individual responds to a noxious stimulus, adding the emotional nature of pain. This factor could explain why patients respond in various ways to the same pain or why the same patient may respond differently to the same noxious stimulus at various times.

In the process of carrying out surgical procedures to alleviate a patient's pain, we manipulate skin, mucosa, bone, or teeth. The resulting pain from these procedures is largely caused by the ensuing acute inflammation. When tissue cells are damaged or destroyed, certain chemical mediators are released that stimulate nociceptors, which in turn generate nerve impulses. These mediators include histamine, potassium chloride, polypeptides (eg, bradykinin and substance P), and serotonin. Each of these substances acts at different levels in the pain pathway peripherally, centrally, or both. Although not capable of directly causing pain, other chemical mediators, such as prostaglandins, sensitize nociceptors by lowering their activation thresholds. Prostaglandins synthesized as a result of cell membrane disruption exert physiologic and pathologic effects. Phospholipids in the cell membrane that contain arachidonic acid ultimately are converted to prostaglandins (ie, PGE_2 and PGF_{2a}), prostacyclin (PGI_2), or thromboxanes (TXA_2).

Prostaglandins can be synthesized as a direct result of the initial noxious stimulus and by the effect of the released chemical pain mediators (ie, histamine, bradykinin, and substance P) on surrounding tissue cell membranes. Once created, PGE_2 and PGF_{2a} sensitize the peripheral nociceptors to produce an exaggerated pain response to stimulation by the specific pain mediators. This prostaglandin-induced

hyperalgesia seems to have a greater effect on the dull, burning, aching pains mediated via unmyelinated C-polymodal fibers.

Leukotrienes are another series of biologically active compounds derived from arachidonic acid. Their role in the inflammatory process also has been assessed. Like the prostaglandins, leukotrienes are not stored in tissue but are synthesized rapidly from leukocytes as a result of the appropriate stimulus. They are important mediators of inflammation and allergic reactions in concert with histamine. For example, leukotriene B_4 is chemotactic for leukocytes, and leukotrienes C_4 and D_4 increase vascular permeability [1].

Postoperative pain management

Postoperative pain from dental and oral and maxillofacial surgical procedures is largely mediated by its peripheral inflammatory component. Centrally activated mechanisms also add to the overall perception of the painful stimulus. To that end, the management of pain should consider the factors necessary to reduce the local and centrally mediated processes that propagate pain. Techniques and medications must be selected that minimize the untoward side effects (eg, gastrointestinal distress, lightheadedness) while fulfilling the previously mentioned goals. This section deals with the techniques most commonly used by oral and maxillofacial surgeons for dealing with postprocedural and traumatically induced pain.

This section reviews the two most commonly used classes of analgesics used by the dental profession: opioids and nonopioids. The opioid class includes analgesic agents, such as morphine, codeine, hydrocodone, and oxycodone. The nonopioid class includes acetaminophen (APAP) and nonsteroidal anti-inflammatory drugs (NSAIDs). An older, frequently used—although no longer completely accurate—taxonomy system labels opioids as centrally acting, whereas nonopioids are peripherally acting. Newer evidence has suggested that although NSAIDs work peripherally by decreasing the sensitivity of nociceptors to painful stimuli induced by heat, trauma, or inflammation, they also function as antihyperalgesics centrally in the dorsal horn and block signals to higher centers. Conversely, opioids thought only to act centrally by impairing a patient's normal sensory awareness and response to noxious stimuli have been found to exert a peripheral analgesic effect when administered to inflamed tissue [4,5].

Nonopioid analgesics

Nonopioid analgesics are a large group of structurally dissimilar organic acids that comprise several different categories. Examples that are clinically relevant to pain management from several different groups are reviewed.

The prototype for the NSAID class of nonopioid analgesics is aspirin, to which all of the newer NSAIDs are compared. The NSAIDs as a class are excellent anti-inflammatories and antipyretics and have analgesic properties; however, not all are specifically indicated for the management of acute pain. Acetaminophen, a para-aminophenol derivative and part of the nonopioid class, is an excellent analgesic and antipyretic, although it has no appreciable anti-inflammatory activity. For this article we only include medications with the indication for acute pain in the drug manufacturer's product literature.

The mechanism of action of the nonopioid analgesics is theorized to be caused by their ability to inhibit prostaglandin synthesis as the result of tissue damage. When prostaglandins are released at the site of tissue injury, they sensitize the nociceptors by lowering their activation thresholds. This activity, coupled with other locally found chemical mediators of pain, such as bradykinin, histamine, and substance P, increases impulse transmission, which results in increased pain perception as a result of inflammation. NSAIDs work by partially inactivating cyclo-oxygenase 1 (COX-1) and cyclo-oxygenase 2 (COX-2), which reduce prostaglandin synthesis and prevent the sensitization and activation of the afferent peripheral nociceptors and transmission of pain impulses to higher centers. COX-1 is present in many cell types throughout the body and is involved in the homeostatic function of prostaglandins, including modulating functions in the gastrointestinal tract, kidney, and circulatory system. In the gastrointestinal tract, prostaglandins help to maintain mucosal integrity by inhibiting acid secretion and stimulating mucus and bicarbonate secretion. In the kidney, renal blood flow is increased, which increases the glomerular filtration rate and regulates tubular salt and water resorption. In the circulatory system, vascular tone and platelet function are modulated by prostaglandins. Conversely, COX-2 is found in a limited number of cells, including leukocytes, macrophages, fibroblasts, and endothelial cells. COX-2-mediated prostaglandins are involved in the inflammatory process. When prostaglandins are produced as a result of tissue injury, they potentiate other inflammatory mediators, including leukotrienes, histamine, and bradykinin, which is the most potent naturally occurring vasodilator. As a result, prostaglandins are involved with hyperalgesia and vasodilatation, vascular permeability, and edema [6].

Adverse effects with nonsteroidal anti-inflammatory drugs

NSAIDs do not cause the respiratory depression seen with opioids or interfere with bowel or bladder function. That does not mean, however, that they are not without potential adverse effects. One of the limiting factors associated with NSAIDs is their therapeutic ceiling effect, which refers to the property of increasing doses of a given medication to have progressively smaller incremental beneficial effect, until at some point the maximum beneficial effect has been reached and only the incidence and severity of adverse side effects increase (ie, gastrointestinal distress). The adverse effects are attributed to the suppression of the prostaglandin-mediated normal physiologic functions of COX-1. The most common adverse side effects of NSAIDs are gastrointestinal, including gastritis, ulceration, and bleeding. In general, the incidence of these negative effects rises with increasing daily dosages of NSAIDs and prolonged usage. Not surprisingly, individuals who have a prior history of peptic ulcer disease seem to be at increased risk for these complications. Postoperatively, attention has been paid to the potential for NSAIDs to increase the possibility of bleeding. NSAIDs lead to reversible inhibition of platelet function, except for aspirin, which is irreversible. Postoperative bleeding in conjunction with NSAID administration rarely has been seen except in select patient populations or persons concomitantly receiving anticoagulants. This combination could lead to clinically significant bleeding. As with all drugs, the risk for adverse events associated with NSAID therapy increases when a patient already is taking other medications for varying medical conditions. The concurrent use of corticosteroids dramatically increases the risk of life-threatening gastrointestinal bleeding. Great caution should be exercised when using NSAIDs during pregnancy. In dealing with pregnant patients, acetaminophen usually is the first choice.

Table 1 reviews some of the more frequently used NSAIDs by oral and maxillofacial surgeons for the treatment of acute pain. Aspirin (acetylsalicylic acid) has been the prototype NSAID since its discovery in Germany in 1897 and marketing in 1899. It has been proved an effective analgesic, anti-inflammatory, and antipyretic numerous times. It is tolerated by a large segment of the population but does suffer from the therapeutic ceiling effect previously described. It is also available as a compounded drug, including various opioids. Aspirin should not be used in children

Table 1
Nonopioid analgesics

Generic	Proprietary names	Pain level	Dose(mg)	Interval (h)	Max. dose/24 h (mg)	Additional comments
Salicylic acid derivatives						
Aspirin	Anacin Bayer Ecotrin Excedrin	Mild	650–1000	4–6	4000	Increased risk of bleeding with excessive alcohol intake (≥3 drinks/d), avoid use with viral infections in children or teenagers, syndrome of asthma, rhinitis, and nasal polyps
Diflusinal	Dolobid	Mild to moderate	500	12	1500	1000 mg loading dose
Para-aminophenol derivatives						
Acetaminophen	Datril Panadol Tylenol	Mild	650–1000	4–6	4000	Increased risk of hepatotxicity with excessive alcohol intake (≥3 drinks/d)
Propionic acid derivatives						
Ibuprofen	Advil Motrin Motrin-IB	Mild to moderate	400	4–6	3200	
Ketoprofen	Ketoprofen	Mild to moderate	25–50	6–8	300	
Naproxen sodium	Anaprox Anaprox DS	Mild to moderate Mild to moderate	275 550	6–8 12	1375 1375	Start 550 mg then 275 mg every 6–8 h Alternate 550 mg bid
Indolacetic acids						
Etodolac	Lodine	Mild to moderate	200–400	6–8	1000 (1200)	Predominantly COX-2 inhibitor
Heteroaryl acetic acids						
Diclofenac	Cataflam	Mild to moderate	50	8	150	Loading dose up to 100 mg, total of 200 mg day one
Ketorolac	Toradol	Moderate to severe	60 IM, 30 IV 30 IM/IV 20 then 10 PO	Single dose 6 4–6	120 120 40	Transition from IV/IM to PO 20 mg, then 10 mg every 4–6 h; total duration of use ≤5d
Coxibs						
Celcoxib	Celebrex	Mild to moderate	200 mg	12	400	400 mg loading dose, then 200 mg if needed selective COX-2 inhibitor

Abbreviations: IM, intramuscular; IV, intravenous; PO, orally.

and adolescents with suspected viral infections because of the possible development of Reye's syndrome [7]. Diflusinal, a newer derivative in the salicylic acid family, is a potent anti-inflammatory and analgesic similar to aspirin but does not have the antipyretic effect. It has a longer onset and duration of action. In terms of potency, 500 mg of diflusinal is comparable to 650 mg of aspirin.

Acetaminophen is currently the first choice for dealing with mild pain in patients unable to tolerate NSAIDs for various reasons. It is similar in efficacy to aspirin as an analgesic and antipyretic but does not have the anti-inflammatory effects. Acetaminophen is also available as a compounded drug containing an opioid analgesic.

The propionic acid derivatives include ibuprofen, ketoprofen, naproxen, and naproxen sodium, all of which have been shown to be effective in controlling postsurgical pain. Ibuprofen is as effective an anti-inflammatory as aspirin with less gastrointestinal distress. All of the propionic acid derivatives cause reversible platelet inhibition. Naproxen and naproxen sodium differ by the addition of a sodium salt, which hastens the onset of action (approximately 1 hour versus 30 minutes). Naproxen sodium is the preferred choice for postoperative pain management. The overall effects are otherwise unchanged. The initial total daily dose should not exceed 1375 mg of naproxen sodium, followed by total daily doses thereafter of up to 1100 mg/d [8].

The indolacetic acid derivatives include etodolac. The effective analgesic dose was 200 to 400 mg, with an onset of action of approximately 30 minutes. The 200-mg dose was comparable with 650 mg of aspirin. Etodolac, 400 mg, was comparable to acetaminophen, 600 mg, with codeine 60 mg. Although not specifically classified as a COX-2 inhibitor, etodolac consistently has shown selective COX-2 inhibition and COX-1–sparing effects across a wide range of assays [9].

Diclofenac and ketorolac are examples of the heteroaryl acetic acid derivatives. Diclofenac potassium is the immediate release formulation. It has a more rapid onset of action (approximately 30 minutes) than its sodium counterpart. An initial loading dose of up to 100 mg followed by two 50-mg doses for a total of 200 mg is allowed on day 1. Thereafter, 50 mg every 8 hours is the dosing schedule [7]. Ketorolac is unique in the nonopioid category as the only current US Food and Drug Administration–approved parenteral NSAID. It can be administered intravenously or intramuscularly and followed up with oral dosing. Although like other NSAIDs it possesses anti-inflammatory, antipyretic, and analge-

sic properties, the latter seem to be the most pronounced. Clinical trials have shown parenterally administered ketorolac to be at least as effective, if not more so, as parenteral opioids in treating moderate to severe postoperative pain. The usual single treatment dose is either 60 mg intramuscularly or 30 mg intravenously. The dose for multiple dose treatment is 30 mg intravenously or intramuscularly every 6 hours, maximum dose 120 mg/d. The oral formulation of 20 mg as loading dose followed by 10 mg every 4 to 6 hours up to 40 mg/d follows. Currently the manufacturer recommends that the oral product be used only after parenteral administration. The total time of administration, including parenteral and oral dosing, should not exceed 5 days [8].

The newest and recently most controversial category of NSAIDs is the coxibs. Because of the voluntary withdrawal by the manufacturers of rofecoxib in September 2004 and valdecoxib in April 2005, celecoxib remains the sole occupant in this category. Celecoxib is distinguished by its classification as a COX-2 inhibitor. It does not adversely affect the continuously produced COX-1 isoenzyme. In theory only the COX-2–mediated prostaglandins involved in the inflammatory process are inhibited. Undesirable side effects, including gastric distress, decreased renal blood flow, reduced vascular tone, and platelet function mediated by COX-1, are left intact. For acute pain the dose is 400 mg as a single dose on the first day followed by an additional 200 mg if needed, then 200 mg twice daily as needed.

Opioid analgesics

Opioid analgesics include all the naturally occurring compounds derived from opium and the synthetic and semi-synthetic derivatives. The opioids work primarily by dulling the perception of pain in the central nervous system. Recent evidence has shown that opioids also have a peripheral effect. Opioid receptors have been found in the dorsal horn of the spinal cord [5]. Studies have shown that when opioids are administered to inflamed tissue they exert a peripheral analgesic effect. Opioids function by binding to specific receptors in the central nervous system and peripheral tissues. These specific receptors have been designated mu, kappa, and delta and are the same receptors with which endogenously produced opioid-like substances (eg, enkephalins, dynorphins, and beta-endorphins) bind. Each of these receptors is associated with several effects, some desired and others unwanted. For instance, the activation of mu receptors is associated with analgesia, a highly desirable trait, but also with respira-

tory depression, a detrimental and potentially fatal side effect.

Opioid classification

Opioids have been categorized by their pharmaco-biologic activity at the different receptors. This classification divides opioids into three groups: agonists, antagonists, and mixed agonist-antagonists. Agonist opioids act as analgesics primarily by binding and triggering the mu and kappa receptors. Examples of agonists are morphine (considered the prototypical opioid), meperidine, codeine, and propoxyphene. The antagonists preferentially bind to all three receptors but do not stimulate them. In doing so, the effects of the agonists are reversed, which is clinically useful as the reversal agents naloxone and naltrexone. The last group, mixed agonist-antagonist, has properties of both of the previously mentioned groups. Certain receptors are triggered (agonist), whereas other receptors are antagonized. Pentazocine, for example, activates the kappa receptor but antagonizes the mu receptors.

Opioid undesirable side effects

Although the primary activity of opioids is the eradication of pain, this class of drugs has multiple effects on numerous bodily functions. Not only is the central nervous system affected but also other peripheral systems, most notably the respiratory and gastrointestinal systems, may be significantly negatively affected. Analgesia, sedation, euphoria, and mental clouding are distinguishing effects of opioids on the central nervous system (Table 2). Analgesia seems to be related primarily to activity at the mu and kappa receptors. Although all opioids stimulate these receptors, the varying degrees of analgesia produced by these compounds are noteworthy. Drowsiness is seen in pain-free patients and patients who are still experiencing pain. Although patients may become drowsy and lethargic, opioids produce analgesia without a loss of consciousness.

Opioid analgesics have a direct depressant effect on the respiratory centers in the brain stem. Reductions in respiratory rate, minute volume, and tidal exchange may occur. These effects are seen at therapeutic doses and are dose related. As the dose increases, respiratory depression also increases. Most opioid overdoses that result in death are secondary to respiratory depression and arrest.

Nausea and vomiting are probably the most common unwanted side effects of opioid adminis-

Table 2
Opioid receptors

Receptor type	Mu	Kappa	Delta
Analgesia	++	+	+/−
Location	Supraspinal	Spinal	Spinal/ supraspinal
Respiratory depression	++	+	+/−
Pupil	Miosis++	Miosis+	
Gastrointestinal motility	Reduced ++		
Smooth muscle spasam	++		+
Euphoria	++		
Sedation	++	+	
Dysphoria		+	+
Hallucinations		+	
Physical dependence	++	+	+
Endogenous ligand	Beta-endorphin	Dynorphins	Enkephalins
Exogenous ligand	Morphine	Pentazocine	Morphine

tration. Direct stimulation of the chemoreceptor trigger zone in the medulla causes nausea and vomiting. These side effects are most prevalent with this initial dose and tend to subside with subsequent dosing. A vestibular component also is implicated because ambulatory patients have a higher incidence of nausea and vomiting compared with patients who remain recumbent.

In the cardiovascular system opioids may cause arteriolar vasodilatation and reduced peripheral resistance at therapeutic doses. These effects are insignificant in recumbent patients. In assuming an upright position, however, orthostatic hypotension and fainting may occur. Cardiac function is minimally affected in normal patients. In patients who have coronary artery disease or myocardial infarction, opioid administration, notably morphine, decreases cardiac work, myocardial oxygen consumption, and left ventricular end-diastolic pressure.

Opioids cause a decrease in propulsive peristaltic activity (motility) of the small and large intestines and reduce digestive secretions along the alimentary canal. The combined delay of the movement of bowel contents through the intestines and desiccation further enhance the constipating effect.

Tolerance and physical dependence are two other issues that must be dealt with when using opioids. Tolerance is defined as when repeated doses of a drug elicit a lesser effect than the initial dose or when increasing doses are needed to obtain the same effect

Table 3
Opioid analgesics

Generic	Proprietary	Pain level	Dose(mg)	Interval (h)	Onset (min)	Additional comments
Agonists						
Morphine sulfate(IV)	Astramorph PF	Moderate to severe	2–10	Every 8 min	1–3	Prototypical opioid
	Duramorph		2–10		1–3	
Morphine sulfate(PO)	MS Contin	Moderate to severe	10–30	4	30	
	Roxanol	Severe	10–30	4	30	
Meperidine HCI(IV)	Demerol	Moderate to severe	50–150	3–4	3–5	Not recommended because of toxic metabolite
Meperidine HCI(PO)	Demerol	Moderate to severe	50–150	3–4	<30	
Fentanyl citrate	Sublimaze	Severe	0.05–0.1	1–2	<1	
Codeine (PO,IM,IV)		Mild to moderate	15–60	4–6	10–30	360 mg/d maximum
Propoxyphene napsylate	Darvon-N	Mild to moderate	100	4	>60	Maximum 600 mg/d, no alcohol
Propoxyphene HCI	Darvon	Mild to moderate	65	4	<60	Maximum 390 mg/d, no alcohol
Mixed agonist-antagonist						
Pentazocine (IM,IV)	Talwin	Moderate to severe	30–60	3–4	2–3	Maximum 360 mg/d
Other						
Tramdol (PO)	Ultram	Moderate to moderately severe	50–100	4–6	60	400 mg/d maximum

as the initial dose. Physical dependence is a condition produced by continual administration of drug so that physiologic and psychological alterations occur so that discontinuation of the drug produces a withdrawal syndrome. Both of these conditions impose major limitations on agonist opioid use. These phenomena are generally only seen with chronic pain conditions, however (ie, cancer pain). Because most oral and facial postoperative pain requires this degree of medication for a relatively short period of time, these problems are rarely encountered. When dealing with patients who already are tolerant of potent doses of opioids (ie, cancer pain patients, methadone patients), nonopioid analgesics would be an appropriate choice. If the pain is severe enough, additional potent opioids or temporary increase in the dose of the current opioid may be necessary.

Review of opioids

Opioids can be administered intravenously, intramuscularly, subcutaneously, orally, rectally, transdermally, and transmucosally. Aside from being used parenterally in office or in hospital, their greatest use is as oral medications. Most opioids are well absorbed orally via the gastrointestinal tract but are subject to the hepatic metabolism first-pass effect. This effect negatively impacts their efficacy.

Table 3 reviews some of the more frequently prescribed opioids used by oral and maxillofacial surgeons for the treatment of acute pain. The naturally occurring alkaloid morphine is considered the prototype opioid. All other opioids are compared with it relative to potency and side effects. Table 4 can be used as a reference starting point when comparing or converting from one opioid to another. The current recommendation is to decrease the calculated starting dose of the new opioid by approximately 25% to allow for patient variability and titrate up to the effective dose. Morphine, however, is not indicated for

Table 4
Equianalgesic dose of opioid agents

Drug	IM/IV (mg)	PO (mg)
Morphine	10	30–60
Meperidine	75	300
Fentanyl	0.1–0.2	N/A
Codeine	120	200
Pentazocine	30	150
Oxycodone	N/A	20–30
Hydrocodone	N/A	30
Propoxyphene napsylate	N/A	200
Tramdol	N/A	100–150

Abbreviations: IM/IV, intramuscular/intravenous; PO, oral.

the treatment of acute dentofacial pain. Codeine is also a naturally occurring alkaloid that is approximately one-twelfth as potent as morphine. Although an opioid, it does have a maximum dose of 60 mg per dose, because beyond that the adverse side effects outweigh the benefits. It is rarely used alone as a postoperative pain medication because it lacks any anti-inflammatory activity.

Accordingly, NSAIDs are an appropriate first choice for mild to moderate pain. Codeine is paired with an NSAID or acetaminophen. Oxycodone and hydrocodone are synthetic derivatives and are similar to morphine and codeine. They are approximately ten and seven times more potent than codeine, respectively. Oxycodone and hydrocodone are also usually paired with a nonopioid analgesic. They also include the associated adverse effects of opioids. Propoxyphene is a relatively weak synthetic opioid agonist structurally related to methadone. When added to a nonopioid (eg, aspirin or acetaminophen) it improves pain relief by only 7.3% [10]. It does, however, have the same adverse side effects as other more potent opioids, including central nervous system depression, physical dependence, and tolerance, but usually only seen at high-dose long-term use. Propoxyphene also has a greatly increased risk of respiratory depression and psychomotor impairment when mixed with alcohol and should not be given to depressed or suicidal patients. It can be used sometimes as a substitute opioid analgesic for patients unable to tolerate the more commonly prescribed opioid agonists, however [7].

Pentazocine is an example of an agonist-antagonist class of opioids. Although it is an agonist at the kappa receptors, it is only a partial agonist or antagonist at the mu opioid receptors. Pentazocine has fewer respiratory depressive effects than pure agonist opioids but can cause marked dysphoria at doses of more than 50 mg orally. Because of its antagonist effect at mu receptors, pentazocine can precipitate opioid withdrawal syndrome in patients who are concurrently using mu agonist opioids. The oral formulation of pentazocine has 0.5 mg of naloxone in its formulation. Orally the naloxone has no clinically significant effect, but if illicitly crushed and taken parenterally, the naloxone antagonizes all opioids. Tramadol is another opioid analgesic that does not fall into the classification system. It is a synthetic agent unrelated to other opioids, and it seems to have actions on the GABAergic, noradrenergic, and serotonergic systems. It seems to work by two different mechanisms: (1) its metabolite, M1, binds to mu opioid receptors; (2) it inhibits the reuptake of serotonin and norepinephrine in the central nervous system.

When used alone, tramadol is not as effective as the compound that includes acetaminophen, which is comparable to ibuprofen as an analgesic (Table 5).

Adjunctive medications

Corticosteroids have been used in oral and maxillofacial surgery for many years. It is well documented that when administered in adequate doses, most of the postoperative edema seen with major oral and maxillofacial surgery is averted. Methylprednisolone, dexamethasone, and methylprednisolone acetate alone and in combination have been used before, during, and after orthognathic surgery. Empirically, it seems that preventing the inflammatory component (edema) of the procedure has led to decreased pain and earlier ambulation, ability to take oral nutrition, and, ultimately, a shorter hospital stay [11]. Methylprednisolone also has been used as a convenient method of prescribing a short tapering course of oral steroids for a patient after an office procedure expected to have a significant inflammatory component (eg, impacted third molars). NSAIDs block prostaglandin production by COX inhibition. Corticosteroids act earlier in the cascade by suppressing arachidonic acid production. By acting at this level, prostaglandins and leukotrienes are inhibited. In addition to their peripheral anti-inflammatory effects, corticosteroids (and NSAIDs) have central antinociceptive properties at the spinal cord level. Romunstad and colleagues [12] reported that a single dose of methylprednisolone after orthopedic surgery demonstrated a greater opioid-sparing effect than the potent NSAID ketorolac. Corticosteroids also have been found to have an antiemetic effect. Despite these positive findings, not enough research has been conducted to lead to widespread clinical use. Hopefully more research will define properly the role of corticosteroids in postoperative patient management.

Approach to postoperative pain management

The most often used techniques by oral and maxillofacial surgeons for pain management center around various pharmaceutical preparations, including analgesics, general and local anesthetics, anxiolytics, sedatives, and hypnotics. Intraoperative pain management may be provided by the surgeon, particularly for office-based procedures, or by the anesthesiologist, as in operating room procedures. For

Table 5
Compounded opioid analgesics

Generic	Proprietary	Pain level	Dose(mg)	Interval (h)	Onset (min)	Additional comments
Agonists						
Codeine+nonopioid	Tylenol #2,#3,#4	Mild to moderately severe	15-30-60	4	10-30	360 mg/d max codeine+300 mg APAP
Hydrocodone+nonopioid	Vicodin	Moderate to moderately severe	5/500	4-6	15-30	Contains 500 mg APAP max 8 tabs/d
	Vicodin-ES	Moderate to moderately severe	7.5/750	4-6	15-30	Contains 750 mg APAP max 5 tabs/d
	Vicodin-HP	Moderate to moderately severe	10/660	4-6	15-30	Contains 660 mg APAP max 6 tabs/d
	Vicoprofen	Not stated	7.5/200	4-6	15-30	Contains 200 mg ibuprofen max 5 tabs/d
Oxycodone+nonopioid	Percocet	Moderate to moderately severe	2.5/325	6	15-30	Contains 325 mg APAP max 12 tabs/d
		Moderate to moderately severe	5/325	6	15-30	Contains 325 mg APAP max 12 tabs/d
		Moderate to moderately severe	7.5/500	6	15-30	Contains 500 mg APAP max 8 tabs/d
		Moderate to moderately severe	10/650	6	15-30	Contains 650 mg APAP max 6 tabs/d
		Moderate to moderately severe	7.5/325	6	15-30	Contains 325 mg APAP max 8 tabs/d
		Moderate to moderately severe	10/325	6	15-30	Contains 325 mg APAP max 6 tabs/d
	Percodan	Moderate to moderately severe	5/325	6	15-30	Contains 325 mg aspirin max 12 tabs/d
Propox napsylate+APAP	Darvocet N-50	Mild to moderate	50/325	4	>60	Plus 325 mg APAP max 600 mg/d, No ETOH
Propox napsylate+APAP	Darvocet N-100	Mild to moderate	100/650	4	>60	Plus 650 mg APAP max 600 mg/d, No ETOH
Propox HCl+ASA+caffeine	Darvon Compound-65	Mild to moderate	65/389/32.4	4	<60	Plus ASA + caffeine max 390 mg/d, No ETOH
Mixed agonist-antagonist						
Pentazocine+naloxone	Talwin NX	Moderate to severe	50/0.5	1-2 tabs, 3-4	15-30	Max 12 tabs/d, naloxone prevents intravenous abuse
Other						
Tramdol+acetaminophen	Ultracet	Not stated	37.5/325	2 tabs, 4-6	<60	8 tabs/ d max

Abbreviation: ETOH, alcohol.

surgery, a combination of agents may be used, including opioids, anxiolytics, and volatile inhalation agents in conjunction with nitrous oxide and oxygen. Having the anesthesiologist administer a potent NSAID (eg, ketorolac) near the end of the operative procedure aids in reducing postoperative inflammation and has an opioid-sparing effect, which makes the patient more comfortable.

Traditionally, postoperative analgesia in the hospital consisted of intravenously or intramuscularly injected opioids on an "as needed" basis. Unfortunately, intermittently administered analgesics yield incomplete relief. It is not possible to predict accurately what dose is needed to provide sufficient analgesia or even how much pain a patient will have postoperatively. Patient-controlled analgesia allows a patient to self-administer small, predetermined doses of potent opioids and titrate the dose to effective analgesia, which is accomplished by using a microprocessor-controlled infusion pump. This technique circumvents the "peak and trough" phenomena seen with conventional intramuscularly administered opioids and allows for stable plasma concentrations to be maintained with less sedation. Opioids with relatively short half-lives are most commonly used. Overdosing is avoided by controlling the bolus size and the total dose allowed to be administered over a given time. A lockout interval is also set to prevent a second dose from being administered before the previous one would have time to reach maximum effect. Patient-controlled analgesia with an opioid is associated with the typical opioid-related adverse effects, such as nausea and vomiting, constipation, urinary retention, pruritus, and respiratory depression, which is the most serious of all. Patients should be monitored for their level of sedation and respiratory rate. The nursing staff should be allowed to administer opioid antagonists (naloxone) with suspected overdosage (Table 6) [12].

In office-based procedures, adding opioids, anxiolytics (eg, benzodiazepines), sedative hypnotics (eg, methohexital, propofol), and dissociative agents (eg, ketamine) in varying combinations allows the practitioner to manage better the emotional component of pain. By using local or regional anesthetic techniques along with these parenteral agents, we are able to decrease the total systemic analgesic requirement and provide for immediate postoperative pain relief. With the introduction of the long-acting local anesthetic agents bupivacaine and etidocaine, we are able to prevent the transmission of noxious stimuli to the central nervous system for 3 to 8 hours, depending on the anesthetic used and injection type (infiltration versus block). In so doing we may reduce the extent of centrally mediated primary and secondary hyperalgesia. It is little or no trouble to administer one of these long-acting local anesthetics at the conclusion of a procedure, which gives the patient enhanced pain relief during the initial postoperative period.

This technique has another advantage because it allows patients to obtain (if they have not done so already) and self-administer their first dose of enteral analgesia before the local anesthetic effect has subsided. In this way patients avoid that first intense painful episode when the local anesthesia wears off. It is far easier to maintain a relatively pain-free level than progress from a painful state to a relatively pain-free condition [13].

Along with this concept of starting analgesia before the onset of pain are two other thoughts. First, it has been established that with outpatient procedures, taking an initial dose of ibuprofen, 400 mg, 30 minutes before a procedure has been shown to postpone the onset and reduce the intensity of postoperative pain [5]. For patients who are allowed nothing orally because of planned intravenous anesthesia, evidence suggests that if an NSAID is taken within 30 minutes after the procedure there is still a benefit to patients postoperatively. Second, taking analgesia on a fixed-dose schedule or "by the clock" as opposed to as needed optimizes pain relief. When taken on a fixed schedule, stable drug levels are attained, which provides for uniform pain relief and tolerance to opioid side effects. When an as-needed schedule is followed, the analgesics are taken in haphazard fashion. The consequence is that patients are always playing "catch up" with their pain. They experience short periods of pain relief followed by likely prolonged periods of pain while they are waiting for the medication to take effect. As-needed dosing is appropriate when referring to "rescue medication" to treat breakthrough pain.

Combining medications not only applies to compounding nonopioids with opioids. Excedrin is a combination of 250 mg aspirin, 250 mg acetaminophen, and 65 mg caffeine per tablet. In this author's experience—both professional and personal—when the maximum dose of an NSAID (eg, ibuprofen,

Table 6
Dose regimens for patient-controlled analgesia

Drug	Bolus dose (mg)	Lock-out (min)
Morphine	0.5–2.5	5–10
Hydromorphone	0.05–0.4	5–10
Fentanyl	0.01–0.05	5–8

naproxen) has been reached but there is either continued or breakthrough pain, the addition of acetaminophen to the NSAID is often sufficient and the addition of opioids as the next step on the "ladder" is often not necessary. This method of maximizing the nonopioid effective dose also applies to the same nonopioid found in the particular oral combination drug being prescribed. Table 5 shows that compounded medications are a combination of an opioid and an NSAID or acetaminophen. The maximum dose of the different combination medications, with the exception of codeine and propoxyphene, is based on the accompanying NSAID or acetaminophen and not the opioid. With that knowledge you can select the appropriate dose of the combination drug to maximize the effect you are seeking. For example, oxycodone, 2.5 mg/325 mg APAP, maximum dosage is 12 tablets, which equals a total oxycodone dose of 30 mg and acetaminophen dose of 3900 mg/d. If you prescribed oxycodone, 10 mg/325 mg APAP, it has a maximum dose of six tablets a day. The total oxycodone dose would be 60 mg and the acetaminophen dose would be only 1950 mg/d. You could prescribe an additional 500 mg of acetaminophen four times throughout the day or six tablets of acetaminophen, 325 mg, one tablet with each dose of oxycodone compound, while getting double the total dose of oxycodone and still not exceed the dose limit of 4 g/d for acetaminophen.

Suggested guidelines for evaluation and management

Preoperative patient evaluation and planning are crucial to perioperative pain management, including type of surgery, the expected severity of postoperative pain, pre-existing medical conditions (eg, cardiac, pulmonary, or gastrointestinal disease, allergies), patient's previous pain experiences, and treatment preferences. The patient and family, if appropriate, should be counseled before as to what to expect, how pain will be treated, and their role in its management. Patient preparation should include reviewing and adjusting existing pain medication and initiating postoperative pain management preoperatively. This preparation may include starting NSAIDs or acetaminophen preoperatively, because researchers believe that these drugs have a dose-sparing effect for systemically administered opioids [14].

Intraoperative techniques could include administration of long-acting local anesthesia at the conclusion of a case.

Postoperatively the multimodal technique for pain management has been advocated by the American Society of Anesthesiologists. The literature supports the administration of two analgesic agents that act by different mechanisms via a single route for providing superior analgesic efficacy with equivalent or reduced adverse effects. An example involves intravenous opioids in conjunction with ketorolac or ketamine. The literature also suggests that two routes of administration, when compared with a single route, may be more effective in providing perioperative analgesia. An example is intravenous opioids combined with oral NSAIDs, COXIBs, or acetaminophen versus intravenous opioids alone. Whenever possible, multimodal pain management techniques should be used. Unless contraindicated, all patients should receive fixed dose, by-the-clock NSAIDs or COXIB or acetaminophen [14]. Local anesthetic blockade at the conclusion of the case also should be considered. The goal is to maximize analgesia while minimizing the adverse side effects. The medications, dose, route, and duration of treatment must be individualized.

Summary

Perioperative pain management requires a multifaceted approach. The local inflammatory injury and the local and centrally mediated responses must be understood and evaluated to be treated appropriately. The different classes of medication and where each one fits into a pain management plan are reviewed. The implementation of multimodal therapy, which combines different techniques, routes of administration, and different drugs, must be managed. The ultimate goals are to provide safe and effective pain management, reduce adverse outcomes, preserve patients' physical and psychological well-being and improve their quality of life with acute pain during the perioperative period.

References

[1] DiGregorio GJ, Barbieri EJ, Sterling GH, et al. Handbook of pain management. 3rd edition. West Chester (PA): Medical Surveillance; 1991.
[2] Clark RG. Manter and Gantz's essentials of clinical neuroanatomy and neurophysiology. 5th edition. Philadelphia: FA Davis; 1978.
[3] Mehlisch DR, Markenson J, Schnitzer TJ. The efficacy of nonsteroidal anti-inflammatory drugs for acute pain. Cancer Control 1999;6(2 Suppl 1):5–9.

[4] Barr ML, Kiernan JA. The human nervous system: an anatomical viewpoint. 5th edition. Philadelphia: JB Lippincott; 1988.

[5] Jackson DL, Roszkowski MT, Moore PA. Management of acute postoperative pain. In: Fonseca RJ, editor. Oral and maxillofacial surgery. Philadelphia: WB Saunders; 2000. p. 114–40.

[6] Ashburn MA, Ready LB. Postoperative pain. In: Loeser JD, Butler SH, Chapman CR, et al, editors. Bonica's management of pain. 3rd edition. Philadelphia: Lippincott Williams & Wilkins; 2000. p. 765–77.

[7] Shapiro RD, Cohen BH. Perioperative pain control. Atlas Oral Maxillofac Clin North Am 1992;4:663–74.

[8] Physicians' desk reference. 59th edition. Montvale (NJ): Thompson PDR; 2005.

[9] Jones RA. Etodolac (lodine): profile of an established COX-2 inhibitor. Inflammopharmacology 2001;9: 63–70.

[10] Goodman F. Review of the efficacy and safety of propoxyphene. Pharmacy Benefits Management Strategic Healthcare Group and the Medical Advisory Panel Department of Veterans Affairs, 2001:1–84.

[11] Bell WH, Proffit W, White R. Surgical correction of dentofacial deformities. Philadelphia: WB Saunders; 1980.

[12] Romunstad L, Breivik H, Niemi G, et al. Methylprednisolone intravenously one day after surgery has sustained analgesic and opioid-sparing effects. Acta Anaesthesiol Scand 2004;48:1223–31.

[13] Silvasti M. Patient-controlled postoperative analgesia: comparison of efficacy, side-effects and safety of various regimens [academic dissertation]. Helsinki: University of Helsinki; 2001.

[14] Task Force on Acute Pain Management. Practice guidelines for acute pain management in the perioperative setting. Anesthesiology 2004;100:1573–81.

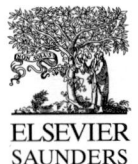
ELSEVIER
SAUNDERS

Oral Maxillofacial Surg Clin N Am 18 (2006) 151–159

**ORAL AND
MAXILLOFACIAL
SURGERY CLINICS
of North America**

Perioperative Treatment of the Patient Taking Anticoagulation Medication

Larry L. Cunningham, Jr, DDS, MD*, M. Todd Brandt, DDS, MD, Eron Aldridge, MD

Department of Oral and Maxillofacial Surgery, University of Kentucky, 800 Rose Street, D-508, Lexington, KY 40536-0297, USA

Prolonged intraoperative and postoperative bleeding is a concern for oral and maxillofacial surgeons who treat patients taking anticoagulation medication. In the United States alone, nearly 2.3 million patients have been found to have atrial fibrillation; of those, 40% receive anticoagulant medications [1]. Anticoagulation medications are often given prophylactically to patients who are at risk of thrombus formation and its sequelae as the result of acquired or hereditary medical disorders, most commonly coronary artery disease, atrial fibrillation, and deep venous thrombosis. Patients who have undergone heart valve replacement, particularly persons who have received mechanical valves, are treated with warfarin. Medical conditions such as cancer, ulcerative colitis, heparin-induced thrombocytopenia, antiphospholipid antibody syndrome, disseminated intravascular coagulation, and hyperhomocystinemia may predispose patients to a hypercoagulable state and the need for anticoagulation therapy. Oral and maxillofacial surgeons also may treat patients with hereditary conditions. Patients who have deficiencies of protein C, protein S, or antithrombin III, patients who have factor V Leiden thrombophilia, and patients who have abnormal plasminogen production may require anticoagulation to prevent thrombotic sequelae.

Patients in a hypercoagulable state who do not receive prophylactic anticoagulation medications are at risk of venous or arterial thrombolic events that may result in substantial morbidity or mortality rates.

These events include cerebrovascular accident, transient ischemic attack, peripheral venous or arterial thrombus or embolus, and clotted arteriovenous grafts. Of these complications, oral and maxillofacial surgeons are probably most familiar with deep venous thrombosis, which is a common occurrence among surgical patients. Its incidence in association with general and orthopedic surgery is 25% to 50% in the absence of any form of prophylaxis [2].

Various pharmacologic methods can be used to treat or prevent complications, such as deep venous thrombosis, or other sequelae related to a hypercoagulable state. Patients who take anticoagulation medications may be seen by oral and maxillofacial surgeons for evaluation and surgery in elective, urgent, and emergent situations. The purpose of this article is to familiarize readers with commonly encountered medications and recently published findings regarding their use by patients at risk of thromboembolic events.

A review of hemostasis

Hemostasis is the cessation of bleeding. To achieve hemostasis, the body maintains a delicate balance between the risk of intravascular thrombus and the risk of hemorrhage. This balance depends on the normal functioning of the vascular endothelium, the coagulation cascade, blood flow, platelets, anticlotting mechanisms, and the fibrinolytic system. It is important to understand the overall concept of hemostasis because multiple medications are used for anticoagulation, each with distinct characteristics and mechanisms by which they disrupt the coagu-

---

* Corresponding author.
E-mail address: llcunn2@email.uky.edu
(L.L. Cunningham, Jr).

1042-3699/06/$ – see front matter © 2006 Elsevier Inc. All rights reserved.
doi:10.1016/j.coms.2005.12.009

oralmaxsurgery.theclinics.com

lation cascade. A complete review of hemostasis is beyond the scope of this article, but the diagrams that cover the intrinsic and extrinsic schemes and the physiologic pathway provide an overview. The process includes primary hemostasis (platelet plug formation), secondary hemostasis (coagulation), and the formation of a stable fibrin clot (Fig. 1).

In general, the coagulation cascade can be described as having three parts: the intrinsic system, the extrinsic system, and the common pathway. Coagulation proteins circulate in the bloodstream in inactive forms. Unlike the subendothelium, the endothelium is devoid of thrombogenic tissue factor and collagen; activation of platelets and the coagulation cascade are prevented.

Maintaining normal, brisk flow through vessels ensures that any activated coagulation proteins are swept away quickly for disposal in the liver. When a vessel wall is injured, however, the coagulation apparatus is stimulated. The intrinsic system begins with the exposure of subendothelial collagen through the defect at the site of injury, which activates platelets and other coagulation proteins. One of the activated

proteins, factor XIIa, cleaves and activates prekallikrein and factor XI into kallikrein and activated factor XIa. These proteins are anchored to the subendothelium by a high molecular weight kininogen. Kallikrein then amplifies the activity of the intrinsic system by activating neighboring molecules of factor XII. Once activated, factor XIa cleaves its anchoring cofactor, high molecular weight kininogen, and diffuses into solution, where it activates factor IX in the presence of calcium. Activated factor IXa forms a complex with activated factor VIIIa and calcium. This complex then binds to the surface of platelets that contain phospholipids, in which the activation of factor X occurs. This event marks the end of the intrinsic pathway and the initiation of the common pathway of the coagulation cascade (Fig. 2) [3].

Unlike the intrinsic system, the extrinsic system initiates the coagulation cascade with components outside the blood. Disruption of the endothelial surface exposes the subendothelium, which expresses tissue factor on its cell surface. Once exposed to the blood, circulating factor VII binds to the tissue factor and forms a tissue factor-factor VII complex that

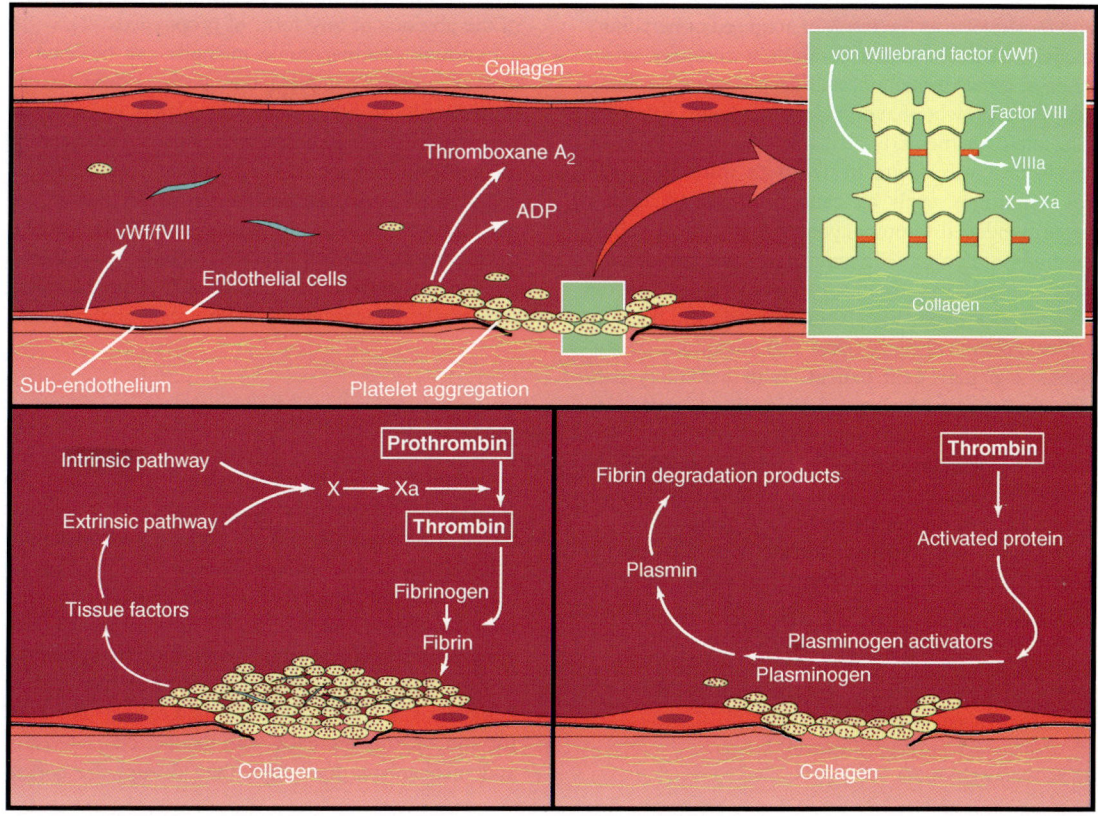

Fig. 1. Normal hemostatic process.

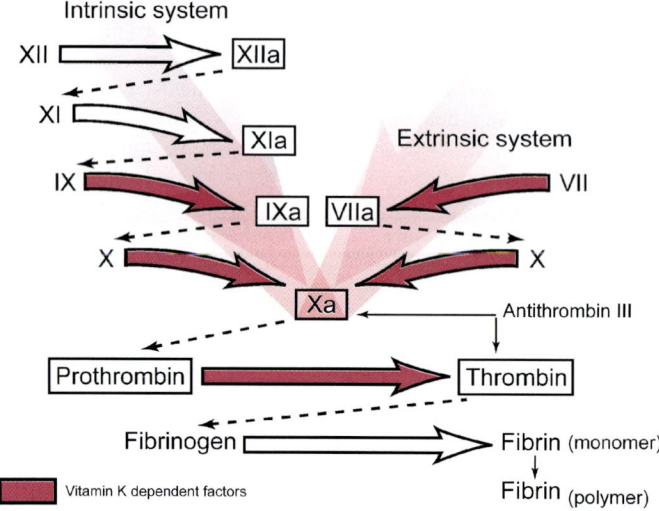

Fig. 2. The classic coagulation cascade.

promotes the autoactivation of factor VII to activated factor VIIa. In the presence of calcium and membrane phospholipids, this complex activates factor X.

The activation of factor X is the point at which the intrinsic and extrinsic pathways converge to form the common pathway of the coagulation cascade. Factor X is activated on the phospholipid-rich surface of activated platelets. Activated factor X forms a complex with its activated cofactor, factor Va, in the presence of calcium; it also converts prothrombin into thrombin [3].

Thrombin is referred to as the primary regulator of the coagulation cascade. Thrombin cleaves fibrinogen to form soluble fibrin monomers, which subsequently polymerize to form an insoluble fibrin clot at the site of injury. Thrombin also activates circulating factor XIII, which catalyzes the formation of cross-links between fibrin molecules. These cross-links provide the necessary structure for a stable fibrin clot. Thrombin also activates surrounding platelets that, in conjunction with the fibrin clot, seal the defect in the vessel wall. Finally, thrombin activates factor V and factor VIII in a positive feedback loop, which further amplifies the activation of the coagulation cascade [4].

Understanding thrombus formation—or the prevention thereof—requires a working knowledge of the three conditions associated with this pathophysiologic process that was first described by Virchow in 1856 [2]. Known as Virchow's triad, the three conditions necessary for thrombus formation are venous or arterial stasis, endothelial wall damage (ie, damage to the intima or inner layer of a vessel), and an

alteration in the blood's coagulability. These conditions produce a hypercoagulable state.

Stasis, the first condition of Virchow's triad, may occur in large and small blood vessels but occurs more commonly in larger vessels, such as the deep veins of the calf [3]. When blood flow is rapid, small quantities of thrombin and other procoagulants are mixed with large quantities of blood and are carried by the blood to the liver, where they are removed mainly by Kupffer cells. When blood flow is too slow, however, these procoagulants accumulate in local concentrations sufficient to initiate clotting [5].

The second condition of Virchow's triad refers to injury to a blood vessel wall. The injury causes disruption of the vessel's endothelial layer, which sets in motion the intrinsic pathway of coagulation. This disruption exposes the underlying collagen to platelets and other coagulation proteins, which are activated by this exposure. Once activated, the platelets spread in shape, and their procoagulant phospholipids become externalized. This change allows the coagulation proteins to assemble on the surfaces of the platelets and accelerates the coagulation reactions. Von Willebrand factor is synthesized and released by endothelial cells and is exposed during this endothelial disruption. During this second condition of Virchow's triad, von Willebrand's factor assists platelets in attaching to collagen; the adherent platelets spread out, and their cytoplasmic granules release substances such as adenosine 5'-diphosphate (ADP), serotonin, and thromboxane A2. These substances cause local vasoconstriction and platelet aggregation, which recruit

more platelets. This initial hemostatic plug is referred to as primary hemostasis; its proper function requires an adequate number of normally functioning platelets, collagen, and von Willebrand's factor, and products of the coagulation cascade, such as thrombin and fibrinogen [4].

Defects of primary hemostasis are recognized in the operating room when normal avascular planes continue to ooze as small capillaries continue to bleed despite the application of pressure and time. Coagulation continues through secondary hemostasis when the platelet plug is stabilized, and a mechanically strong clot composed of fibrin, platelets, and erythrocytes is formed.

Cross-linking of fibrin further strengthens the clot, which then contracts. Propagation of the clot is limited by three different mechanisms. First, tissue factor pathway inhibitor limits the initiation of coagulation. Second, the protein C pathway is activated by thrombomodulin, which binds excess thrombin. Along with the cofactor protein S, this pathway inactivates factors Va and VIIa of the coagulation cascade, which limits amplification of the clot. Finally, thrombin is inactivated by antithrombin III, which limits propagation of the clot [4]. Chemotactic factors then stimulate phagocytic leukocytes to clean up debris in the region of injury. Platelet-derived growth factor, released from degranulating platelets, stimulates vascular repair. When the continuity of the endothelium has been restored, the fibrinolytic system is activated and the occluding thrombus is lysed [4].

The final element of Virchow's triad, the hypercoaguable state, reflects an imbalance between procoagulant and anticoagulant tendencies. Patients who undergo oral or maxillofacial surgery may have medical conditions that cause hypercoagulable state, such as cancer, ulcerative colitis, heparin-induced thrombocytopenia, antiphospholipid antibody syndrome, disseminated intravascular coagulation, hyperhomocystinemia, Factor V Leiden thrombophilia, abnormal plasminogen production, and deficiencies in antithrombin, protein C, and protein S.

Because of the wide variety of diseases among surgical patients, it is important to understand where the coagulation factors are synthesized. Most of them are produced in the liver. In fact, hepatic synthesis has been confirmed for fibrinogen, factor V, and the group of factors that require vitamin K for synthesis, namely, factor II (prothrombin), factor VII, factor IX, factor X, protein C, and protein S [4]. Factor XIII is involved in fibrinogen cross-linkage and is synthesized partially in megakaryocytes and partially in the liver.

Factor VIII is believed to be produced at several sites. Although liver transplantation has corrected factor VIII deficiency among patients with hemophilia A, for example, factor VIII concentrations actually may be increased rather than decreased among patients with severe liver disease. This increase is probably an acute phase response [4]. Fibrinogen is the precursor of fibrin, from which fibrin clots are built. Fibrinogen is produced by the liver and is an acute phase reactant. An inflammatory stimulus increases the hepatic output of fibrinogen to as much as eight times its normal level [4].

Platelets are the disk-shaped fragments of megakaryocyte cytoplasm that are initially found in bone marrow. These fragments adhere to the site of injury, become activated, and stimulate further aggregation. Once platelets have been activated, they change their shape, release the contents of their granules, and expose receptor sites that provide a surface for activation and assembly of the coagulation complexes. As mature cells, platelets circulate in the blood at a constant level, and approximately 33% of the platelet pool is sequestered in the spleen. These sequestered platelets are freely exchangeable with those in the blood and can be released in large numbers in response to epinephrine or exercise. It is important to remember that among patients who have hypersplenism, an increase in the sequestration of platelets may result in thrombocytopenia. Likewise, among patients who have undergone splenectomy, the entire platelet pool is contained within the circulation, and thrombocytopenia may persist to some degree after this procedure [4].

Preoperative evaluation

Every preoperative evaluation begins with a comprehensive medical history, regardless of the type of surgery planned. Questioning should assess each patient's individual bleeding risk by emphasizing past and current usage and dosage of medications, including vitamins, herbal remedies, over-the-counter drugs, and prescription medications. Patients often forget to mention medications that they are currently taking. During the interview process, questions should focus on medical conditions that would warrant the use of anticoagulants or other medications that could cause prolonged bleeding after surgery, such as nonsteroidal anti-inflammatory drugs. Once the history has been obtained, bleeding risk should be assessed by a consideration of medical conditions, medications, previous surgical history or complications, and the type of surgery planned. Although individually these factors may not arouse suspicion before surgery, their combination in certain

situations may pose a serious preoperative risk of immediate or delayed hemorrhage.

For example, dentists and physicians view a simple extraction as minor surgery, after which prolonged bleeding would not be expected. When this "minor surgery" is combined with a history of poorly monitored anticoagulation use that results in inadvertent overmedication of a patient, a lack of preoperative laboratory assessment, and a preoperative diagnosis of advanced periodontal disease, the outcome can change drastically.

In any clinical situation, numerous steps can be taken preoperatively to reduce the risk of bleeding intraoperatively and postoperatively. In addition to a proper history that details medication usage and underlying medical conditions that may increase the effects of anticoagulant medication or contribute to prolonged bleeding, a detailed, focused physical examination should be performed. Certain anatomic considerations and disease processes can predispose a patient to bleeding complications. Surgery that requires a maxillary osteotomy or a neck dissection poses a greater risk than surgery that does not traverse such anatomic structures and does not increase the risk of severing a vessel that may or may not be amenable to ligation or cautery. Inflammation at the proposed surgical site may lead to fibrinolysis and prolonged bleeding. Excessive operative trauma also may predispose a patient to postoperative bleeding, especially from oral soft tissues.

Once a patient's history has been obtained and the type of surgery and its potential operative complications have been considered fully, clinicians should assess each patient's risk of intraoperative or postoperative bleeding and determine whether preoperative laboratory assessment is indicated. This determination does not depend entirely on the type or dose of anticoagulant medication but also is influenced by the type of surgery to be performed and a patient's preoperative diagnosis. Laboratory assessment may include determining hemoglobin or hematocrit, platelet count, prothrombin time (PT), partial thromboplastin time (PTT), an Ivy bleeding time, platelet function analysis, International Normalized Ratio (INR), or some combination of these factors.

Surgeons must assess a patient's coagulation status preoperatively. Surgeons commonly use a few basic measures that deserve a brief explanation. For the purposes of this article we categorize these measures as tests of primary hemostasis or tests of secondary hemostasis. Tests of primary hemostasis include determination of the platelet count, bleeding time, and platelet function and screening for von Willebrand's disease. Tests of secondary hemostasis include

determination of the PTT, PT, and thrombin time and mixing studies and tests for inhibitors, disseminated intravascular coagulation, and factor XIII deficiency.

Testing for primary hemostasis begins with determination of the platelet count. For this test, the blood must be collected in citrated tubes without exposure to ethylenediaminetetra-acetic acid, which may cause platelet clumping and an inaccurate count.

In the absence of overt thrombocytopenia, determination of bleeding time is a means of assessing platelet dysfunction as a cause of symptoms. Traditionally this is known as an Ivy bleeding time. A blood pressure cuff is placed on the upper arm and inflated to 40 mm Hg. A small wound is made on the forearm, filter paper is applied to the site, and the blood is pulled away by capillary action while bleeding time is measured at 20-second intervals. A prolonged bleeding time indicates a problem with platelet function or perhaps with capillary integrity [6].

Although some hospitals and laboratories still use the Ivy bleeding time to assess platelet function, a more recently developed test is the platelet function analysis. This laboratory test simulates the process of platelet adhesion and aggregation after a vascular injury in vitro. Using separate test cartridges known as the collagen/epinephrine test and the collagen/ADP test, the platelet function analysis is reported as a closure time. A closure time above the normal range may indicate the need for further testing to determine any possible causes of platelet dysfunction, including acquired, inherited, or induced by platelet-inhibiting medications. The collagen/epinephrine test determines if the platelet dysfunction is induced by intrinsic platelet defects, von Willebrand's disease, or exposure to platelet-inhibiting agents. The collagen/ADP test is used to determine if an abnormal collagen/epinephrine test was caused by either the effect of acetyl salicylic acid or medications that contain acetyl salicylic acid.

Screening for von Willebrand's disease screen is appropriate for a patient with a history of bleeding, a normal platelet count, and prolonged bleeding time.

Finally, platelet function studies, such as secretion and aggregation in response to agonists, can implicate platelet dysfunction as a cause of bleeding. Such studies are not indicated for the initial evaluation of anticoagulation status, however.

Tests of secondary hemostasis include the determination of PT (often reported as INR). For this test, calcium and thromboplastin (a mixture of tissue factor and phospholipid membrane fragments) are added to citrated blood, and the time required for a clot to form is measured. This test measures the extrinsic pathway of the coagulation cascade. The PT

is prolonged by deficiencies in factors II (prothrombin), V, VII, and X and in fibrinogen. The PT is used to monitor the anticoagulation status of patients who are taking warfarin [4].

The determination of PTT measures the slower intrinsic pathway. In vitro, this pathway requires all of the clotting factors except factor VII. Likewise, in vitro, a reliable result can be obtained only when the concentrations of factor XII, prekallikrein, and high molecular weight kininogen are normal. These concentrations are not believed to be as important in vivo as they are in vitro, because patients who lack these factors do not bleed abnormally [4]. The PTT is used to monitor anticoagulation with heparin. When PT and PTT are used as tools for measuring anticoagulation, the results are generally not prolonged until factor levels fall to less than 30% of normal [4]. Thrombin time measures the time to clot formation after thrombin is added to anticoagulated blood. This test is a good measure of quantitative and qualitative deficiencies in fibrinogen.

Mixing studies should be one of the initial tests of coagulation status. A prolonged PT or PTT may indicate either a factor deficiency or the presence of an inhibitor. If the test plasma is mixed with an equal amount of normal plasma, deficient factors are restored to at least 50% of normal levels. These levels are sufficient to normalize the clotting results, but an excess of inhibitors remains, and test results are not correct. In the event that mixing studies fail to correct a prolonged coagulation time, confirmatory testing for the specific inhibitors should be conducted.

Another test that may be clinically appropriate is screening for disseminated intravascular coagulation. This test is especially helpful in differentiating disseminated intravascular coagulation from liver failure.

Finally, specific tests can be used to determine which of several inherited thrombophilic conditions may be present, such as abnormalities in antithrombin III activity, protein C level and activity, or protein S level and activity. When patients have a history of venous thromboses and a positive family history of such events, depending on patient age it may be appropriate to evaluate for inherited causes of the hypercoagulable state [6].

The two most common types of chronic anticoagulation medications that may be used by patients seen by oral and maxillofacial surgeons are warfarin and antiplatelet therapy. Understanding the mechanism or pathophysiology of anticoagulation and the indications for which medicated patients are being treated greatly aids in decisions regarding the treatment of these patients.

Warfarin therapy

Patients may require warfarin therapy for such diagnoses as atrial fibrillation, pulmonary embolism, myocardial infarction, stroke, and deep venous thrombosis or because they have prosthetic heart valves. Warfarin causes anticoagulation by inhibiting the vitamin K–dependent coagulation factors II, VII, IX, and X. Its duration of action is 2 to 5 days. Warfarin is 99% bound to plasma proteins. The addition of other medications that are also protein bound may result in decreased binding of warfarin, which increases the level of anticoagulation. PT or INR is checked regularly so that therapeutic levels of the drug can be maintained in the blood.

Several studies have evaluated dentoalveolar surgery among anticoagulated patients. Souto and colleagues [7] prospectively studied bleeding complications in 92 patients who were chronically treated with acenocoumarol for valvular heart disease or cardiac valve prosthesis and who were scheduled for dental extractions (one or two teeth). At the time of surgery, the INR of all patients was between 2 and 3. Patients were assigned to one of six groups. For three groups, the acenocoumarol dosage was decreased before surgery and one of three antifibrinolytic therapies was initiated: oral epsilon-amino-caproic acid (4 g orally) before surgery, tranexamic acid as a mouthwash, or oral epsilon-amino-caproic acid as a mouthwash. The other three groups used the same antifibrinolytic therapies but maintained the normal dosage of acenocoumarol. There was no statistically significant difference between groups on the basis of gender, age, gingival hypertrophy, surgical trauma, or number of extracted teeth. The authors concluded that the most desirable treatment was no change in the dose of anticoagulation medication and topical treatment with tranexamic acid for 2 days after surgery. They also determined that heparin administration was an additional uncontrollable risk factor for hemorrhagic complications.

Blinder and colleagues [8] studied three types of local hemostasis after extractions performed on patients who were maintained on coumarin therapy. Reasons reported for anticoagulation included valvular disease, atrial fibrillation, ischemic heart disease, and venous thromboembolism. Patients in group one were treated with a gelatin sponge in the extraction site and sutures; patients in group two were treated with a gelatin sponge, sutures, and tranexamic acid mouthwash for 4 days; patients in group three were treated with fibrin glue, gelatin sponges, and sutures. Reasons for extraction were severe periodontitis and deep caries. The patients' preoperative INRs ranged

from 1.5 to 4. There was no statistically significant difference in postoperative bleeding between groups. Postoperative bleeding was associated with advanced periodontal disease but was not associated with an elevated INR. All postoperative bleeding episodes (13/150 patients) were controlled with local measures.

Blinder and colleagues [9] studied the association of INR and bleeding complications after dental extractions. In a study of 249 patients who underwent 543 extractions, the authors separated the INR values into five ranges: 1.5 to 1.99, 2.0 to 2.49, 2.5 to 2.99, 3.0 to 3.49, and higher than 3.5. After the extractions, patients were treated with gelatin sponges and sutures at the extractions sites. Prolonged postoperative bleeding occurred among 12% of patients, but there was no statistically significant difference in bleeding time between the five groups.

The invasiveness of the procedure is important in the determination of treatment for anticoagulated patients. Simple extractions can be accomplished without cessation of anticoagulation therapy. The use of gelatin sponges and sutures after simple extractions has been shown to control postoperative bleeding in patients with INRs as high as 3.5 [8,9]. For more invasive procedures, conventional therapy has included hospitalization, heparinization, and daily monitoring of PT, PTT, and INR. Such procedures are typically required for 3 to 4 days before surgery so that a patient's INR can normalize. Heparin administration is discontinued 6 hours before surgery and resumed postoperatively. Warfarin administration is also resumed postoperatively, and heparin administration can be discontinued when the INR reaches the therapeutic level [10,11].

The condition for which a patient is treated is also important in the decision about the anticoagulation process. For example, the risk of stroke in a patient treated for atrial fibrillation is lower than the risk of thrombus in a patient treated for a mechanical heart valve. These patients might be treated differently with regard to discontinuation of anticoagulation therapy.

An interesting study by Pham and colleagues [12] examined the risks associated with discontinuing warfarin therapy for high-risk patients who were being treated for intracranial hemorrhage. Indications for anticoagulation were prosthetic heart valves (group 1), atrial fibrillation and cardioembolic stroke (group 2), and recurrent transient ischemic attack or and ischemic stroke (group 3). The probability of an ischemic stroke 30 days (Kaplan-Meier curve) after the discontinuation of warfarin was 2.9% for group 1, 2.6% for group 2, and 4.8% for group 3. The authors concluded that cessation of warfarin therapy for 1 to 2 weeks is

associated with a comparatively low probability of embolic events in patients at high risk for embolism.

A review of 28 patients by Ananthasubramaniam and co-workers [13] led to similar conclusions. All patients had mechanical heart valves and were receiving chronic anticoagulation therapy. This therapy was discontinued because of severe bleeding complications. The mean duration of warfarin cessation was 15 days. Four deaths occurred: two were thought to be related to the initial diagnosis, one was caused by intracerebral bleeding, and one was caused by massive hematemesis. Telephone follow-up at 6 months found that no clinically recognized thromboembolic events had occurred in 19 of 21 patients.

Another strategy that can be used to treat patients undergoing long-term anticoagulation is decreasing a patient's INR to 1.5 to 2.0 without discontinuing treatment entirely. No study has shown that the risk of bleeding is significantly increased when the INR is kept in this range. Larson and colleagues [14] reported the outcomes of 93 patients treated in this way. Most of the patients, all of whom were chronically treated with warfarin, were at high risk of thromboembolic events during the perioperative period. Of the surgical procedures for which the INRs were adjusted, 58% were considered to be substantially invasive (joint replacement, vascular surgery). For 35 patients, warfarin was supplemented with heparin (administered intravenously or subcutaneously) or with low molecular weight heparin (LMWH) (administered subcutaneously) because the INR fell below 1.5. The mean INR was 2.1 on the day before and 1.8 on the day of surgery (range, 1.2–4.9). Complications were four minor bleeding episodes, two major bleeding episodes (2% rate of major bleeding), two events of thromboembolism (one death), and the need for 34 transfusions. Most of the transfusions occurred in patients who received autogenous units of previously donated blood for joint replacement surgery. The theoretical advantage of continuing warfarin therapy and maintaining the INR between 1.5 and 2 is the rebound phenomenon and the hypercoagulable state that occurs when warfarin therapy is stopped and started [14].

Antiplatelet therapy

Multiple medications are used as antiplatelet therapy. Patients may be treated with antiplatelet drugs for various reasons. Antiplatelet therapy has been shown to be effective in decreasing the risk of myocardial infarction and nonfatal stroke among patients who have peripheral vascular disease [15,16].

Clopidogrel, a commonly administered antiplatelet drug, inhibits ADP-induced platelet fibrinogen binding. Clopidogrel has been identified as an independent risk factor for re-exploration after coronary artery bypass graft surgery [17]. In one study, the risk of surgical re-exploration because of postoperative bleeding was 6.1% for patients treated with clopidogrel but only 1% for patients not treated with the drug ($P = 0.058$) [17]. The rate of transfusions was also higher for patients treated with clopidogrel. The findings of this study were confirmed in 2005 by Kapetanakis and associates [15], who demonstrated that patients taking clopidogrel and undergoing coronary artery bypass graft surgery had a higher risk of intraoperative hemorrhage, the need for transfusions with various blood products (platelets, packed red blood cells, and fresh frozen plasma), and the need for re-operation to control bleeding.

In only a few instances would maxillofacial surgery be needed within 3 weeks of the insertion of a coronary artery stent. Should major maxillofacial surgery be indicated during this 3-week period, however, antiplatelet therapy should not be stopped. Sharma and colleagues [18] reviewed the records of patients who underwent major noncardiac surgery after coronary stenting. They found that the risk of cardiac complications and death was greatest during the 3 weeks after stent placement; six of seven deaths occurred among patients whose antiplatelet therapy had been discontinued.

Many patients may receive a combination of antiplatelet drugs (eg, aspirin and clopidogrel) [16,19]. This combination has been shown to cause a synergistic antiplatelet action; in other words, the risk of bleeding complications is much higher in association with combined therapy than in association with single-drug therapy. No large trials have been performed to evaluate the risk of bleeding complications in association with combined antiplatelet therapy. A recent survey of vascular surgeons showed that most did not stop the administration of antiplatelet drugs preoperatively [20]. One might assume that the risk of bleeding complications would be much higher in association with vascular procedures (carotid endarterectomy or infrainguinal bypass) than in association with routine exodontia. For more invasive maxillofacial procedures, a surgeon may consider continuing the administration of aspirin alone. The small studies that have been reported indicate that the risk of myocardial infarction and stroke is lower for patients who continue to receive antiplatelet therapy than for patients who stop such therapy. The results also suggest that the risk additional surgery for a bleeding

complication is higher when antiplatelet therapy is not discontinued, however [20].

Other platelet-inhibiting medications are aspirin and ticlopidine. Aspirin inhibits the activity of cyclooxygenase, and ticlopidine inhibits ADP-induced platelet fibrinogen binding. Platelets are affected for the life of the cell, and complete reversal of antiplatelet activity does not occur until after approximately 2 weeks. It has been recommended that the administration of antiplatelet drugs should be discontinued 7 to 9 days before surgery, if indicated, so that sufficient numbers of normal circulation platelets can be regenerated [11].

Low molecular weight heparins

An alternative to heparin for anticoagulation during warfarin cessation is the administration of LMWH. LMWHs are administered subcutaneously, have a bioavailability of more than 90%, and offer a predictable and reproducible anticoagulant response [21]. There is no need to monitor the anticoagulation activity of the drugs [22]. LMWHs are not totally reversed by protamine, as is regular heparin [21]. The mechanism of action of this group of drugs is via binding to antithrombin III, which increases the ability of antithrombin III to inactivate factor Xa and factor II [22].

LMWHs have been used as bridging therapy for patients taking warfarin. The reported incidence of major bleeding episodes in patients treated with this therapy ranges from 0% to 10% [14,23,24]. An advantage of this bridging therapy is that it avoids the need for postoperative hospitalization while the INR returns to normal [24]. Although LMWHs are approved only for prophylaxis of venous thromboembolism, they may be considered as an alternative to intravenously administered heparin.

Summary

Patients who are undergoing chronic anticoagulation therapy and require maxillofacial surgery present a challenge to oral and maxillofacial surgeons. Typical treatment previously required prolonged hospital stays, complicated medication adjustments, multiple laboratory tests, and a high level of anxiety. A thorough surgeon continues to elicit a detailed history, perform a thorough physical examination, and consult with a patient's internist or cardiologist. A growing body of literature indicates that routine dental extractions can be completed with only local measures for hemostasis, without cessation of anti-

coagulation medications and without the risk of thromboembolic events.

For patients who need more invasive surgery (eg, patients who have suffered trauma), options include discontinuation of warfarin with heparin bridging, LMWH bridging, and maintaining the INR between 1.5 and 2.0. Patients who receive antiplatelet therapy and require invasive maxillofacial surgery can be treated with single-drug therapy with the use of local measures for hemostasis or can be considered for aspirin therapy alone if on two-drug therapy.

References

[1] Dunn AS, Turpie AG. Perioperative management of patients receiving oral anticoagulants: a systematic review. Arch Intern Med 2003;163(8):901–8.

[2] Solomon JM, Schow SR. The potential risks, complications, and prevention of deep vein thrombosis in oral and maxillofacial surgery patients. J Oral Maxillofac Surg 1995;53(12):1441–7.

[3] Wakefield TW. Hemostasis. In: Greenfield LJ, Oldham KT, Mulholland MW, editors. Surgery: scientific principles and practice. Philadelphia: Lippincott, Williams & Wilkins; 2001. p. 86–107.

[4] Scott-Conner CEH, Spence RK, Shander A, et al. Hemostasis, thrombosis, hematopoiesis, and blood transfusions. In: O'Leary JP, editor. The physiologic basis of surgery. Philadelphia: Lippincott, Williams & Wilkins; 2002. p. 531–47.

[5] Guyton AC, Hall JE. Hemostasis and blood coagulation. In: Guyton AC, Hall JE, editors. Textbook of medical physiology. WB Saunders: Philadelphia; 2002. p. 419–29.

[6] Andritsos L, Yusen RD, Eby C. Disorders of hemostasis. In: Green GB, Harris IS, Lin GA, et al, editors. The Washington manual of medical therapeutics. Philadelphia: Lippincott, Williams & Wilkins; 2004. p. 398–422.

[7] Souto JC, Oliver A, Zuazu-Jausoro I, et al. Oral surgery in anticoagulated patients without reducing the dose of oral anticoagulant: a prospective randomized study. J Oral Maxillofac Surg 1996;54(1):27–32 [discussion 323].

[8] Blinder D, Manor Y, Martinowitz U, et al. Dental extractions in patients maintained on continued oral anticoagulant: comparison of local hemostatic modalities. Oral Surg Oral Med Oral Pathol Oral Radiol Endod 1999;88(2):137–40.

[9] Blinder D, Manor Y, Martinowitz U, et al. Dental extractions in patients maintained on oral anticoagulant therapy: comparison of INR value with occurrence of postoperative bleeding. Int J Oral Maxillofac Surg 2001;30(6):518–21.

[10] Mehra P, Cottrell DA, Bestgen SC, et al. Management of heparin therapy in the high-risk, chronically anti-coagulated, oral surgery patient: a review and a proposed nomogram. J Oral Maxillofac Surg 2000;58(2): 198–202.

[11] Sear JW, Higham H. Issues in the perioperative management of the elderly patient with cardiovascular disease. Drugs Aging 2002;19(6):429–51.

[12] Phan TG, Koh M, Wijdicks EF. Safety of discontinuation of anticoagulation in patients with intracranial hemorrhage at high thromboembolic risk. Arch Neurol 2000;57(12):1710–3.

[13] Ananthasubramaniam K, Beattie JN, Rosman HS, et al. How safely and for how long can warfarin therapy be withheld in prosthetic heart valve patients hospitalized with a major hemorrhage? Chest 2001;119(2):478–84.

[14] Larson BJ, Zumberg MS, Kitchens CS. A feasibility study of continuing dose-reduced warfarin for invasive procedures in patients with high thromboembolic risk. Chest 2005;127(3):922–7.

[15] Kapetanakis EI, Medlam DA, Boyce SW, et al. Clopidogrel administration prior to coronary artery bypass grafting surgery: the cardiologist's panacea or the surgeon's headache? Eur Heart J 2005;26(6):576–83.

[16] Robless P, Mikhailidis DP, Stansby G. Systematic review of antiplatelet therapy for the prevention of myocardial infarction, stroke or vascular death in patients with peripheral vascular disease. Br J Surg 2001; 88(6):787–800.

[17] Yende S, Wunderink RG. Effect of clopidogrel on bleeding after coronary artery bypass surgery. Crit Care Med 2001;29(12):2271–5.

[18] Sharma AK, Ajani AE, Hamwi SM, et al. Major noncardiac surgery following coronary stenting: when is it safe to operate? Catheter Cardiovasc Interv 2004; 63(2):141–5.

[19] Payne DA, Hayes PD, Jones CI, et al. Combined therapy with clopidogrel and aspirin significantly increases the bleeding time through a synergistic antiplatelet action. J Vasc Surg 2002;35(6):1204–9.

[20] Smout J, Stansby G. Current practice in the use of antiplatelet agents in the peri-operative period by UK vascular surgeons. Ann R Coll Surg Engl 2003; 85(2):97–101.

[21] Harder S, Klinkhardt U, Alvarez JM. Avoidance of bleeding during surgery in patients receiving anticoagulant and/or antiplatelet therapy: pharmacokinetic and pharmacodynamic considerations. Clin Pharmacokinet 2004;43(14):963–81.

[22] Johnson Leong C, Rada RE. The use of low-molecular-weight heparins in outpatient oral surgery for patients receiving anticoagulation therapy. J Am Dent Assoc 2002;133(8):1083–7.

[23] Spandorfer JM, Lynch S, Weitz HH, et al. Use of enoxaparin for the chronically anticoagulated patient before and after procedures. Am J Cardiol 1999;84(4): 478–80, A10.

[24] Tinmouth AH, Morrow BH, Cruickshank MK, et al. Dalteparin as periprocedure anticoagulation for patients on warfarin and at high risk of thrombosis. Ann Pharmacother 2001;35(6):669–74.

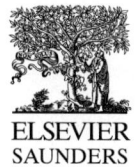

ELSEVIER
SAUNDERS

Oral Maxillofacial Surg Clin N Am 18 (2006) 161 – 171

ORAL AND
MAXILLOFACIAL
SURGERY CLINICS
of North America

Perioperative Management of the Patient with Hematologic Disorders

Guillermo E. Chacon, DDS*, Carlos M. Ugalde, DDS

Section of Oral and Maxillofacial Surgery, Anesthesiology, and Oral and Maxillofacial Pathology,
The Ohio State University Medical Center, 305 West 12ᵗʰ Avenue, Box 182357, Columbus, OH 43218-2357, USA

Surgeons of all specialties have an unavoidable interaction with the ability of a patient to heal physical wounds. Whether traumatic or surgically induced, wound healing is a complex process that must occur uninterrupted to achieve what is popularly known as surgical success. Once injury is induced to the tissue, a series of events are triggered aimed at repairing the sequelae of the insult. This orchestrated set of events always starts with the control of any bleeding that may occur at the surgical site. Once injury to tissues takes place and bleeding starts, the body's first step in the intricate process of wound healing is to stop blood loss and stabilize the wound to permit the subsequent series of steps to take place. For this to happen in a predictable fashion, a patient's ability to control and stop bleeding is critically important. This process of bleeding control is called hemostasis. Unfortunately, not all patients possess intact hemostatic ability. What is even more critical is that in some instances, the disorder presents such benign manifestations that an individual may be undiagnosed until a revealing event takes place, such as major trauma or surgery. This occurrence presents a serious problem for the treating surgeon if the first manifestation of the disease is identified on the operating room table. It is important to carry out the preoperative health history in an inquisitive fashion to unmask any underlying condition with which a patient may present.

According to the National Hemophilia Foundation, the incidence of bleeding disorders can be as frequent as 1 in every 10,000 patients [1]. A bleeding disorder is any condition in which an inherited or acquired blood deficiency caused by the absence or inactivity of an essential blood protein or factor causes the body to form unstable blood clots that allow bleeding to continue for a longer period of time than the normal accepted parameters. Depending on the severity of the condition, the clinical implications can range from the nagging wound that continues to ooze and inconvenience a patient for an extended period of time to a serious life-threatening blood volume depletion.

When plasma coagulation factor concentrations are in the range of 5% of normal, neither spontaneous hemarthrosis nor spontaneous bleeding occurs [2]. With trauma or minor surgery, however, severe bleeding may ensue unless coagulation factor levels approach 40% to 50% of normal serum levels for a given coagulation factor. Conversely, major surgery requires 100% of normal clotting activity to prevent intraoperative and postoperative complications as a result of excessive blood loss. After major surgery, replacement of essential coagulation factors is continued for at least 10 days. Oral surgery or minor surgery requires an additional 5 to 7 days of factor replacement [3].

Hemostasis

Hemostasis is the process the body launches for the prevention of blood loss after injury has been caused to the tissues. This process involves a series of complex reactions that are intricately linked with

* Corresponding author.
E-mail address: chacon.4@osu.edu (G.E. Chacon).

1042-3699/06/$ – see front matter © 2006 Elsevier Inc. All rights reserved.
doi:10.1016/j.coms.2005.12.010

each other and occur almost simultaneously. For the purpose of this discussion, we divide these stages of hemostasis into four phases: vascular phase, platelet phase, coagulation phase, and fibrinolytic phase. The process to stop loss of blood is triggered by soft tissue trauma that involves the endothelial wall of blood vessels, and the end product is a clot that acts as a mechanical stop or seal that eventually stops bleeding. The final phase of this process is followed by a fibrinolytic phase, which prevents uncontrolled coagulation beyond the site of injury and dissolves the clot [4,5].

Vascular phase

Normal endothelial cells have a thromboresistant surface that prevents clot formation and allows blood to flow through the vasculature without interruption. Certain proteins contained within the vessel wall also act in the prevention of intravascular coagulation. Thrombomodulin is a molecule contained in the endothelium that inhibits coagulation by activating the natural anticoagulant protein C to bind free thrombin. The endothelium also is capable of stimulating blood clot breakdown or fibrinolysis through the production of tissue-type plasminogen activator [4–6].

The vascular phase of hemostasis starts immediately after a blood vessel is injured. An almost instantaneous reflex of the vessel wall produces constriction of its lumen, which in turn decreases blood flow to the site and reduces the amount of blood that is lost. The injured cells secrete ADP and von Willebrand factor (vWF), which promote platelet adhesion to the subendothelial tissue leading toward the platelet phase. The efficiency of the vascular phase depends to a great extend on the size of the lumen of the injured vessel and the volume and flow of the blood carried through it. Smaller vessels in the venous system are more likely to undergo constriction that allows for spontaneous sequencing of the hemostatic process. Larger vessels in the arterial system in particular require surgical intervention and mechanical clamping to stop blood loss.

Platelet phase

Platelets are cellular components of blood anatomically characterized by the absence of a nucleus. These anuclear cells have an average lifespan in the circulation of approximately 8 to 12 days. The ultracellular structure of platelets includes multiple components that are critical for adequate platelet function, including the glycocalyx, plasma membrane, microfilaments, tubules, and granules. Platelet

receptors, such as glycoprotein Ib, which interacts with vWF, and glycoprotein IIb, which binds with fibrinogen, are located in the plasma membrane [7]. If vascular injury exposes the underlying collagen, platelets adhere to the exposed subendothelial tissue as a result of contact activation to begin forming the platelet plug. During this phase, platelets release granules that help attract more platelets to the site and aid in stabilization of the immature plug. This process is referred to as platelet degranulation. The granules released in this process include dense granules, alpha granules, and lysosomes. Platelets also release serotonin, ADP, and thromboxane A_2 as part of the degranulation process. These substances function as strong platelet chemotactic agents and promote aggregation, continued degranulation, and further vasoconstriction, which lead to the formation of a stable platelet plug. Changes in the platelet membrane receptors plus the conversion of coagulation factors strengthen the platelet plug with fibrin, which leads it into a proper and stable blood clot [8,9].

Coagulation phase

Classic model of coagulation

Although it is possible to single out the events of hemostasis, which helps in our understanding of it (eg, platelet agglutination and formation of fibrin), it must be realized that this whole process occurs synergistically [10]. The discovery of thrombin by Schmidt in 1872 [11] and the initial work of Morawitz [12], which focused on delineating the scheme in which blood undergoes clotting, contributed to what is known currently about this process.

Coagulation is a sequential process that involves multiple components in a series of events often referred to as a cascade. Phospholipids, calcium ions, and plasma proteins are the main components involved in this stage of hemostasis [8]. Most of the proteins involved in this process are synthesized in the liver, including fibrinogen, prothrombin, and factors V, VII, IX, X, XI, XII, and XIII. Some of these proteins also depend on the presence of vitamin K to function properly. Vitamin K–dependent factors include factors II, VII, IX, and X. The coagulation cascade is divided into two pathways: the extrinsic and the intrinsic pathways. These pathways converge to form the common pathway at the level in which factor X is activated and ends with the formation of fibrin (Fig. 1).

Extrinsic pathway. The extrinsic pathway is activated by tissue factor (TF), which is released as a result of subendothelial tissue exposure of the injured

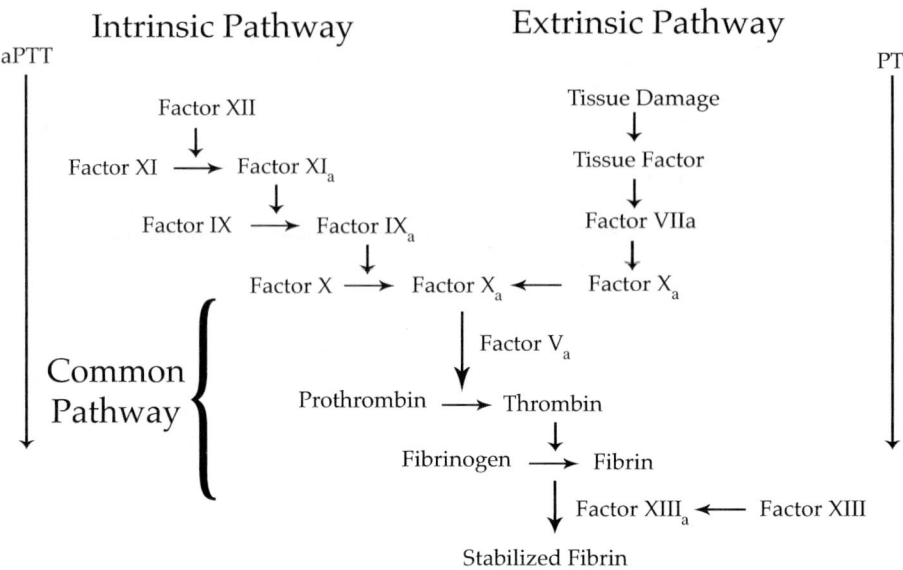

Fig. 1. Classic model of coagulation.

vessel. This factor, which is extrinsic to the coagulation system, activates factor VII to VIIa. Factor VIIa in the presence of ionized calcium activates factor X. The laboratory test used to measure the function of this pathway is the prothrombin time (PT). Normal PT is 11 to 15 seconds. Although this test is sensitive, it is not specific in determining the cause of an abnormal result. An abnormal result can be caused by low levels of blood proteins (clotting factors), a decrease in activity of any of these factors, the absence of any of the factors, or the presence of a substance that blocks the activity of any of these factors.

Intrinsic pathway. The intrinsic pathway starts with contact activation with elastin, collagen, platelets, prekallikrein, high molecular weight kininogens, or plasmin. Factor XII is activated followed by further activation of factor XI and factor IX. Finally, the intrinsic pathway leads to the common pathway when factor IXa activates factor X under the presence of ionized calcium, platelet factor III, and factor VIIIa. The screening laboratory test of choice for this pathway is the activated partial thromboplastin time (aPPT). The normal aPPT is 25 to 35 seconds.

Common pathway. The common pathway consists of the convergence point of the intrinsic and the extrinsic pathways. Factor X is transformed to factor Xa and, along with factor V, activates prothrombin (factor II) to thrombin (factor IIa). Thrombin is an enzyme with four key functions: (1) removal of small fibrinopeptides from the large fibrinogen precursor, which favors the polymerization of fibrinogen into strands of fibrin, (2) activation of factor XIII to XIIIa (XIIIa is the fibrin-stabilizing factor, which in the presence of calcium ions interlinks fibrin strands), (3) activation of platelets, and (4) activation of protein C (an antithrombotic plasma enzyme).

At the same time that thrombin activates fibrinogen to form fibrin, it also stimulates the production of more factor VIII and activates factor XIII, which is responsible for cross-linking the fibrin monomers and stabilizing the clot [9].

Cell-based model of coagulation

The in vivo process of coagulation occurs in a synergistic fashion rather than in a sequentially separated cascade of events. Hoffman and colleagues [13–15] determined that this classic model inadequately explains how coagulation happens. Many questions about disorders in this process are left unanswered as to whether coagulation truly consists of an intrinsic and extrinsic pathway. For example, why does the extrinsic pathway not compensate for the lack of factor VIII and IX? Why do patients who lack activators of the intrinsic pathway (factor XII, high molecular weight kininogens, prekallikrein) not present with major clinical bleeding but reflect a prolonged aPPT? In an attempt to answer these and other relevant questions, investigators came to the conclusion that there is an interrelationship between intrinsic and extrinsic pathways, and they developed a model to explain how coagulation occurs in vivo. The

model consists of three interrelated processes: initiation, amplification, and propagation. It is also based on the evidence that coagulation takes place in two cell surfaces: TF-bearing cells and platelets (Fig. 2).

Initiation phase. The initiation phase takes place on the surface of the TF-bearing cell, which, under normal circumstances, is isolated from the blood. When tissue injury occurs, plasma is allowed to come in contact with these TF-bearing cells and functions as a receptor for factor VII. The TF in plasma activates factor VII and forms the FVIIa/TF complex, which in turn activates small amounts of factors IX and X. Factor Xa interacts with its cofactor Va and forms thrombin. The amount of thrombin formed at this point is not enough to form a fibrin clot. It is enough to promote platelet activation and factor VIII formation as part of the amplification phase, however. The FVIIa/TF complex not bound to the cell surfaces can become easily inhibited by the TF pathway inhibitor and antithrombin III.

Amplification phase. The small amount of thrombin produced in the initiation phase activates platelets and triggers the production of a large amount of factor VIII. In this process, the activation of the platelets exposes the receptor sites for more coagulation factors. The factor VIIIa is activated by

dissociation of the FVIII/vWF complex, which allows vWF to promote more platelet adhesion and aggregation. Factors V and XI are activated on the platelet surface. The role of factor XI is to increase the amount of factor IXa on the platelet surface to increase the amount of surface available for factor Xa in the propagation phase. At the end of this phase the final product is an activated platelet with factors Va, VIIIa, and XIa on its surface.

Propagation phase. Factor IXa activated during the initiation phase diffuses from the TF-bearing cell to the activated platelets surfaces and binds to factor VIIIa to form FVIIIa/FIXa complex (tenase) on the platelet surface. Factor Xa cannot move from TF environment. It must be brought directly to the platelet surface. In this phase, plasma factor X is activated by factor IX, and factor Xa associates with its cofactor Va on the platelet surface to create complex FXa/Va (prothrombinase), which is capable of producing sufficient thrombin to create cleavage of fibrinogen to form the fibrin clot.

Fibrinolytic phase

The fibrinolytic phase is a vital component of hemostasis. Its main function is to avoid thrombotic occlusion of the blood vessel and propagation of the

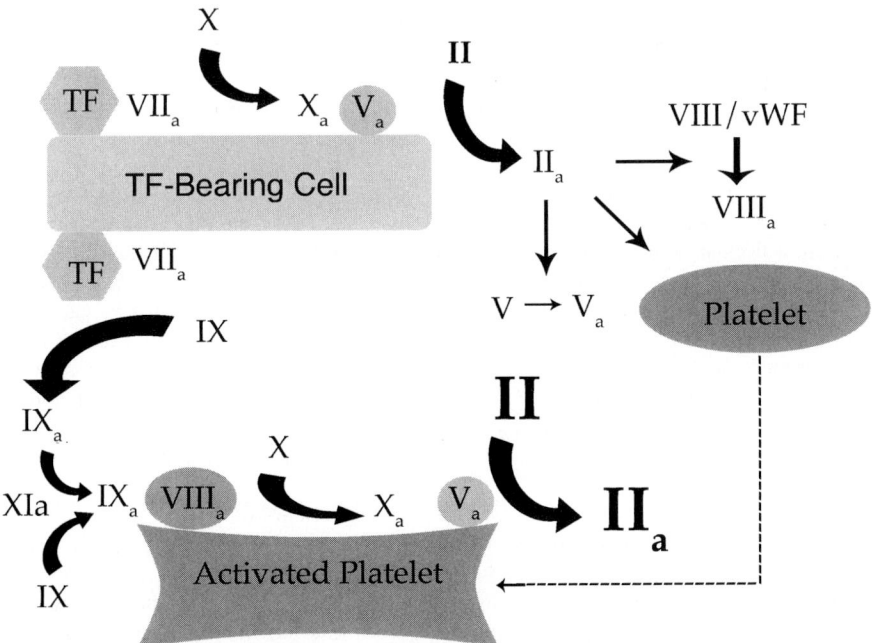

Fig. 2. Cell-based model of coagulation. (*Adapted from* Hoffman M. Remodeling the blood coagulation cascade. J Thromb Thrombolysis 2003;16(1–2):18; with permission.)

coagulation throughout the entire vascular system. The process starts early during the coagulation process and consists of the activation of plasminogen, a normal plasma protein that is converted into plasmin by the action of enzymes called plasminogen activators. The most important plasminogen activator is tissue-type plasminogen activator, which is found in the vascular endothelium. Plasmin is broken down into small fragments called fibrin degradation products that exert an anticoagulant effect. The action of this fibrinolytic system is regulated by naturally occurring inhibitors and antiplasmins [8,9].

Screening laboratory tests

Laboratory tests are useful in identifying specific problems of the hemostasis process. These tests help to establish a diagnosis but cannot predict actual bleeding during surgery.

Ivy bleeding time

This test is performed by placing a blood pressure cuff on a patient's arm and inflating it to 40 mm Hg. A small incision is made on the patient's arm, and every 30 seconds the blood is blotted gently with filter paper until bleeding has stopped. The filter paper must not touch the wound. This test is intended to measure platelet function, but it is neither sensitive nor specific. For this reason, its use is declining and at some institutions has been eliminated completely. Platelet counts <100,000/microL, low hematocrit, aspirin, other platelet inhibitory drugs, and certain other medications can prolong the bleeding time. Many variables influence the result, including skin thickness, temperature, blood vessel characteristics, type of blade, orientation of the incision (horizontal versus vertical), location of the incision, handedness, and other features.

Prothrombin time

PT evaluates the formation of thrombin and fibrin through the extrinsic pathway. The test consists of adding thromboplastin as an activating agent to the sample. The factors measured in this test are I, II, V, VII, and X. Some of them are vitamin K dependent, such as factors II, V, and VII, which are also depressed by warfarin sodium. The normal value range is 11 to 15 seconds [8].

International normalized ratio

The accuracy of the PT is known to be system dependent. Because of this dependency, the World Health Organization has addressed this system variability problem by (1) the establishment of primary and secondary international reference preparations of thromboplastin and (2) the development of a statistical model for the calibration of thromboplastins to derive the International Sensitivity Index (ISI) and the INR. The INR uses the ISI to equate all thromboplastins to the reference thromboplastin through the following equation

$$INR = (patient\ PT/mean\ normal\ PT)^{ISI}$$

Thus, the INR can be calculated using the working PT ratio once the ISI of the thromboplastin is known. Documented differences in PT results in several interlaboratory trials led the International Committee on Thrombosis and Hemostasis to make a joint recommendation in 1983 to express all PTs as INRs and request that manufacturers indicate the ISI of their thromboplastin reagents [16].

Activated partial thromboplastin time

The aPTT measures the time required to generate thrombin and fibrin via the intrinsic and common pathway. The normal aPTT ranges from 25 to 35 seconds. The clinical application of these tests involves screening for deficiency of prekallikrein, high molecular weight kininogens, and factors I, II, V, VIII, IX, X, XI, and XII, XI, IX.

PTT reagent (phospholipid with an intrinsic pathway activator, such as silica, celite, kaolin, ellagic acid) and calcium are added to patient plasma, and the time until clot formation is measured in seconds. Phospholipid in the PTT assay is called "partial thromboplastin" because TF is not present. TF is present with phospholipid in (complete) thromboplastin reagents that are used for PT assays [17]. The aPTT is also the test of choice for controlling heparin therapy.

Platelet count

The circulating platelet count can be determined accurately in a blood sample using an electronic particle counter or manual methods. Examination of a stained blood film provides a rapid estimate of platelet numbers. Normally, there are 8 to 20 platelets per 100× (oil) immersion field in a properly prepared smear (in which the erythrocytes barely touch or just overlap). At least ten different fields should be ex-

amined carefully for platelet estimation. The average number (eg, 14) can be multiplied by a factor of 20,000 to arrive at an approximation of the quantitative platelet concentration. If an average number of 14 platelets is multiplied by 20,000, the approximate platelet concentration would be 280,000 or 280 X 10^9/L. Although estimation of platelets from a blood smear does not replace an actual quantitative measurement, it should be done as a cross-check of the quantitative measurement [18].

Platelet function analyzer 100

The platelet function analyzer 100 was developed as a platelet function screen with the idea of having a more reliable way to assess function than with bleeding time. This test mimics the clotting process in vitro and allows for a more accurate determination of platelet function. Once blood is drawn from a patient, a sample is placed in a test cartridge. A vacuum is applied to the test cartridge through a thin glass to draw the blood. This fine tube is coated previously with collagen and with either epinephrine or ADP. This coating activates the platelets present in the sample and promotes adherence and aggregation. The time it takes for a clot to form and occlude it to prevent further blood flow is measured and reported as a closure time. An initial screen is performed with collagen/epinephrine coating. If the closure time is normal, the likelihood of platelet dysfunction is almost nonexistent. The collagen/ADP test is performed only to confirm an abnormal collagen/epinephrine test. If both test results are abnormal, it is likely that the patient has a platelet dysfunction and further testing for inherited or acquired conditions is indicated. If the collagen/ADP test results are normal, then the abnormal collagen/epinephrine test results may be the result of aspirin ingestion. This is the most common reason why the result may be altered in an otherwise healthy patient with no history of bleeding disorders.

Perioperative management

As with many other disease entities, prevention in the management of patients who have bleeding disorders is the best way to complete surgical treatment on this patient group without regrets and complications. The number of patients with these types of deficiencies is not necessarily uncommon. In 1989, Rhodus and colleagues [19] reported that 2.3% of 1500 adult patients with medically compromising conditions treated in a dental school had

significant bleeding problems. Surgical management of individuals with these conditions can be as simple as using topical agents and sutures for routine procedures. More complex cases may require combined attention with a hematologist and possible in-hospital treatment and postoperative stay.

The rainbow of hematologic disorders is vast, and one could dedicate a complete book to that topic. In the interest of time and space, however, we limit this discussion to the most commonly found entities that oral and maxillofacial surgeons may encounter in their practice.

Inherited coagulation disorders

Hemophilia A

Classic hemophilia (hemophilia A) is an X-linked recessive disorder that results in deficiency of plasma factor VIII coagulant activity [20]. It is the most severe of all inherited bleeding disorders and accounts for eight of every ten cases of hemophilia diagnosed every year. Women are carriers of this trait. Fifty percent of the male offspring of female carriers have the disease, and 50% of their female offspring are carriers. In contrast to this, all female children of a male parent with hemophilia are carriers of the trait.

Its severity is classified according to the level of activity of factor VIII present. Factor VIII levels between 50% and 150% are considered normal. Patients are considered as having mild hemophilia A cases if their factor VIII level is between 5% and 30%. Individuals whose factor level approaches the bottom end of this range rarely have unprovoked bleeding episodes, but surgery or injury may cause uncontrolled bleeding, which can be fatal. Milder cases of hemophilia may not be diagnosed at all, although some patients whose clotting activity is 10% to 25% of normal may have prolonged bleeding after surgery, dental extractions, or a major injury. Generally, the first bleeding episode occurs before 18 months of age, often after a minor injury. A child who has hemophilia bruises easily. Even an intramuscular injection can cause bleeding that results in a large hematoma. Moderate cases are those with levels between 1% and 5%, and severe cases correspond to factor VIII level of less than 1% [21]. This last group of patients is significantly more prone to spontaneous bleeding. Recurring bleeding into the joints and muscles ultimately can lead to crippling deformities with significant functional limitations for patients. Bleeding can elevate the floor of the mouth and push

the base of the tongue against the posterior pharyngeal wall until it blocks the airway, which makes breathing difficult. Minor head trauma can trigger substantial intracranial hemorrhage, which can cause brain damage and death [1].

During routine minor surgical procedures (ie, simple extractions, small biopsies), minor cases can be managed with a combination of topical agents to stimulate early formation of a blood clot followed by systemic administration of an antifibrinolytic agent. Topical products routinely used in our clinic include absorbable collagen wound dressing (Collaplug), absorbale gelatin sponge (Gelfoam), absorbable oxidized cellulose (Surgicel), and topical thrombin (Thrombin-JMI). Patients typically follow their surgical treatment with oral administration of epsilon aminocaproic acid. This drug acts as an effective inhibitor of fibrinolysis by inhibiting plasminogen activator substances and, to a lesser degree, through antiplasmin activity. It has the advantage of rapid absorption after oral administration, which makes self-administration at home a viable option for this patient group. The typical protocol calls for an initial dose of 5 g, followed by hourly 1-g doses, not to exceed 30 g in a 24-hour period. Tranaxemic acid acts in a similar way and can be used for this purpose.

In patients who have mild to moderate levels of the disorder, 1-deamino-8D-arginine vasopressin (DDAVP) can be used to raise factor VIII to hemostatic levels [22,23]. This synthetic analog of the antidiuretic hormone vasopressin causes release of von Willebrand's factor from storage sites in the endothelial cells, which increases factor VIII levels twofold to threefold. The biggest advantage for this patient subset is that it substitutes plasma-derived coagulation products and avoids the risk for infection with blood-borne viruses. The recommended dose is 0.3 μg/kg in 50 mL of normal saline given intravenously over 15 to 30 minutes or subcutaneously. Peak effect occurs 30 to 60 minutes after administration, with an average duration of 4 hours. Dosing can be repeated every 12 hours for three to four doses [20,24]. Over the last few years, the use of high-concentration intranasal DDAVP spray has made this therapy even more user friendly. Seremetis and Aledort [25] reported 90.2% rating of excellent or good results in a group of 184 patients who used this treatment modality.

Patients with more severe levels of hemophilia A require factor VIII replacement before any surgical procedure. Available clotting factor concentrates consist mainly of recombinant products (Recombinate, Bioclate, and Helixate) and plasma-derived products (Hemophil-M, Hyate C, and Koate DVI).

These concentrates are intended to provide patients with a plasma level of at least 50% for minor surgical procedures and 80% to 100% for major surgery [2,26]. Patients are routinely dosed 1 hour before surgery, with redosing at 12 and 24 hours postoperatively. The main disadvantages of this therapy include risk of transmission of viral diseases [27], development of inhibiting antibodies that neutralize factor VIII, and cost (care of an average person who has hemophilia from age 3 to 50 is estimated at $5 million) [28].

Use of topical agents at the time of surgery is also highly recommended. This therapy can be augmented by the use of cryoprecipitate, DDAVP, or antifibrinolytic therapy [29].

Hemophilia B

Hemophilia B (also called "Christmas disease" after Stephen Christmas, a British boy in the twentieth century who was first diagnosed with it) is a bleeding disorder that results from a deficiency in clotting factor IX (plasma thromboplastin component) and is inherited as an X-linked recessive trait. It is one fourth as prevalent as factor VIII, but clinically they cannot be differentiated [30]. A factor IX assay is required to separate the two. Classification and clinical problems are the same as for hemophilia A.

Replacement therapy for mild deficiencies consists of fresh frozen plasma (one unit factor IX/mL) or prothrombin complex concentrates (factors II, VII, IX, and X). Factor IX replacement therapy for more severe cases is the same as that for factor VIII, with the huge advantage that inhibitors to factor IX are rare. The desired factor IX level for minor surgery is 30% to 50%, with levels more than 50% carrying the risk of thromboembolic disease and disseminated intravascular coagulation.

Unlike factor VIII, which is maintained within the circulatory system, factor IX enters the extravascular spaces [31]. It exhibits a two-phase disappearance: (1) rapid initial disappearance (half-life of 4.5 hours) that occurs as an equilibrium with the extravascular spaces and (2) second-phase disappearance (half-life of 32 hours) [32]. Local hemostatic measures are indicated, and Amicar (epsilon aminocaproic acid) can be used with plasma replacement therapy but is contraindicated with prothrombin complex concentrates [33].

von Willebrand's disease

In 1926, Erik von Willebrand first described a hemorrhagic disorder characterized by a prolonged bleeding time and an inheritance pattern that distin-

guished the disease from classic hemophilias. Unlike hemophilia, von Willebrand's disease is not sex-linked and is autosomal dominant. It can occur via a number of genetic abnormalities or it can be an acquired disorder. The deficit is in von Willebrand's factor, more specifically with vWF gene on chromosome 12, but in some patients the coexistence of an impaired response to plasminogen activator and telangectasia suggests the presence of a regular defect or more extensive endothelial abnormalities.

Von Willebrand's factor binds and stabilizes factor VIII in circulation and mediates platelet adhesion. The amount of bleeding seen in a patient with this disorder can vary from day to day. Often administration of desmopressin before a procedure, which causes the release of von Willebrand's factor and plasminogen activator from the endothelial cells, suffices to prevent bleeding [34]. When patients who have von Willebrand's disease are given a single injection of desmopressin (0.4 µg/kg body weight), there is a considerable increase in platelet reactivity. On flow cytometry, increased glycoprotein Ib/IX expression in the platelets was found after the desmopressin injection when phycoerythrin-marked anti-CD62 antibodies were used. Apart from the rise in the vWF, this could explain the increased platelet reactivity [35]. A hematologist, through dosing and measurements of factor levels, determines the correct dosage of desmopressin necessary for each patient. As with hemophilia, supplemental topical agents might be useful.

There are more than 20 distinct clinical and laboratory subtypes of von Willebrand's disease. Most of these variants can be catalogued in three different broad subtypes, however, of which 70% to 80% are considered to be type 1. Type 1 is characterized by a partial quantitative decrease of qualitatively normal vWF and factor VIII. Typically, a proportional reduction in vWF activity, vWF antigen, and factor VIII exists.

Approximately 15% to 20% of patients who have von Willebrand's disease have type 2, which is a variant of the disease with primarily qualitative defects of vWF. It can be either autosomal dominant or recessive. Of the five known type 2 subtypes (ie, 2A, 2B, 2C, 2M, 2N), type 2A is the most common. Type 2A is inherited as an autosomal dominant trait and is characterized by normal to reduced plasma levels of factor VIIIc and vWF. Analysis of vWF multimers reveals a relative reduction in intermediate and high molecular weight multimer complexes. These abnormalities are likely the result of in vivo proteolytic degradation of the vWF. The ristocetin cofactor activity is greatly reduced, and the platelet

vWF reveals multimeric abnormalities similar to those found in plasma [36].

Type 2B is also inherited as an autosomal dominant trait. This type is characterized by a reduction in the proportion of high molecular weight vWF multimers, whereas the proportion of low molecular weight fragments is increased. These patients have a hemostatic defect caused by a qualitatively abnormal vWF and intermittent thrombocytopenia. The platelet count may fall further during pregnancy, in association with surgical procedures, or after the administration of desmopressin. Measurements of factor VIIIc and vWF in plasma are variable; however, studies involving the use of titered doses of ristocetin reveal that aggregation of normal platelets is enhanced and induced by unusually small amounts of the drug [37].

In individuals who have type 2C, which is inherited as a recessive trait, the proportion of high molecular weight multimers is reduced and the individual multimers are qualitatively abnormal. Increases in small multimers also are evident in most cases of type 2C. Ristocetin cofactor activity may be decreased out of proportion to reductions in vWF.

A small number of patients who have type 2M disease have laboratory results similar to certain patients who have type 2A. Type 2M is characterized by a decreased platelet-directed function that is not caused by a decrease of high molecular weight multimers. Laboratory findings show decreased vWF activity, but vWF antigen, factor VIII, and multimer analysis are found to be within reference range [38].

Type 2N von Willebrand's disease is also rare and is characterized by a markedly decreased affinity of vWF for factor VIII, which results in factor VIII levels reduced to approximately 5% of the reference range. Other vWF laboratory parameters are usually normal. The factor VIII binding defect in these patients is inherited in an autosomal-recessive manner.

Type 3 is the most severe form of von Willebrand's disease. In the homozygous patient, it is characterized by marked deficiencies of vWF and factor VIIIc in the plasma, the absence of vWF from platelets and endothelial cells, and a lack of the secondary transfusion response and the response to DDAVP [39,40]. It is also characterized by severe clinical bleeding and is inherited as an autosomal-recessive trait. Consanguinity is common in kindreds with this variant. Less severe clinical abnormalities and laboratory abnormalities may be identified in occasional heterozygotes; however, such cases are difficult to identify. Multimeric analysis of the small amount of vWF present yields variable results, in some cases revealing only small multimers [41].

Platelet aggregation disorders

There are three clearly identified groups of platelet dysfunction disorders depending on their etiology. These hematologic alterations can be acquired, drug-induced, or hereditary. Acquired platelet function defects can occur as a result of a blood plasma inhibitory substance, which is the case in conditions such as myeloproliferative syndromes, uremia, paraprotein disorders, liver disease, and pernicious anemia [8]. The most common mechanism of drug-induced platelet dysfunction is through interference with the membrane or membrane receptor sites. The most common offenders in this group are aspirin chlorpromazine, cocaine, xylocaine, cephaloptin, ampicillin, penicillin, and alcohol. Hereditary platelet dysfunctions can be subdivided into surface membrane defects (eg, Bernarrd-Soulier syndrome, Glanzmann's thrombasthenia, collagen receptor defect, and platelet-type von Willebrand's disease) and defects of granule storage (eg, alpha granule deficiency–Gray platelet syndrome, dense granules–Wiskott-Aldrich syndrome, Hermanky-Pudlak syndrome, Chédiak-Higashi syndrome, and thrombocytopenia-absent radius baby syndrome).

Bleeding disorders that result from platelet abnormalities also can be the result of a low number of circulating platelets or thrombocytopenia, which is almost always an acquired condition. The normal laboratory value is anywhere from 150 to 400 $\times$ 10^9/L. Bleeding is rarely a problem if the platelet count is above 50, however. The platelet shortage can be caused by bone marrow depression after irradiation, the administration of certain drugs or chemicals, or a deficiency of B_{12} complex or folic acid. Specifically, thrombocytopenic disorders may be caused by decrease platelet production, increased platelet destruction, increased platelet use, or platelet dilution [42]. The most common causes for a low platelet count include idiopathic thrombocytopenic purpura, hypersplenism, and disseminated intravascular coagulation [43].

During the acute management of trauma patients, massive blood loss and replacement can create a problem with platelet function. Adult patients with platelet counts of 100,000 who have received 15 to 20 U of blood can develop severe bleeding because of thrombocytopenia. In some cases of massive bleeding, other factors may contribute to thrombocytopenia besides the relationship between blood transfused and platelet count. These factors include soft tissue damage, severe hypotensive shock, hypoxemia, and sepsis. The most useful parameter for estimating the need for platelet transfusion under these circumstances is simply looking at the platelet count. Bleeding times and other platelet function tests under emergency conditions either in the operating room or in the emergency department are impractical and often do not reflect clinical bleeding problems [44].

Preoperative correction of the causative agent for thrombocytopenia is the main goal for elective surgical patients. Under emergency conditions, however, the main goal is to maintain ideal platelet count level (ie, >100,000/uL).

There are two types of platelet concentrates used for transfusion: (1) pooled platelet units (usually six) harvested from individual random, whole blood donations, which are commonly called a "six pack" and (2) a unit from a single donor harvested by apheresis. The number of platelets in each type is comparable; both types of platelets are suspended in plasma. Platelets may be stored a maximum of 5 days; shortages of this blood component are much more common than with other components [45]. The dose of platelets needed depends on the change desired in the platelet count. In general, a pool of six whole blood platelets (six pack) or a single unit of apheresis platelet increases the count by approximately 30,000/μL for a 70-kg person.

Patients who are Rh negative, especially if they have child-bearing potential, should receive platelets from Rh-negative donors whenever possible to prevent alloimmunization. If this is not possible, 300 μg Rh immunoglobulin should be administered intramuscularly after the transfusion (no later than 72 hours after the transfusion) [46].

Prophylactic transfusion is not recommended in idiopathic thrombocytopenic purpura or untreated disseminated intravascular coagulation. There is evidence of increased risk of thrombosis if platelets are transfused into patients who have thrombotic thrombocytopenic purpura and heparin-induced thrombocytopenia. Patients who have thrombocytopenia from septicemia or hypersplenism are not likely to respond to platelet transfusions [47].

Two other common causes for increased bleeding during the acute management of trauma patients are hypothermia and acidosis. Hypothermia associated with severe trauma is correlated with significant worse prognosis than either trauma or hypothermia alone [48]. Isolated hypothermia of 32.2°C leads to a 23% mortality rate, whereas trauma-induced hypothermia of less than 32°C is associated with 100% mortality [49–51]. The primary risk of hypothermia is abnormal bleeding. Several factors have been proposed to contribute to this coagulopaththy, including reduced activity of coagulation enzymes and platelets, activation of fibrinolysis, and endothelial injury [52].

Acidosis is also associated with worse survival in trauma and surgical patients because of metabolic derangements that may develop. Excess lactic acid production associated with tissue hypoxia is the best recognized cause. It is the end product of anaerobic metabolism, and its level is related to oxygen availability [53]. Acidosis can impair coagulation and worsen the risk of serious hemorrhage. Massive transfusion can exacerbate acidosis caused by the decreased pH of banked blood, which makes it a cyclic problem [54].

Summary

Bleeding at the time of surgery has the potential to become a serious complication. Careful patient assessment and review of history are of the utmost importance if this situation is to be avoided on the operating table. Unfortunately, many patients, particularly younger individuals with little to no previous exposure to surgery, are unaware of underlying bleeding disorders that they may have. Understanding the basic pathophysiology and management of these conditions becomes critical for the treating surgeon. For patients who have known conditions, close interconsultation with the treating hematologists and careful observation of preoperative, intraoperative, and postoperative established protocols reduces the risk of complications for patients and makes the possibility of success a reality for these individuals.

References

[1] National Hemophilia Foundation. Types of bleeding disorders. Available at: www.hemophilia.org. Accessed February 10, 2005.

[2] Peterson SR, Joseph AK. Inherited bleeding disorders in dermatologic surgery. Dermatol Surg 2001; 27:885–9.

[3] Kasper C, Boylen L, Ewing N, et al. Hematologic management of hemophilia A for surgery. JAMA 1985;253:1279–83.

[4] Lake CL, Moore RA. Normal hemostasis. In: Lake CA, Moore RA, editors. Blood: hemostasis, transfusion, and alternatives in the perioperative period. New York: Lippincott Williams & Wilkins; 1995. p. 3–16.

[5] Little JW, Falace DA, Miller C, et al. Bleeding disorders. In: Dental management of the medically compromised patient. 6th edition. St. Louis: Mosby; 2002. p. 332–64.

[6] Rodgers GM. Endothelium and the regulation of hemostasis. In: Lee GR, Foerster J, Lukens J, et al, editors. Wintrobe's clinical hematology. 10th edition.

[7] Stenberg PE, Hill RJ. Platelets and megacaryocytes. In: Lee GR, et al, editors. Wintrobe's clinical hematology. 10th edition. Philadelphia: Lippincott Williams & Wilkins; 1999. p. 615–60.

[8] Turgeon ML. Principles of hemostasis and thrombosis. In: Clinical hematology: theory and procedures. 4th edition. Philadelphia: Lippincott Williams & Wilkins; 2005. p. 339–68.

[9] Salem RF. Normal hemostasis. In: Blood conservation in the surgical patient. Baltimore (MD): Williams & Wilkins; 1996. p. 3–16.

[10] Davie EW, Fujikawa K, Kisiel W. The coagulation cascade: initiation, maintenance, and regulation. Biochemistry 1991;30:10363–70.

[11] Schmidt A. Neue untersuchung über die faserstoffgerinnung. Pfluegers Archiv fur die Gesamte Physiologie des Menschen und der Tiere 1872;6:413–20.

[12] Morawitz P. Die chemie der blutgerinnung. Ergeb Physiol 1905;4:307–22.

[13] Hoffman III M. A cell-based model of hemostasis. Thromb Haemost 2001;85(6):958–65.

[14] Hoffman M. Remodeling the blood coagulation cascade. J Thromb Thrombolysis 2003;16(1–2):17–20.

[15] Hoffman M, Mannucci P. Coagulation module. In: Hemostasis management modules. Available at: Hemsotasiscme.org. Accessed January 15, 2005.

[16] Hirsch DR, Goldhaber SZ. Contemporary use of laboratory tests to monitor safety and efficacy of thrombolytic therapy. Chest 1992;101:98–105.

[17] Massachusetts General Hospital. Pathology service, laboratory medicine. Available at: www.mgh.harvard.edu/labmed/lab/coag/handbook. Accessed February 28, 2005.

[18] Turgeon ML. Clinical hematology: theory and procedures. 4th edition. Baltimore (MD): Lippincott Williams & Wilkins; 2005. p. 348.

[19] Rhodus NL, Bakdash MB, Little JW, et al. Implications of the changing medical profile of a dental school patient population. J Am Dent Assoc 1989;119(3):414–6.

[20] Patton LL, Ship JA. Treatment of patients with bleeding disorders. Dent Clin North Am 1994;38(3):465–82.

[21] Rodgers GM, Greenberg CS. Inherited coagulation disorders. In: Lee GR, Foerster J, Lukens J, et al, editors. Wintrobe's clinical hematology. 10th edition. Philadelphia: Lippincott Williams & Wilkins; 1999. p. 1682–732.

[22] Mannucci PM, Ruggeri ZM, Pareti FI, et al. 1-Deamino-8-d-arginine vasopressin: a new pharmacological approach to the management of haemophilia and von Willebrand diseases. Lancet 1977;23;1(8017):869–72.

[23] Warrier I, Lusher JM. DDAVP: a useful alternative to blood components in moderate hemophilia and von Willebrand disease. J Pediatr 1983;102:228–33.

[24] De La Fuente B, Kasper CK, Rickles FR, et al. Response of patients with mild and moderate hemo-

philia A and von Willebrand disease to treatment with desmopressin. Ann Intern Med 1985;103:6–14.

[25] Seremetis SV, Aledort LM. Desmopressin nasal spray for hemophilia A and type I von Willebrand's disease. Ann Intern Med 1997;126:744–5.

[26] Piot B, Sigaud-Fiks M, Huet P, et al. Management of dental extractions in patients with bleeding disorders. Oral Surg Oral Med Oral Pathol Oral Radiol Endod 2002;93:247–50.

[27] Frieck W, Lamb M. Viral safety of clotting factor concentrates. Semin Thromb Hemost 1993;19:54–61.

[28] Hoyer LW. Factor VIII inhibitors. Curr Opin Hematol 1995;2:365–71.

[29] Gill JC. Transfusion principles for congenital coagulation disorders. In: Hoffman R, Benz E, Shattil S, et al, editors. Hematology: basic principles and practice. Philadelphia: Churchill-Livingstone; 2000. p. 2282–5.

[30] Shapiro AD, McKown CG. Oral management of patients with bleeding disorders. Part I: medical considerations. J Indiana Dent Assoc 1991;70:28–31.

[31] Johnson WT, Leary JM. Management of dental patients with bleeding disorders: review and update. Oral Surg Oral Med Oral Pathol Oral Radiol Endod 1988;66:297–303.

[32] Kasper CK. Hereditary disorders of coagulation. In: Powell D, editor. Recent advances in dental care for the hemophiliacs. Los Angeles (CA): Hemophilia Foundation of Southern California; 1979. p. 16–28.

[33] Goldsmith JC. Medical management of dental patients with bleeding disorders. J Iowa Med Soc 1981;71(7): 291–7.

[34] Schardt-Sacco D. Update on coagulopathies. Oral Surg Oral Med Oral Pathol Oral Radiol Endod 2000;90:559–63.

[35] Gordz S, Mrowietz C, Pindur G, et al. Effect of desmopressin (DDAVP) on platelet membrane glycoprotein expression in patients with von Willebrand's disease. Clin Hemorheol Microcirc 2005;32(2):83–7.

[36] Geil JD. Von Willebrand disease. Available at: www. emedicine.com. Accessed August 20, 2005.

[37] Batlle J, Torea J, Rendal E, et al. The problem of diagnosing von Willebrand's disease. J Intern Med Suppl 1997;740:121–8.

[38] Lee CA, Brettler DB, editors. Guidelines for the diagnosis and management of von Willebrand disease. Haemophilia 1997;3:1–25.

[39] Werner EJ. von Willebrand disease in children and adolescents. Pediatr Clin North Am 1996;43(3):683–707.

[40] Werner EJ, Abshire TC, Giroux DS, et al. Relative value of diagnostic studies for von Willebrand disease. J Pediatr 1992;1:34–8.

[41] Zhang Z, Blomback M, Anvret M. Understanding von Willebrand's disease from gene defects to the patients. J Intern Med Suppl 1997;740:115–9.

[42] Staffileno Jr H, Ciancio S. Bleeding disorders in the dental patient: causative factors and management. Compendium 1987;8(7):501, 504–7.

[43] Wray D, Stenhouse D, Lee D, et al. Blood disorders and their management in clinical practice. In: Textbook of general and oral surgery. London: Churchill-Livingstone; 2003. p. 36–45.

[44] Weaver DW. Differential diagnosis and management of unexplained bleeding. Surg Clin North Am 1993; 73(2):353–61.

[45] Schiffer CA, Anderson KC, Bennett CL, et al, American Society of Clinical Oncology. Platelet transfusion for patients with cancer: clinical practice guidelines of the American Society of Clinical Oncology. J Clin Oncol 2001;19(5):1519–38.

[46] British Committee for Standards in Haematology, Blood Transfusion Task Force. Guidelines for the use of platelet transfusions. Br J Haematol 2003; 122(1):10–23.

[47] Sacher RA, Kickler TS, Schiffer CA, et al, College of American Pathologists, Transfusion Medicine Resource Committee. Management of patients refractory to platelet transfusion. Arch Pathol Lab Med 2003;127(4):409–14.

[48] Wolberg AS, Meng ZH, Monroe DM, et al. A systemic evaluation of the effect of temperature on coagulation enzyme activity and platelet function. J Trauma 2004; 56:1221–8.

[49] Jurkovich GJ, Greiser WB, Luterman A, et al. Hypothermia in trauma victims: an ominous predictor of survival. J Trauma 1987;27:1019–24.

[50] Danzl DF, Pozos RS, Auerbach PS, et al. Multicenter hypothermia survey. Ann Emerg Med 1987;16(9): 1042–55.

[51] Peng RY, Bongard FS. Hypothermia in trauma patients. J Am Coll Surg 1999;188(6):685–96.

[52] Hoffman M. The cellular basis of traumatic bleeding. Mil Med 2004;169(12 Suppl):5–7.

[53] Meng ZH, Wolberg AS, Monroe DM, et al. The effect of temperature and pH on the activity of factor VIIa: implications for the efficacy of high-dose factor VIIa in hypothermic and acidotic patients. J Trauma 2003; 55:886–91.

[54] Cosgriff N, Moore EE, Sauaia A, et al. Predicting life-threatening coagulopathy in the massively transfused trauma patient: hypothermia and acidosis revisited. J Trauma 1997;42(5):857–61 [discussion: 861–2].

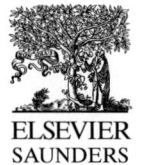

ELSEVIER
SAUNDERS

Oral Maxillofacial Surg Clin N Am 18 (2006) 173 – 184

ORAL AND
MAXILLOFACIAL
SURGERY CLINICS
of North America

Infection, Host Resistance, and Antimicrobial Management of the Surgical Patient

Ladi Doonquah, MD, DDS[a,b,c,*], Leleka Doonquah, MD[d,e]

[a]University Hospital of the West Indies, Kingston, Jamaica
[b]University of the West Indies, Kingston, Jamaica
[c]Private Practice, Decatur, GA, USA
[d]Providence Hospital, Washington, DC, USA
[e]Family and Medical Counseling Services, Washington, DC, USA

Chemotherapeutic management of the microbial milieu that impacts patients undergoing surgery is profoundly important in surgery involving the head and neck region. This region is a repository for a diverse population of microbes, which stand ready to invade the underlying structures once the barriers have been breached. This article evaluates human resistance to these microorganisms and reviews conditions that may increase susceptibility in patients undergoing surgery.

Nosocomial infections are a continuing danger in the care of surgical patients. These infections place a severe strain on the health care system [1] and contribute significantly to patient morbidity and mortality. They are the source of tremendous financial cost to the society, directly and indirectly. Pneumonias, urinary tract infections, blood-borne infections, and wound infections are the most commonly seen nosocomial infections. Wound infections are now designated *surgical site infections* (SSIs) [2]. This article outlines the current thinking regarding perioperative prevention of nosocomial infections, in particular SSIs [3,4], and provides specific criteria that practicing surgeons can use in treating surgical patients.

The discovery of microorganisms' role in surgical infections and of specific measures used to combat

their sequela, such as aseptic technique and antibiotic administration, has helped advance the field of surgery significantly. The accidental discovery of penicillin by Sir Alexander Flemming in 1928 is considered a pivotal event that helped lay the foundation for more extensive and invasive surgical practices.

Microorganisms

The microbial flora in the patient undergoing oral and maxillofacial surgery is intrinsic to that site and is usually considered to be nonpathogenic. The presence of this intrinsic population of microbes serves several purposes, including decreasing and preventing colonization and invasion of other pathologic organisms. This function helps provide a secure and effective defense at the mucosal surface, thereby enabling local host resistance to infection.

The intrinsic microbial flora in the adult oral cavity and surrounding tissues is diverse, consisting of protozoa, yeast, viruses, and bacteria. This flora includes gram-positive cocci; gram-positive rods and filaments; gram-negative cocci; gram-negative rods and filaments; spirochetes; fungi and yeasts; viruses; and protozoa. The more common organisms that are implicated in SSIs of the head and neck region are gram-positive cocci, such as staphylococci and streptococci, and anaerobic gram-negative rods. For surgery that involves grafts or flaps taken from lower regions of the body, aerobic gram-negative bacilli such as *Escherichia coli* may be a factor.

* Corresponding author. 2855 Candler Road, Suite #5, Decatur, GA 30034.
E-mail address: ldoonquah@mindspring.com (L. Doonquah).

Surgeons working in the head and neck region must have a thorough knowledge of these microbes and their effects.

Gram-positive cocci

Streptococci are facultative and are the most abundant group of gram-positive cocci found in the saliva and the dorsum of the tongue. Viridans streptococci are predominantly found in the oral cavity and are divided into four subspecies. These are *mitis*, *mutans*, *salivarius*, and *anginosus* [5]. This group of organisms tends to be more pathogenic in patients who are immunocompromised and neutropenic.

The *mitis* subspecies is predominantly α-hemolytic and resides mostly in the pharynx and oral cavity. The organisms include *Streptococcus mitis*, *S sanguis*, *S oralis*, and *S gordonii*.

The *mutans* subspecies is predominantly nonhemolytic. These include *S salivarius* and *S vestibularis*. The *anginosus* subspecies can be nonhemolytic, α-hemolytic, or β-hemolytic. They include *S salivarius* and *S vestibularis* and can be nonhemolytic, α-hemolytic, or β-hemolytic. Their usual habitat is the oral cavity and upper respiratory tract. *S intermedius* and *S anginosus* are usually isolated in association with deep-seated abscesses [5].

Other gram-positive cocci such as peptostreptococci, which is anaerobic and present at different sites in the oral cavity, can contribute to odontogenic and other soft tissue abscesses. Enterococci and staphylococci are found in the oral cavity and must be considered in infectious complications in patients undergoing surgery.

Gram-positive rods and filaments

The *Actinomyces* organisms are branched filamentous facultative anaerobes that usually inhabit the oral cavity. They include *A israelii*, *A viscosus*, *A naeslundii*, and *A odontolyticus*. Diphtheroid organisms are found in abundance in the oral cavity. They are pleomorphic and are found predominantly on the dorsum of the tongue and the sulcus, and in plaque. They typically are not known to cause disease in the oral cavity [6]. Lactobacilli are normally present in small quantities in the oral cavity and are usually not pathologic but have been shown to contribute to dental caries [5,6].

Gram-negative cocci

Veillonella organisms are anaerobic and can be located on the tongue and in the saliva. The most common of these are *V parvula*, *V atypia*, and *V dispar*.

Gram-negative rods and filaments

Bacteroides, Fusobacterium, Prevotella, Capnocytophaga, Campylobacter, Eikenella, Actinobacillus, Selenomonas, and *Porphyromonas* [5] are gramnegative facultative rods and filaments. The numbers tend to increase in the presence of gingivitis.

Spirochetes

Treponema is the predominant genus that occupies the oral cavity. It is usually found in the gingival crevice and is responsible for acute necrotizing ulcerative gingivitis [5,6].

Fungi and viruses

Candida albicans is the most common yeast found in the oral cavity. Its presence alone can affect the normal oral milieu. Herpes simplex virus is present in a large portion of the population. It normally remains dormant in the trigeminal ganglion and presents in the oral cavity during an acute outbreak, and should be considered when assessing an infection in a patient who is immunocompromised [7].

Protozoa

Entamoeba gingivalis and *Trichomonas tenax* are nonpathogenic protozoa typically found in the oral cavity.

Local factors

Several factors can influence the pathogenicity of these microbes. These include saliva, diet, changes in the local microenvironment, and the presence of other microorganisms. Saliva is an important factor that influences the microbial flora in the oral cavity. Changes in the pH, temperature, flow, and dietary content (eg, minerals, vitamins, proteins) of the saliva influence the number and type of microorganisms present in the oral cavity and surrounding tissues, which affect how the body responds to infection. The saliva's extensive contents regulate the microbial flora of the oral cavity. The minerals in the saliva, which regulate pH, provide a buffer and act as cofactor to the salivary enzymes. The organic components of the saliva include vitamin C, amino acids, carbohydrates, proteins, and glycoproteins. These

components serve as nutrients to the local microorganisms, add viscosity, and impact adherence and aggregation [8,9].

The host's diet can also influence the oral microbial flora. This diet provides a readily accessible nutritional supply to the microorganisms and can have an effect on the numbers and types of organisms present in the oral cavity. Most microorganisms prefer a diet high in carbohydrates. For example, *S mutans* organisms increase in the presence of a high sucrose diet. Other microorganisms, such as actinomycetes and diphtheroids, convert the simple carbohydrates into a storage form for later use. A high-protein or high-lipid diet rather than one high in carbohydrates tends to cause a reduction of acidogenic flora such as Lactobacillus.

Infection

Infections may arise when a change occurs in the intrinsic microbial flora. Such change can be caused by invasion of the host cell by pathologic microorganisms or another form of disruption in the immune system. The infectious process occurs in four distinct steps: adherence, colonization, multiplication, and penetration. Adherence is the initial step in the process, which occurs when the host is exposed to the microbe and the microbe adheres itself to the host cell. The major mechanism of adherence seems to be recognition of specific receptors on the host cell surface by the microbe [10]. Pili and other microbial cell structures assist the microorganism in adhering to the cell.

The next step in the infectious process is colonization of the host by the microbe. The microorganism seems to rely on this process for survival and thus must overcome the host's natural resistance. Colonization can occur without infection. The third step in the infectious process is multiplication. To further survive, the microbe must be able to reproduce within the host. The microbe does this by avoiding phagocytosis. Extracellular pathogens avoid phagocytosis by producing capsules, fimbriae, or pili. Facultative intracellular pathogens, such as *Mycobacterium tuberculosis*, avoid phagocytosis by preventing fusion of the phagosome and lysosome. Other pathogens avoid this phagocytic process by producing lytic enzymes and antioxidants (eg, catalase in staphylococci) [11].

During multiplication the nutritional needs of the microbes are extremely high. They seek nutrients from several sources, including extracellular enzymes like kinases, nucleases, and proteases. Other microorganisms produce specific compounds that stimulate nutritional support; for example, *E coli* produces a porphyrin-like substance that binds iron for nutritional growth and stimulation.

The fourth and final stage of the infectious process is penetration. This step occurs when the microorganism invades the host-cell tissues by attaching to the mucous membrane and crossing the epithelial cell layer. The host responds to this invasion through a series of cell-signaling events [12]. This process is aided by pinocytosis and activation of several enzymes, such as hyaluronidase and protein kinases [12].

Host resistance

The healthy host is naturally resistant to infection. This changes when the host becomes exposed to a highly virulent microorganism or the amount of exposure exceeds a critical number per volume of tissue. The natural barriers to infection, otherwise known as resistance, are typically classified as mechanical, chemical, and immunologic. Mechanical barriers physically inhibit microorganisms from attaching to and penetrating the host cells. These barriers include the skin, hair, mucous membranes, and other physiologic secretions. The skin is the primary physical barrier to infection. Penetration through this layer is almost impossible for many microorganisms. The hair protects the skin and mucous membranes from the invading microbes. The mucous coating provides another mechanical barrier against the microorganisms. Specialized epithelial ciliated cells help remove microbes from the upper respiratory tract. Other physiologic functions that assist the mechanical barrier include sneezing, coughing, and vomiting.

Chemical and biochemical inhibitors provide the chemical barrier to invading microorganisms. These inhibitors are usually found in bodily secretions. Sebaceous gland secretions and perspiration help maintain a harsh acidic environment on the skin. The salt and fatty acid contents inhibit the growth of many microorganisms.

Immunologic barriers to infection are usually complex and involve numerous factors. Humoral and cell-mediated immunity are the two factors of concern in the surgical patient. After entering a host, the pathologic microorganism, or its major antigens, is taken up by macrophages. The antigen is then expressed on the macrophage surface with the major histocompatibility complex proteins and is presented to T lymphocytes. Surgery itself often causes a dis-

turbance of this native microbial habitat and can lead to complications in the outcome of the procedure. This disturbance can be a change in temperature, pH, or oxygen tension; an increase or decrease in blood flow; an increase or decrease in nutritional support; or a displacement of the normal bacterial flora to a different site.

When the body is exposed to an infection it responds peripherally and systematically. The classic signs and symptoms of the host peripheral response to infection are well-known as *rubor, calor, dolor,* and *tumor*. Systematically the response may consist of fever, chills, rigors, headaches, and anorexia. The peripheral and systematic responses are caused by the complement pathway activation by the microbial pathogens. The systemic inflammatory response syndrome manifests if the infection persists uncontrolled. If untreated, this infection can become a sepsis syndrome, leading to life-threatening septic shock and multiorgan dysfunction syndrome. This response to infection and inflammation is somewhat beneficial to the host fighting an infection. However, if this response is excessive, it can be detrimental. What these beneficial effects are and exactly where the threshold for the adverse effects begins are unknown.

Humoral immunity is host defense provided by antibodies that are produced by β-lymphocytes against specific antigenic components of the affecting microorganism. In most infectious diseases, the host response depends on processing of antigens by the macrophage antigen–presenting cells. Initially, IgM antibodies respond to the infection, followed by IgG. IgM activates the byproducts of the classical pathway of complement C3a, which acts as an opsonin, and C5a, which acts as an anaphylatoxin. This activation facilitates phagocytosis through the C3a receptor of the phagocytic cell and enhances leukocyte migration to the site of infection. IgG acts as an opsonin by binding to the microorganism at the antibody-combining site. Circulating secretory IgA acts locally to impair microbial colonization and invasion at the mucosal surface.

Cell-mediated host immunity is primarily caused by sensitized T lymphocytes that have been activated by the antigens of the offending microorganism.

Comorbid conditions

Several conditions, listed in Box 1, may increase the risk for nosocomial infections in surgical patients by affecting their immunocompetence. This compromised immunocompetence may be seen in neonates,

---

> **Box 1. Medical conditions associated with increased risk of infection**
>
> Diabetes
> Renal failure
> Cirrhosis
> Drug abuse
> Corticosteroid use
> Immunocompromised states (eg, HIV, organ transplantation)
> Malnutrition
> Age extremes
> Autoimmune disorders
> Malignancy
> Obesity
> Existence of remote infections

---

elderly patients, malnutrition states, alcoholism, cirrhosis, diabetes, renal failure, dialysis, corticosteroid use, and drug abuse. The immunosuppression causes a breakdown of the physical barriers to infection, which are the first line of defense, and also causes immunologic cell dysfunction. Patients who have diabetes not only have a prolonged healing time because of their poor intracellular nutritional state but also are at increased risk for infections caused by *C albicans, P aeruginosa,* and *S aureus*. These circumstances are caused by depressed T-lymphocyte function and breaches in the first line of defense, the mucosal membrane.

Neonates are susceptible to numerous infections because of their immature host defense mechanism. They have no intrinsic microflora, which decreases their resistance to new pathogens. They also have a poor mucosal barrier to infection. Complement factors and cytokines such as interferon gamma are present in low concentrations [13,14]. The granulocytes and monocytes have decreased chemotactic activity and phagocytic function, impairing the ability to kill pathogenic microorganisms [15–17].

Studies have shown that age older than 60 years is an independent risk factor for nosocomial infection [18]. The quality of the skin and mucous membranes (the first line of defense) is decreased and the production of most cytokines and hematopoietic growth factors is reduced in elderly patients. This reduced production is manifested by the blunted neutrophil response to infection and the lack of fever some patients experience during an acute infection. Aging causes a 20% to 30% decrease in circulating T-lymphocytes [19], thus putting the elderly patient at increased risk for infections.

The patient infected with human immunodeficiency virus is at increased risk for nosocomial infections and a complicated recovery course if their CD4+ T-lymphocyte count is below 200 cells/µL. The organisms of concern include staphylococci and streptococci, in addition to pneumocystis and *M avium* complex.

Poor nutritional status is often underestimated as a potential cause of complications in patients undergoing surgery, especially in elderly patients or those who have an underlying serious illness. Protein-energy malnutrition can lead to infections such as tuberculosis; bacterial and viral respiratory tract infections; aspergillosis; candidiasis; and pneumocystosis [20]. These infections are caused by deficiencies in several aspects of the host's defense mechanism, such as thinning of the mucosa and decreased production of lysozyme and secretory IgA [21]. Neutrophils are also deficient in patients who have protein-energy malnutrition, resulting in a poor chemotactic response and impaired phagocytosis. Malnutrition also causes impaired cell-mediated immunity apparently because of a deficiency in T-helper lymphocyte function [22]. Deficiency in micronutrients influences the host's response to infection [23]. Vitamin A deficiency leads to an impaired humoral immunity. Zinc deficiency is usually seen in patients who are hospitalized and receiving total parental nutrition, and in those who have sickle cell disease. These patients have decreased cell-mediated immunity and are therefore at increased risk for infections caused by microbes such as *Pneumocystis jiroveci* (formerly *P carnii*), *M avium* complex, and fungi [24].

Alcoholics have a depressed host response to infections. They are at risk for developing bacterial pneumonia because of a decrease in their first and second lines of defense. Patients who have chronic renal failure experience poor wound healing because of impairment of the delayed-type hypersensitivity reaction. These patients are at increased risk for developing serious infections caused by *Listeria monocytogenes*, *Klebsiella*, and *Yersinia*.

Patients taking therapeutic doses of glucocorticosteroids may experience impaired resistance to infections. This impairment is manifested by defective phagocytic and cell-mediated functions, making these patients susceptible to SSIs.

Postsurgical infections

Several nosocomial infections impact negatively on the surgical patient [3]. Practices that can lower the incidence of these infections should be used in managing these patients. Planning should begin before hospitalization and must include identification of infection risks [25,26]. Preadmission optimization of the patient's medical and nutritional status should be paramount. Once the patient is hospitalized, every effort should be made to prevent nosocomial infections specifically. Aseptic technique should be used in placing all intravascular catheters, especially central and arterial lines, and proper and frequent care of the sites through dressing changes and antibiotic ointment use is important. Urinary catheters must be placed aseptically and should remain in place for as short a time as possible. Postoperative atelectasis and improper hygiene of tracheostomy sites predispose patients to pulmonary infections. Early ambulation and encouragement of deep breathing and coughing are important. Adequate suction and toileting of the tracheostomy site assists proper respiratory function, thus decreasing the chance for infection.

Infections caused by surgical interventions that develop within 30 days of the procedure are classified as SSIs by the Centers for Disease Control and Prevention (CDC) [2]. Two categories of SSIs, organ–space and incisional, are illustrated in Fig. 1. Incisional SSIs were termed a *postoperative wound infections*, whereas organ–space SSIs refer to infections involving organs and spaces in the deeper recesses of the body. Incisional SSI is further subdivided into superficial incisional and deep incisional SSIs. Superficial incisional SSIs are typical skin and subcutaneous infections that do not involve underlying fascia and muscle. Deep incisional SSIs usually involve underlying fascia and muscle and are more challenging to treat. Organ–space SSIs are infections of body cavities or organs.

The prevention of SSIs consists of a multipronged approach. Attention to every category of prevention is important [4]. Wider selection and increasing effectiveness of new antibiotics have caused some surgeons to rely too much on chemoprophylaxis to stem the scourge of SSIs. As Nguyen and colleagues [27] point out, this reliance places the patient at increased risk for adverse effects and does not decrease infection rates.

Several areas must be addressed together with antimicrobial administration to reduce the rate of SSI. Enhancing the status of all existing medical conditions; improving nutritional status; creating an infection-averse surgical environment; performing proper, efficient, and timely surgical techniques; adequately preparing the site of surgery; and maintaining normal perioperative patient physiology are all important and must be given adequate consideration.

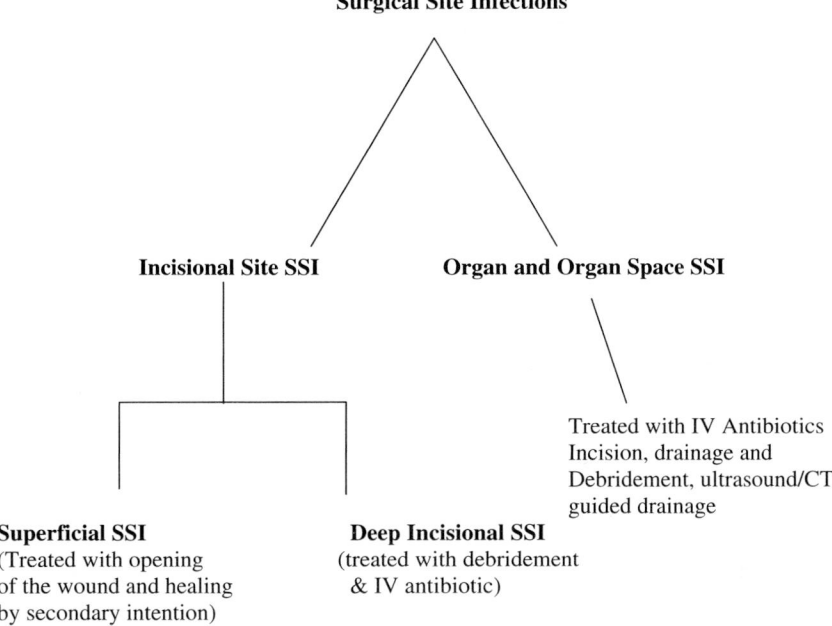

Fig. 1. Ultrasound/CT guided drainage when indicated.

Operations are classified into four categories according to the likelihood of microbial introduction and presence: (1) clean, (2) clean-contaminated, (3) contaminated, and (4) dirty. Prevention strategies are based on proper categorization of the wound by all involved health care personnel [28]. Chemoprophylaxis is primarily used for surgeries classified as clean-contaminated, contaminated, or dirty. Generally patients who may be immunocompromised have significant comorbid illnesses or local mitigating wound factors, and therefore prophylaxis should be considered in clean cases. Unfortunately, because of pressures such as the possibility for malpractice litigation, a large segment of clean cases in healthy patients are now being treated inappropriately with prophylactic antibiotics. However, antibiotic prophylaxis should be targeted toward situations of specific risk.

Perioperative environment

In the modern hospital or outpatient operating suite, patients often believe that proper methods are consistently applied to maintain aseptic technique. However, this is not always the case and the breaches that occur can negatively impact the patient [29,30]. Maintaining an operative environment that is at low

risk for introduction of microbes should be a priority for surgeons. Specific systems to locate and correct problems must be developed and maintained. Improper or lack of hand washing before and after patient contact; inadequate surgical scrub; poor barrier techniques; inadequate skin preparation; and poor operating room (OR) ventilation all contribute to the development of postsurgical infections. Some studies suggest that increased traffic and excessive talking in the OR suite are associated with increased infection rates. Such breaches in the aseptic chain promote the development of SSIs.

Use of preoperative antimicrobial showers and shampoo has been shown [31] to lower the amount of surface microorganisms and should be considered in major head and neck surgery, especially where distant flaps and grafts are used for reconstruction. Shaving before surgery significantly increases wound inoculation rates and should be avoided. If shaving is absolutely required, it should be performed in the OR suite before surgery and a clipping method should be used if possible.

Presurgical antimicrobial rinses or ointments may be used in intraoral, transconjunctival, and intranasal incisions, particularly when grafts or biomaterials are being placed. Although studies do not conclusively show that these agents are effective in reducing infections [32–36], their use in transoral placement

of dental and facial implants is increasing. Houston and colleagues [36] showed that patients undergoing cardiac surgery treated preoperatively with chlorhexidine oral rinse experienced a reduced incidence of nosocomial pneumonia. Further extensive studies in other types of surgery must be performed if this finding is to be extrapolated to other disciplines. Patients who have poor oral hygiene and periodontal disease should undergo dental cleaning and scaling before transoral procedures involving placement of grafts, implants, or distraction devices, and definitely before segmental osteotomies.

Proper control of the surgical environment is critical to the prevention of infection.

Surgical technique

Meticulous surgical technique is a primary bulwark against the development of infections. Surgeons sometimes are of the opinion that poor technique can be overcome by appropriate use of antibiotics, which is obviously not true [27]. Delicate and correct handling of tissue; proper suturing with the correct sutures; elimination of dead space; avoidance of excessive temperatures when using motorized instruments on bone; correct use of drains with active closed circuits and remote exit points; effective debridement; and copious use of irrigation are all important [37]. Surgery must be completed in a timely fashion because increased surgical time leads to increased infection rates.

Chemoprophylaxis of Infections

The following are important principles of antimicrobial prophylaxis in preventing SSIs:

1. The surgical procedure should have a significant risk for infection;
2. The antibiotic should be appropriate and targeted;
3. The dosage and timing of administration must be effective;
4. Prophylactic antibiotics should not be the only method used to prevent SSIs.

Various studies have substantiated the perioperative use of antibiotics for reducing the incidence of post-surgical infections [38–41]. The different categories of surgical wounds (ie, clean, clean-contaminated, contaminated, and dirty) must be remembered when establishing the indication to treat. Perioperative administration of antibiotics is recommended for clean-contaminated, contaminated, and dirty cases. Contaminated and dirty cases require a postsurgical therapeutic regime of antibiotics. Chemoprophylaxis should be considered for clean cases that involve an existing medical illness, such as diabetes, alcoholism, and various other immunocompromised states.

Clean and clean-contaminated operations that entail the placement of implants and extensive bone grafting and that last longer than 3 hours should involve antibiotic prophylaxis. All patients who have an established infection should undergo a full post-operative therapeutic course.

The quantity of antibiotic given is determined by the type of drug, patient's weight, and length of surgery. The antibiotic chosen must be directed toward the possible contaminants that exist at the surgical site and the usual microorganisms that have been implicated in previous postsurgical infections. The cost of administration should be reasonable. Bacteriocidal antibiotics are preferred for prophylaxis, and some bacteriostatic drugs such as clindamycin can be used at higher dosages that render them bacteriocidal to the present microbes. Antibiotics should not be used to try and cover every conceivable organism at the site. This use is inappropriate, ineffective, and expensive, and may contribute to increased toxic side effects. More importantly, this approach leads to continued development of drug-resistant strains. Several new antimicrobials are now available. The tendency is to use the new agents and abandon the old. However, many penicillin-based preparations and their analogs are still efficacious in managing conditions in the maxillofacial region and should be considered before new medications are used.

For preoperative administration the antibiotics should be in the tissues in an adequate concentration before incision. Most experts recommend intravenous administration of the antibiotic 30 to 40 minutes before incision for major surgical cases [42]. The amount initially given should be four times the minimum inhibitory concentration and should be repeated on a schedule based on one to two times the half-life of the particular antibiotic used, not on the regular dosing regime. The goal is to keep the tissue concentration of the antibiotic at therapeutic levels throughout the operation. To get the best results, physicians must have a thorough comprehension of antibiotics and how they should be administered in chemoprophylaxis [43].

The choice of antimicrobial therapy is based on what organisms usually cause infections at the specific anatomic location. The microorganism presently varies from the head and neck region where

most procedures occur, to the upper and lower trunk and extremities where flaps and graft are harvested for reconstruction. In the head and neck region the major causative organisms are anaerobic gram-positive cocci such as streptococci and pepto-streptococci; gram-negative rods such as bacteroides and fusobacterium; aerobic streptococci and staphylococci; and aerobic gram-negative bacilli [6]. When grafts or flaps from the lower trunk and extremities are used, E coli and staphylococci are possible pathogens. The antibiotic regime should be tailored to the implicated organisms.

Minor oral surgery

For minor outpatient procedures, such as biopsies, placement of dental implants, impacted teeth, and other dentoalveolar surgical treatment, the debate continues. For healthy patients, no chemoprophylaxis is recommended for most of these procedures [44,45]. However, for more extensive minor intraoral procedures, such as difficult impacted teeth, extensive osseous reconstruction, long complicated implantation involving graft placement, and endodontic surgery, preoperative antibiotics should be given [46–49]. Patients who have existing medical conditions that impair their ability to fight infections should also be given preoperative antibiotics. If a coexisting infection is present, then postoperative therapeutics should be administered. The choice of whether to give oral or parenteral antibiotics in the outpatient setting is based on factors such as the indications, convenience, and facilities available. Whatever the route, the goal must be to get the tissue levels of the antibiotic at an appropriate level before incision. Longer-acting antibiotics encourage greater patient compliance in patients who require a postoperative oral regime.

Oral antibiotics should be given 1 hour before the procedure when indicated. Giving only postoperative oral antibiotics in minor, outpatient, uncomplicated oral surgery is nonsensical [50,51]. This practice does not achieve the first goal of antibiotic prophylaxis, which is to have the medication present in the tissue at the start of surgery, and has questionable efficacy in preventing infection. Lastly, but significantly, the risk for infection in minor cases that have no existing infection is too low to warrant routine chemoprophylaxis.

For patients undergoing minor oral surgery that requires prophylaxis, the choice should be penicillin, cephalexin, or amoxicillin orally. Clindamycin or erythromycin is indicated in patients who are allergic to penicillin. For intravenously administered penicil-lin, ampicillin or ampicillin/sulbactam is sufficient, or clindamycin in patients who are allergic to penicillin.

Major maxillofacial surgery

For major maxillofacial cases that involve osseous manipulation (eg, orthognathic surgery, osteotomies of the craniofacial complex, major jaw reconstruction) and skin incisions, a first-generation cephalosporin such as cefazolin by itself or in combination with clindamycin or an extended-spectrum penicillin combination is appropriate for prophylaxis [48,52,53]. Cleft lip and palate surgery should not require chemoprophylaxis in healthy patients. Surgery involving the temporomandibular joint, whether open or arthroscopic, should not require prophylaxis provided no implant or graft is placed. If implants or a graft is placed, a first-generation cephalosporin is appropriate.

Antibiotic prophylaxis should be considered for all compound facial fractures, especially gunshot wounds and fractures with gross contamination. Some authors have suggested antibiotics are not needed because the face has an excellent blood supply. However, many experts have shown that antibiotics are appropriate with extensive use of internal fixation devices [54,55]. The antibiotic of choice in mandibular fractures is penicillin or its derivatives and clindamycin in patients who are allergic to penicillin. For midfacial and craniofacial fractures, an extended-spectrum penicillin such as amoxicillin/clavulanate, ampicillin/sulbactam, or a first-generation cephalosporin is an option. Compound fractures treated beyond 72 hours should get a postoperative therapeutic course [54]. For closed fractures, such as coronoid or condylar fractures, no prophylaxis is needed.

Surgery for infections ranging from fascial space infections to osteomyelitis not only qualify for antibiotic prophylaxis but should receive a therapeutic regimen. The culture and sensitivity results determine the medication used. Empiric therapy could begin with penicillin, clindamycin, or ciprofloxacin and adjusted later based on culture results.

Cosmetic procedures such as rhytidectomy, rhinoplasty, blepharoplasty, brow lift, liposuction, skin resurfacing, and placement of facial implants may be considered for antimicrobial prophylaxis depending on factors such as age of patient, comorbid illness, contact with oral or nasal cavities, length of surgery, and placement of implants. If any of these indications arise, a first-generation cephalosporin is the appropriate choice in procedures involving skin incisions [56–59]. However, few studies exist regarding antibiotic prophylaxis in cosmetic maxillofacial surgery,

Box 2. Antibiotic prophylaxis

Minor oral surgery (dentoalveolar surgery, implants, bone grafts, sinus lifts, distraction osteogenesis, and cystectomy, and surgery involving immunocompromised patients)

Penicillin
Amoxicillin
Amoxicillin/clavulanate
Clindamycin
Erythromycin

Major maxillofacial surgery (orthognathic, craniofacial, and cosmetic surgeries; osseous reconstruction; distraction osteogenesis; surgery involving the temporomandibular joint and facial fracture)

Cefazolin
Ampicillin/sulbactam
Clindamycin
Cefazolin/clindamycin
Cefazolin/metronidazole
Ciprofloxacin

Head and neck surgery (maxillectomy, parotidectomy, mandibulectomy, neck dissection, commando, graft and flap reconstruction)

Cefazolin
Cefazolin/clindamycin
Cefazolin/metronidazole
Ampicillin/sulbactam
Ticarcillin/clavulanate
Piperacillin/tazobactam
Ciprofloxacin

Box 3. Specific measures used to reduce surgical site infection rates and the CDC-recommended category

Surgical scrub 2 to 5 minutes: category 1B
Sterile gowns and sheets: category 1A
Head and facial hair covering and masks: category 1A
Limit shaving: category 1A
Antiseptic shower and shampoo: category 1B
Skin preparation: category 1B
Normothermia: NR
Stop smoking: category 1B
Remote infection delay: category 1A
Surgical technique: category 1B
Antibiotic prophylaxis: category 1A
Aseptic placement of catheters: category 1A
Clean soiled environmental surfaces: category 1B
Hand wash before and after dressing changes: category 1B
Maintain sterile dressing for 24 to 48 hours: category 1B

Category 1A: Strongly recommended and strongly supported by well-designed experimental, clinical or epidemiological studies.

Category IB: Strongly recommended and supported by some experimental, clinical or epidemiological studies and strong theoretical rationale.

Category II: Suggested for implementation and supported by suggestive clinical or epidemiologic studies, or theoretical rationale.

NR: No recommendation. The issue is unresolved. Insufficient evidence or no consensus regarding efficacy exists.

Adapted from Mangram AJ, Horan TC, Parson ML, et al. Guideline for prevention of surgical site infection Infect Control Hosp Epidemiol 1999;20:247–80.

so the recommendations are not necessarily based on hard data.

Head and neck surgery

In the case of major head and neck surgery, clean cases such as parotidectomy and excision of submandibular gland are treated differently. These and other similar procedures that do not violate the oral cavity and last less than 3 hours should not require antibiotics. However, major resections (eg, mandibulectomies, maxillectomies, neck dissection, com-

mando procedures) with the placement of flaps and or grafts require antibiotic prophylaxis [60–63]. The antibiotic of choice would be a first-generation cephalosporin or extended-spectrum penicillin combination such as ampicillin/sulbactam or piperacillin/tazobactam. Cefazolin in combination with an antibiotic specifically targeted to cover anaerobic microorganisms, such as metronidazole or clindamycin, is also a good alternative. The fluoroquinolones are also an option. A postoperative course is indicated especially if drains are placed and reconstruction of the floor of mouth is performed.

These choices, outlined in Box 2, have been designed to include simple, effective, and inexpensive antibiotics. The more powerful broad-spectrum antibiotics should be reserved for serious established infections to preserve the selections available and reduce the generation of drug-resistant organisms.

Outcome analysis

Various methods have been delineated for preventing SSIs, and continuous assessment of the efficacy of each method is important [64,65]. Rigorous peer review studies, and not just anecdotal evidence, should support each activity. The CDC has established recommendations for reducing SSI rates, some of which are listed in Box 3 [4]. These practices are assessed based on the evidence supporting them and are assigned a recommended category that reflects the status of supporting literature [4]. Existing medical practices for preventing SSI, their cost/benefit ratio, and their ultimate necessity should be continuously assessed [66].

Summary

Several factors impact the welfare of the surgical patient [62,63]. Development of infections after surgery significantly increases the morbidity and, unfortunately, the occasional mortality of patients. Infections prolong hospitalization and may increase operative interventions.

Several factors have been outlined that can contribute to bad outcomes. Assessment and positive manipulation of the factors that can be altered is critical. Prevention efforts must be broad-based and headed by the surgical group, and should involve all members of the health care team. This practice will improve surgical outcomes, redound to patients' benefit, directly decrease the cost of health care, and impact positively on the economic well-being

of the patients and their family. Measures to combat and prevent SSIs are therefore very critical in the overall management of oral and maxillofacial surgical patients.

References

[1] Kirkland KB, Briggs JP, Trivette SL, et al. The impact of surgical site infection in the 1990s: attributable mortality, excess length of hospitalization and extra costs. Infect Control Hosp Epidemiol 1999;20:725–30.

[2] Horan TC, Gaynes RP, Martone WJ, et al. CDC definitions of nosocomial surgical site infections, 1992: a modification of CDC definitions of surgical wound infections. Infect Control Hosp Epidemiol 1992;13:606–8.

[3] Brachman PS, Dan BB, Haley RW, et al. Nosocomial surgical infections: incidence and costs. Surg Clin North Am 1980;60:15–25.

[4] Mangram AJ, Horan TC, Pearson ML, et al. Guideline for prevention of surgical site infection, 1999. Infect Control Hosp Epidemiol 1999;20:247–80.

[5] Whiley RA, Brighton D. Current classification of the oral streptococci. Oral Microbiol Immunol 1998;13:195–216.

[6] Schuster GS. The microbiology of oral and maxillofacial infections. In: Topazian RG, Goldberg MH, editors. Oral and maxillofacial infections. 3rd edition. Philadelphia: WB Saunders; 1994. p. 39–78.

[7] Tanner A, Maiden MF, Macuch PJ, et al. Microbiota of health, gingivitis and initial periodontitis. J Clin Periodontol 1998;25:85–98.

[8] Kleinberg I. Dynamics of the oral ecosystem. In: Nolte WA, editor. Oral microbiology. St Louis (MO): C.V. Mosby Company; 1982. p. 229.

[9] Nolte WA. Defense mechanisms of the mouth. In: Nolte WA, editor. Oral microbiology. St. Louis (MO): C.V. Mosby Company; 1982. p. 193.

[10] Hultgren SJ, Abraham S, Caparon M, et al. Pilus and non-pilus bacterial adhesions: assembly and function in cell recognition. Cell 1993;73:887–901.

[11] Moors MA, Portnoy DA. Identification of bacterial genes that contribute to survival and growth in an intracellular environment. Trends Microbiol 1995;3:83–5.

[12] Bliska JB, Galan JE, Falkow S. Signal transduction in the mammalian cell during bacterial attachment and entry. Cell 1993;73:903–20.

[13] Adamkin D, Stitzel A, Urmson J, et al. Activity of the alternative pathway of complement in the newborn infant. J Pediatr 1978;93:604–8.

[14] Wilson CB, Lewis DB. Basis and implications of selectively diminished cytokine production in neonatal susceptibility to infection. Rev Infect Dis 1990;12(Suppl 4):410–20.

[15] Marodi L, Jzernicky J, Csorba S, et al. Chemotactic

and random movement of cord blood granulocytes. Experienta 1984;40:1407–10.

[16] Marodi L, Csorba S, Nagy B. Chemotactic and random movement of human newborn monocytes. Eur J Pediatr 1980;135:73–85.

[17] Marodi L, Leijh PDJ, Van Furth R. Characterization and functional capacities of human cord blood granulocytes and monocytes. Pediatr Res 1984;18: 1127–31.

[18] Saviteer SM, Samsa GP, Rutala WA. Nosocomial infections in the elderly. Increased risk per hospital day. Am J Med 1988;84:661–6.

[19] Saltzman RL, Peterson PK. Immunodeficiency of the elderly. Rev Infect Dis 1987;9:1127–39.

[20] Chandra RK. Nutrition and the immune system. Proc Nutr Soc 1993;52:77–83.

[21] Keusch GT, Wilson CS, Waksal SD. Nutrition, host defenses and the lymphoid system. In: Gallin JI, Fauci AS, editors. Advances in host defense mechanisms, volume 2. New York: Raven Press; 1983. p. 275–359.

[22] Salimonu LS, Ojo Amaize E, Williams AIO, et al. Depressed natural killer cell activity in children with protein calorie malnutrition. Clin Immunol Imunopathol 1982;24:1–7.

[23] West CE, Romout JHW, Van der Zijp AJ, et al. Vitamin A and immune function. Proc Nutr Soc 1991;50: 251–62.

[24] Chandra RK, McBean LD. Zinc and immunity. Nutrition 1994;10:79–80.

[25] Haley RW, Culver DH, Morgan WM, et al. Identifying patients at high risk of surgical wound infection: A simple multivariate index of patient susceptibility and wound contamination. Am J Epidemiol 1985; 121:206–15.

[26] Culver DH, Horan TC, Gaynes RP, et al. Surgical wound infection rates by wound class, operative procedure, and patient risk index. Am J Med 1991; 91(Suppl 3B):S152–7.

[27] Nguyen D, Macleod WB, Phung DC, et al. Incidence and predictors of surgical site infections in Vietnam. Infect Control Hosp Epidemiol 2001;22(8):485–92.

[28] Devaney L, Rowell KS. Improved surgical wound classification-why it matters. AORN J 2004;80(2): 208–9, 212–23.

[29] Nichols RL. The operating room. In: Bennett JV, Brachman PS, editors. Hospital infections. 3rd edition. Boston: Little, Brown and Co; 1992. p. 461–73.

[30] Favero MS, Bond W. Sterilization, disinfection, and antisepsis in the hospital. In: Balows A, Hausler Jr WJ, Hermann KL, et al, editors. Manual of clinical microbiology. 5th edition. Washington (DC): American Society of Microbiology; 1991. p. 183–200.

[31] Garibaldi RA. Prevention of intraoperative wound contamination with chlorhexidine shower and scrub. J Hosp Infect 1988;11:5–9.

[32] Darouiche RO. Antimicrobial approaches for preventing infections associated with surgical implants. Clin Infect Dis 2003;15;36(10):1248–9.

[33] Simons JP, Johnson JT, Yu VL, et al. The role of topical antibiotic prophylaxis in patients undergoing contaminated head and neck surgery with flap reconstruction. Laryngoscope 2001;111(2):329–35.

[34] Montan PG, Setterquist H, Marcusson E, et al. Preoperative gentamicin eye drops and chlorhexidine solution in cataract surgery. Experimental and clinical results. Eur J Ophthalmol 2000;10(4):286–92.

[35] Bandhauer F, Buhl D, Grossenbacher R. Antibiotic prophylaxis in rhinosurgery. Am J Rhinol 2002;16(3): 135–9.

[36] Houston S, Hougland P, Anderson JJ, et al. Effectiveness of 0.12% Chlorhexidine gluconate oral rinse in reducing prevalence of nosocomial pneumonia in patients undergoing heart surgery. Am J Crit Care 2002;11(6):567–70.

[37] Leach J. Proper handling of soft tissue in the acute phase. Facial Plast Surg 2001;17(4):227–38.

[38] Burke JF. Preventative antibiotic management in surgery. Annu Rev Med 1973;24:289.

[39] Larsen RA, Evans RS, Burke JP, et al. Improved perioperative antibiotic use and reduced surgical wound infections through use of computer decision analysis. Infect Control Hosp Epidemiol 1989;10: 316–20.

[40] Silver A, Eichorn A, Kral J, et al. Timeliness and use of antibiotic prophylaxis in selected inpatient surgical procedures. The Antibiotic Prophylaxis Study Group. Am J Surg 1996;171:548–52.

[41] Bratzler DW, Houck PM, Richards C, et al. Use of antimicrobial prophylaxis for major surgery: baseline results from the National Surgical Infection Prevention Project. Arch Surg 2005;140(2):174–82.

[42] Classen DC, Evans RS, Pestotnik SL, et al. The timing of prophylactic administration of antibiotics and the risk of surgical-wound infection. N Engl J Med 1992; 326(5):281–6.

[43] Ehrenkranz NJ. Antimicrobial prophylaxis in surgery: mechanisms, misconceptions, and mischief. Infect Control Hosp Epidemiol 1993;14(2):99–106.

[44] Martin MV, Kanatas AN, Hardy P. Antibiotic prophylaxis and third molar surgery. Br Dent J 2005;198(6): 327–30.

[45] Kanatas AN, Rogers SN, Martin MV. A survey of antibiotic prescribing by maxillofacial consultants for dental extractions following radiotherapy to the oral cavity. Br Dent J 2002;192(3):157–60.

[46] Rikhotso E, Ferretti C. Prophylactic antibiotic use in oral surgery—a review of current concepts. SADJ 2002;57(10):408–13.

[47] Foy SP, Shugars DA, Phillips C, et al. The impact of intravenous antibiotics on health-related quality of life outcomes and clinical recovery after third molar surgery. J Oral Maxillofac Surg 2004;62(1):15–21.

[48] Lindeboom JA, van den Akker HP. A prospective placebo-controlled double-blind trial of antibiotic prophylaxis in intraoral bone grafting procedures: a pilot study. Oral Surg Oral Med Oral Pathol Oral Radiol Endod 2003;96(6):669–72.

[49] Binahmed A, Stoykewych A, Peterson L. Single

preoperative dose versus long-term prophylactic antibiotic regimens in dental implant surgery. Int J Oral Maxillofac Implants 2005;20(1):115–7.

[50] Poeschl PW, Eckel D, Poeschl E. Postoperative prophylactic antibiotic treatment in third molar surgery—a necessity? J Oral Maxillofac Surg 2004;62(1): 3–8.

[51] Bulut E, Bulut S, Etikan I, et al. The value of routine antibiotic prophylaxis in mandibular third molar surgery: acute-phase protein levels as indicators of infection. J Oral Sci 2001;43(2):117–22.

[52] Lazzarini L, Brunello M, Padula E, et al. Prophylaxis with cefazolin plus clindamycin in clean-contaminated maxillofacial surgery. J Oral Maxillofac Surg 2004; 62(5):567–70.

[53] Baqain ZH, Hyde N, Patrikidou A, et al. Antibiotic prophylaxis for orthognathic surgery: a prospective, randomised clinical trial. Br J Oral Maxillofac Surg 2004;42(6):506–10.

[54] Maloney PL, Lincoln RE, Coyne CP. A protocol for the management of compound mandibular fractures based on the time from injury to treatment. J Oral Maxillofac Surg 2001;59(8):879–84.

[55] Southwell-Keely JP, Russo RR, March L, et al. Antibiotic prophylaxis in hip fracture surgery: a metaanalysis. Clin Orthop Relat Res 2004;(419): 179–84.

[56] Fatica CA, Gordon SM, Zins JE. The role of preoperative antibiotic prophylaxis in cosmetic surgery. Plast Reconstr Surg 2002;109(7):2570–3 [discussion 2574–5].

[57] Huether MJ, Griego RD, Brodland DG, et al. Clindamycin for intraincisional antibiotic prophylaxis in dermatologic surgery. Arch Dermatol 2002;138(9): 1145–8.

[58] Perrotti JA, Castor SA, Perez PC. Antibiotic use in aesthetic surgery: a national survey and literature review. Plast Reconstr Surg 2002;15;109(5):1685–93 [discussion 1694–5].

[59] Gaspar Z, Vinciullo C, Elliott T, et al. Antibiotic prophylaxis for full-face laser resurfacing: is it necessary? Arch Dermatol 2001;137(3):313–5.

[60] Simons JP, Johnson JT, Yu VL, et al. The role of topical antibiotic prophylaxis in patients undergoing contaminated head and neck surgery with flap reconstruction. Laryngoscope 2001;111(2):329–35.

[61] Penel N, Fournier C, Roussel-Delvallez M, et al. Prognostic significance of wound infections following major head and neck cancer surgery: an open non-comparative prospective study. Support Care Cancer 2004;12(9):634–9.

[62] Rodrigo JP, Surez C, Bernaldez R, et al. Efficacy of piperacillin-tazobactam in the treatment of surgical wound infection after clean-contaminated head and neck oncologic surgery. Head Neck 2004;26(9): 823–8.

[63] Carroll WR, Rosenstiel D, Fix JR, et al. Three-dose vs extended-course. Arch Otolaryngol Head Neck Surg 2003;129(7):771–4.

[64] Cantaneo C, Silveira CA, Simpionato E, et al. The preparation of the surgical team: significant aspect in the control of environmental contamination. Rev Lat Am Enfermagem 2004;12(2):283–6.

[65] Malone DL, Genuit T, Tracy JK, et al. Surgical site infections: reanalysis of risk factors. J Surg Res 2002; 103(1):89–95.

[66] Akalin HE. Surgical prophylaxis: the evolution of guidelines in an era of cost containment. J Hosp Infect 2002;50(Suppl A):S3–7.

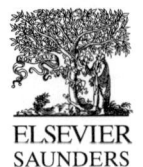

ELSEVIER SAUNDERS

Oral Maxillofacial Surg Clin N Am 18 (2006) 185 – 193

ORAL AND MAXILLOFACIAL SURGERY CLINICS of North America

Perioperative Considerations of the Patient on Cancer Chemotherapy

Orrett E. Ogle, DDS[a],*, Manaf Saker, DMD[b]

[a]Woodhull Medical and Mental Health Center, Oral and Maxillofacial Surgery, 760 Broadway, Room 3C-320, Brooklyn, NY 11206, USA
[b]Private Practice, Suite 207, 385 South Maple Avenue, Ridgewood, NJ 07450, USA

Chemotherapeutic treatment of cancer has made great progress over the past 25 years and is frequently used as an important component of combined-modality therapy with surgery and radiation. Individuals undergoing cancer treatment with chemotherapeutic drugs frequently experience oral complications that may require oral surgical intervention. This article reviews the categories of drugs that are used and their side effects, and possible management strategies for patients undergoing cancer treatment with chemotherapy drugs in oral surgery practice.

Chemotherapy is indicated for patients who have cancer that is not curable by regional modalities, and is currently the best adjuvant to local therapy for several human malignancies. *Adjuvant chemotherapy* is chemotherapy that follows surgery, and has the theoretical advantage of destroying any residual or metastatic cells, thus improving survival rate. *Neoadjuvant chemotherapy*, also called *primary* or *induction therapy*, is chemotherapy that is given before surgery. It offers the oncologist the ability to monitor drug sensitivity in the intact primary tumor and allows them to make a judgment about the definitive local therapy. For patients who prefer an organ-preserving strategy, the oncologist may be able to predict the success of chemotherapy alone. Neoadjuvant chemotherapy is very applicable as a first-line treatment for breast cancer where surgery will result in significant cosmetic defects and the need for extensive reconstruction.

The perioperative considerations of patients undergoing chemotherapy are related primarily to the multiplicity of noxious adverse effects presented by the various drugs. Although some tumors are treated with a single medication, most chemotherapy regimens involve the use of several antineoplastic drugs (combination therapy). The most effective regimens consist of drugs that are individually effective against the neoplasm and have nonoverlapping toxicities, thereby allowing administration of full doses of all drugs [1]. The side effects of each drug used for combined therapy will be manifested individually.

Some rudimentary knowledge of how these agents work and their side effects is needed for one to best understand the factors involved in the perioperative management of patients undergoing chemotherapy. All chemotherapeutic agents act by interfering with cell division and are most active against rapidly dividing cells. Malignant tissues consist of rapidly dividing cells that are characterized by rapid synthesis of DNA, and nondividing cells with slower DNA replication. Most of the drugs used in chemotherapy work by affecting either enzymes or substrates acted on by enzyme systems that relate to DNA synthesis or function. For treating cancer, most agents exploit kinetic differences between normal and malignant cells by acting preferentially on the cells

* Corresponding author.
E-mail address: orrett.ogle@woodhullhc.nychhc.org (O.E. Ogle).

that are dividing at a faster rate [1]. Consequently, malignant cells are destroyed faster than normal cells at the tumor site. However, normal cells that have a high proliferative capacity rivaling malignant cells (eg, bone marrow, gastrointestinal [GI] mucosa, oral mucosa, skin, hair follicles) are also severely affected. Therefore, the side effects of chemotherapeutic agents include myelosuppression (neutropenia, thrombocytopenia, and anemia), GI disturbance (nausea, vomiting, and diarrhea), mucosal ulceration (GI and oral ulcers), and skin and hair follicle problems (dermatitides and alopecia). Cardiotoxicity, hepatotoxicity and renal toxicity are also associated with some of the agents. Most perioperative management involves these side effects.

Types of chemotherapy drugs

Chemotherapeutic drugs (Table 1) are classified according to how they work. The main categories are alkylating agents, plant alkaloids, antimetabolites, antitumor antibiotics, enzymes, random synthetics, and hormones [2].

Alkylating agents

Alkylating drugs [3] undergo electrophilic chemical reactions that result in the formation of covalent links (alkylation) with various nucleophilic substances, primarily DNA. The 7-nitrogen atom of guanine residues in DNA is particularly susceptible to the formation of a covalent bond that results in a miscoding of DNA information or opening of the purine ring with damage to the DNA molecule. The alkylating agent can act on the DNA molecule at any stage of cell division.

Side effects
Alkylating agents are very potent bone marrow suppressants, with lymphocytopenia occurring within 24 hours. Hemolytic anemia, alopecia, nausea, and vomiting occur commonly. Alkylating agents also inhibit plasma cholinesterase activity, which can cause prolonged skeletal muscle paralysis after administration of succinylcholine. Pneumonitis and pulmonary fibrosis may also occur.

Plant alkaloids

Plant alkaloids, referred to as *Vinca alkaloids*, arrest cells in the metaphase of mitosis by binding to tubulin and thereby inhibiting microtubular function. Useful Vinca alkaloids derived from the periwinkle plant are vinblastine and vincristine, whereas paclitaxel is an extract of the bark of the Pacific yew. Despite their structural similarity, no cross-tolerance exists among them.

Side effects
Myelosuppression (neutropenia, thrombocytopenia, and anemia) is the most common side effect and appears 7 to 10 days after the start of therapy. Other common side effects are symmetric peripheral sensory–motor neuropathy, ataxia, and transient depression. Autonomic neuropathy with orthostatic hypotension, bowel motility dysfunction, and cranial nerve involvement (weakness of extraocular muscles and laryngeal nerve paralysis with hoarseness) are seen in 10% of patients. Syndrome of inappropriate antidiuretic hormone secretion occurs with vincristine.

Antimetabolites

Antimetabolites [3] act as fraudulent analogs of vital physiologic substrates that inhibit the synthesis of DNA or its nucleotide building blocks. They include analogs of folic acid (methotrexate), pyrimidine (cytosine arabinoside), and purine (6-mercaptopurine). These drugs interact directly with specific enzymes, leading to inhibition of that enzyme and subsequent synthesis of an aberrant DNA molecule that functions abnormally. These drugs are all immunosuppressants.

Side effects
Side effects are dependent on the analog used.

Methotrexate. With methotrexate, side effects are most commonly seen in the GI tract (ulcerative stomatitis and diarrhea) and bone marrow (neutropenia and thrombocytopenia). Hemorrhagic enteritis and death from intestinal perforation are other common side effects. Renal toxicity (10%) and pulmonary toxicity (8%) may also occur. Methotrexate is sometimes used to treat psoriasis and rheumatoid arthritis.

Cytosine arabinoside. Myelosuppression (neutropenia, thrombocytopenia, and anemia) is the most common side effect of cytosine arabinoside, but GI disturbance, stomatitis, and hepatic dysfunction also occur less frequently.

Mercaptopurine. The principal side effect of mercaptopurine is gradual bone marrow depression re-

Table 1
Chemotherapeutic agents

Alkylating agents	Antineoplastic antibiotics	Antimetabolites	Hormonal agonists/antagonists	Mitotic inhibitors	Immunomodulators	Miscellaneous antineoplastics
Busulfan (Myleran)	Bleomycin (Blenoxane)	Capecitabine (Xeloda)	Anastrozole (Arimidex)	Etoposide (VePesid)	Aldesleukin (Proleukin injection)	Altretamine (Hexalen)
Carboplatin (Paraplatin for injection)	Dactinomycin (Cosmegen for injection)	Cladribine (Leustatin injection)	Bicalutamide (Casodex)	Teniposide (Vumon injection)	Levamisole (Ergamisol)	Asparaginase (Elspar)
Carmustine (BiCNU for injection)	Daunorubicin (Cerubidine, DaunoXome)	Cytarabine (Cytosar-U, Tarabine PFS, DepoCyt)	Diethylstilbestrol (Stilphostrol)	Vinblastine (Alkaban-AQ, Velban, Velsar)		Docetaxel (Taxotere injection)
Chlorambucil (Leukeran)	Doxorubicin (Adriamycin, Rubex, Doxil)	Floxuridine (FUDR for injection)	Estramustine (Emcyt)	Vincristine (Oncovin injection, Vincasar PFS)		Hydroxyurea (Hydrea)
Cisplatin (Platinol, Platinol-AQ)	Idarubicin (Idamycin)	Fludarabine (Fludara for injection)	Flutamide (Eulexin)			Interferon alpha (Roferon, Intron, Alferon)
Cyclophosphamide (Cytoxan, Neosar)	Mitomycin (Mutamycin for injection)	Fluorouracil (Adrucil, Efudex, Fluoroplex)	Goserelin (Zoladex)			Irinotecan
Ifosfamide (Ifex for injection)	Mitoxantrone (Novantrone for injection)	Mercaptopurine (Purinethol)	Leuprolide (Lupron injection)			Mitotane (Lysodren)
Lomustine (CeeNU)	Pentostatin (Nipent)	Methotrexate (Folex for injection, Rheumatrex)	Megestrol (Megace)			Paclitaxel (Paxene, Taxol)
Mechlorethamine (Mustargen for injection)	Plicamycin (Mithracin)	Thioguanine (Tabloid)	Nilutamide (Nilandron)			Procarbazine (Matulane)
Melphalan (Alkeran)			Tamoxifen (Nolvadex)			
Pipobroman (Vercyte)			Testolactone (Teslac)			
Polifeprosan 20 with Carmustine (Glidel wafer)			Toremifene (Fareston)			
Streptozocin (Zanosar for injection)						
Thiotepa (Thioplex for injection)						
Uracil Mustard						

sulting in thrombocytopenia, granulocytopenia, and anemia. Anorexia, nausea, and vomiting are also common side effects. Jaundice associated with bile stasis, and occasionally hepatic necrosis, have been reported in 30% of patients.

Antitumor antibiotics

Antitumor antibiotics [3] are natural products of certain soil fungi. Their effects are produced by the formation of stable complexes with DNA, thereby inhibiting DNA synthesis, RNA synthesis, or both. Like antibiotics used for their antimicrobial activities, these antitumor antibiotics all act differently. Some commonly used antibiotics are actinomycin D (dactinomycin) and bleomycin. Actinomycin D binds to DNA in rapidly proliferating cells, blocking RNA polymerase and thus the transcription of DNA. Bleomycin is made up of water-soluble glycopeptides that differ from one another in their terminal amine moiety (more than 200 congeners are present) and cause fragmentation of DNA.

Side effects
Anthracycline chemotherapy agents (doxorubicin and mitoxantrone), which are used in 32% of women who undergo chemotherapy for breast cancer, are associated with greater odds of neutropenia, thrombocytopenia, infection, fever, delirium, and unspecified adverse effects of systemic therapy [4].

Enzymes

L-asparaginase is an enzyme with useful chemotherapeutic effects [3]. It depletes cells of the nonessential amino acid asparagine. Most human tissues have the capacity to synthesize asparagine through L-asparagine synthetase. Some tumor cells, particularly those of T-cell lineage, lack asparagine synthesis capability and require exogenous asparagine to proliferate. Consequently, depletion of circulating pools of asparagine by L-asparaginase results in inhibition of protein synthesis and ultimately cell death.

Side effects
Unlike other chemotherapeutic drugs, asparaginase has minimal effects on bone marrow; oral and GI mucosa; and hair follicles. However, it carries the risk for coagulopathy (increased prothrombin time) because of its hepatotoxicity. This hepatotoxicity is clinically evident in 10% to 20% of patients, and 50% have biochemical evidence of liver dysfunction.

Random synthetics

Synthetic chemotherapeutic drugs [3] include cisplatin, hydroxyurea, and procarbazine.

Cisplatin is an inorganic platinum-containing complex (a heavy metal) that enters cells through diffusion and disrupts the DNA helix. It causes DNA breaks and cross-links complimentary DNA strands that prevent replication. Renal toxicity is prominent and can lead to renal failure. Myelosuppression is also seen, along with ototoxicity (manifested by tinnitus), peripheral sensory neuropathies, nausea, and vomiting.

Hydroxyurea acts on the enzyme ribonucleoside diphosphate reductase to interfere with DNA synthesis. Myelosuppression, nausea, and vomiting are the major side effects.

Procarbazine inhibits DNA synthesis. Myelosuppression, nausea, and vomiting are the major side effects. Sedative effects and depression are prominent. This drug is a weak monoamine oxidase inhibitor, so tricyclic antidepressants should be used concurrently with caution. Synergism occurs with barbiturates, narcotics, phenothiazines, and sedatives, and therefore intravenous sedation must be administered carefully.

Hormones

Hormones [3], including corticosteroids, progestin, antiestrogens, and antiandrogens, slow the growth of some cancers that depend on hormones.

Corticosteroids
Corticosteroids possess lympholytic effects and suppress mitosis in lymphocytes. They are used to treat acute lymphoma in children (not adults).

Progestins
Progestins are used for endometrial carcinoma because they slow the overstimulation of the endometrium that causes neoplastic changes.

Estrogens and androgens
Malignant changes in the breast and prostate often depend on hormones for their continued growth. For example, prostatic cancer is stimulated by androgens, so giving estrogen (diethylstilbestrol) will slow the growth of the tumor cells. Estrogens and androgens are valuable in the treatment of advanced breast cancer. Malignant tissues that are responsive to estrogens contain receptors for that hormone, whereas malignant tumors lacking these receptors are unlikely to

respond hormonal manipulation. Hypercalcemia is often associated with androgen or estrogen therapy and is sometimes treated with bisphosphonates.

Antiestrogens

Tamoxifen binds to estrogen receptors and inhibits continued growth of estrogen-dependent tumors. It is used for palliative treatment of advanced breast cancer in women who are postmenopausal. Side effects are hot flashes, nausea, and vomiting.

Antiandrogens

Flutamide is a nonsteroidal antiandrogenic drug used for prostate cancer. It prevents androgen binding to androgen receptors. Side effects are skeletal muscle weakness, osteoporosis, and methemoglobinemia (at levels >35%, pulse oximetry readings will approach 85%).

Perioperative care

Most people do not experience serious long-term problems from chemotherapy and are acceptable surgical risks approximately 6 to 8 weeks after drug therapy is completed [5]. However, chemotherapy can occasionally cause permanent changes or damage to the heart, lungs, and kidneys that increase the surgical risks. Preoperative evaluation should consist of a thorough history and physical examination, focusing on the clinical presence of any negative drug side effects that could increase morbidity and mortality. Routine laboratory testing should include complete blood count, serum electrolytes, and urinalysis. Depending on the drug used or being used, or other clinical findings or symptoms, an liver function test, chest radiograph, ECG, and platelet function test may also be required.

Management of specific problems

Bone marrow suppression

Bone marrow suppression is a major side effect of nearly all widely used agents. It manifests as neutropenia, anemia, and thrombocytopenia. The myelosuppression is reversible and should be close to normal 6 to 8 weeks after drug use is stopped. The surgeon should therefore allow 6 to 8 weeks after chemotherapy for bone marrow to regrow. Neutropenia and thrombocytopenia are the two major perioperative concerns for the oral surgeon. If the

absolute neutrophil count (ANC) is 1500/mm^3 or less, the patient is considered to have neutropenia and the clinical sequela manifests as infection, most commonly of the mucous membranes. Platelet counts less than 50,000 present coagulation problems with tooth extractions.

Neutropenia

Neutropenia is defined in terms of the ANC, which is determined by multiplying the percentage of bands and neutrophils on a differential by the total white blood cell (WBC) count [6]. An abnormal value would be anything less than 1500 cells/mm^3. African Americans have a lower normal ANC value of 1000 cells/mm^3, but a normal total neutrophil count. (Studies have shown that Africans and Afro-Caribbeans had lower total WBC, neutrophil, and platelet counts than Caucasians and Africans had lower counts than Afro-Caribbeans [7].) The severity of neutropenia is categorized as mild for ANC values of 1000 to 1500 cells/mm^3, moderate for values of 500 to 1000 cells/mm^3, and severe for values less than 500 cells/mm^3 [8]. The risk for bacterial infection is related to the severity and duration of the neutropenia.

Patients who have mild neutropenia do not require prophylactic antibiotics for routine oral surgery. Moderate neutropenia requires the judgment of the practitioner. The authors believe that prophylactic antibiotics should be given for invasive procedures such as tooth extraction, followed by a 7-day course of antimicrobials to prevent secondary infections. The antibiotic should cover the normal oral flora. Severe neutropenia (absolute counts <500/mm^3) is a definite indication for prophylactic antimicrobials for oral surgical procedures. Ciprofloxacin plus amoxicillin-clavulanate are the recommended antibiotics for adult patients who have cancer and severe neutropenia and are at low risk for complications [9]. Although it is not specific for oral surgery, this regimen would also target the opportunistic organisms that may invade after exodontia, which provides a portal of entry for infectious organisms. Individuals who have lower counts and higher risk require vancomycin therapy [9]. The American Heart Association prophylactic antibiotic regimen should be considered for patients who have central venous catheters. Meticulous attention must also be given to aseptic techniques in the perioperative period to avoid iatrogenic infections that could be lethal [3].

The use of colony-stimulating factors to stimulate the production of neutrophils is not routine, but should be considered in cases involving significant

neutropenia ($<200/mm^3$), or when the risk for postsurgical infection is high because of a preexisting dental infection or extensive surgery. Two of these growth factors that stimulate production of WBCs in the bone marrow are the granulocyte-macrophage colony-stimulating factor (GM-CSF), sargramostim, and the granulocyte colony-stimulating factor (G-CSF), filgrastim.

Sargramostim is a recombinant human GM-CSF (rhu GM-CSF) produced by recombinant DNA technology in a yeast (Saccharomyces cerevisiae) expression system. It is a hematopoietic growth factor that stimulates proliferation and differentiation of hematopoietic progenitor cells [10,11]. Sargramostim is administered through intravenous injection over 2 hours.

Filgrastim is also an amino acid protein manufactured by recombinant DNA technology produced by Escherichia coli into which the human G-CSF gene has been inserted. The protein has an amino acid sequence identical to the natural sequence predicted from human DNA sequence analyses except for the addition of an N-terminal methionine necessary for expression in E coli. Because it is produced in E coli, the product is nonglycosylated and thus differs from G-CSF isolated from a human cell. The recommended starting dose of filgrastim is 5 µg/kg/d, administered as a single daily injection through subcutaneus bolus injection, short intravenous infusion (15 to 30 minutes), or continuous subcutaneous or intravenous infusion [12]. Both agents should be administered daily for up to 2 weeks until the ANC has reached $10,000/mm^3$.

Thrombocytopenia

Chemotherapy-induced thrombocytopenia typically occurs 6 to 10 days after administration of the chemotherapy drugs. The type and dose of chemotherapy affect how low the platelet count drops and how long it takes for the patient to recover. The risk for bleeding and the magnitude of risk are closely correlated with the severity and duration of the thrombocytopenia. The risk for excessive bleeding with invasive procedures occurs at counts below $50,000/mm^3$. Currently, platelet transfusion is the primary method for managing thrombocytopenia [13]. Traditionally, the "trigger" value (ie, the laboratory value below which a transfusion is automatically prescribed) for platelet transfusion for a surgical procedure is $50,000/mm^3$ [14,15]. However, because transfusions are associated with complications, the clinician must carefully evaluate all options (including local hemostatic methods) when considering a platelet transfusion because the benefits should outweigh the risk or complications of transfusion.

The need for transfusion of platelets before minor procedures in patients who have quantitative or qualitative platelet abnormalities is controversial. For open minor procedures, such as a single tooth extraction where the bleeding can be directly observed and controlled through local means, experts have suggested that the transfusion guidelines should be more restrictive than for major operative procedures. Scientific evidence is currently inadequate to determine the platelet count below which the risk for surgical bleeding increases [15]. In patients not undergoing surgery, spontaneous bleeding is uncommon with platelet counts greater than $20,000/mm^3$, and some studies suggest that patients who have thrombocytopenia and are undergoing surgery have low complication rates [16]. The recommendations of the College of American Pathologists regarding safe platelet counts are based on evidence that may not be applicable to all patients undergoing surgery, particularly those undergoing minor procedures. In the absence of evidence, therefore, the task force on transfusion believes platelet transfusion for values less than $50,000/mm^3$ is justified because of the increased risk for complications caused by bleeding in patients undergoing surgery [17].

Platelet transfusion

The goal of a platelet transfusion in surgery is to prevent or stop bleeding. The usual therapeutic dose for transfusion is one platelet concentrate per 10 kg of body weight. A single unit of random-donor platelets (RDPs) contains a minimum of 5.5×10^{10} platelets suspended in 50 mL of plasma. Single-donor platelets (SDPs) are collected by apheresis and contain a minimum of 3.0×10^{11} platelets suspended in 200 to 600 mL of plasma. Comparative studies have shown that the post-transfusion increments, hemostatic benefit, and side effects are similar with either product. Thus, these products can be used interchangeably in routine circumstances, but pooled platelet concentrates are less costly. SDPs from selected donors are preferred when histocompatible platelet transfusions are needed. Both preparations can be stored for up to 5 days after collection at 20°C to 24°C with good maintenance of platelet viability [18].

Platelets are ABO and Rh typed. Although ABO-identical or -compatible units are preferred, they are not absolutely required because the volume of plasma in the product is usually not clinically significant.

Apheresis units may contain 350 mL of plasma, but passive transfer of antibodies rarely results in hemolysis. Cross-matching is also not necessary because the volume of red blood cells (RBCs) is less than 2 mL in each platelet component. However, because 1 mL of RBCs is capable of causing alloimmunization to the D antigen, Rh compatibility is recommended in women of childbearing age to prevent D antibody formation and potential hemolytic disease of the newborn [19]. Leukoreduction (filtration) of platelets is frequently performed to remove the WBCs responsible for alloimmunization and cytomegalovirus transmission.

Dosage

RDPs are dosed at 1 unit per 10 kg of body weight. Stable patients who are not refractory to platelet transfusions can be expected to have a platelet count increase between 5000 and 7000 per unit. SDPs are dosed at one apheresis unit per transfusion episode, which is generally equivalent to 6 to 8 units of pooled RDPs [19].

A standard adult therapeutic pack has the platelets from six blood units and contains more than 240×10^9 platelets. Transfusion of one pack will, on average, raise the platelet count by 20,000 to 40,000/mm^3 in an adult. Platelets must be given through a fresh blood transfusion set, a special platelet transfusion set [20], or devices such as the Alaris infusion pump (ALARIS Medical Systems, San Diego, California).

Complications of platelet transfusion

Reactions from platelet transfusion range from mild allergic reactions to life-threatening anaphylaxis. Febrile reactions are the most common, occurring in 1 in every 100 transfusions, but most do not represent significant clinical problems and generally subside within 30 minutes after transfusion is stopped. Allergic reactions occur in approximately 1% of platelet transfusions. These reactions are generally mild and respond to antihistamines [19]. Clinically, the most significant complications are the immunomodulatory effects of alloimmunization, immunosuppression, and graft-versus-host disease, all of which are rare [18].

In an attempt to reduce the complications from platelet transfusion and decrease their cost, several thrombopoietic cytokines and growth factors have been clinically evaluated in the past 20 years. Interleukin-11 (oprelvekin) is approved for treating thrombocytopenia. It is a thrombopoietic growth factor that directly stimulates the proliferation of hematopoietic stem cells and megakaryocyte progenitor cells and induces megakaryocyte maturation, resulting in increased platelet production. Oprelvekin prevents severe thrombocytopenia and reduces the need for platelet transfusions after myelosuppressive chemotherapy in adult patients who have nonmyeloid malignancies. Daily subcutaneous dosing for 14 days has been shown to increase the platelet count in a dose-dependent manner. Platelet counts begin to increase relative to baseline between 5 and 9 days after the start of dosing. After treatment is stopped, platelet counts continue to increase for up to 7 days then return toward their original value within 14 days [21]. The therapeutic index of oprelvekin is currently limited [22]. Although not very practical, this product may be applicable in elective oral surgery to decrease the need for and cost of platelet transfusion in minor procedures.

Coagulation defects not caused by thrombocytopenia may be caused by mechlorethamine, mithramycin, and L-asparaginase, which are toxic to the liver. Patients treated with these drugs should be screened with a coagulation profile, and abnormalities should be corrected appropriately.

Cardiotoxicity is associated with Adriamycin, daunorubicin, and cisplatin. Cardiomegaly or pleural effusion may be seen on the chest radiograph. Congestive heart failure should be treated in the standard fashion with digitalis, diuretics, and oxygen. Mortality from anesthesia is high in this group. Within 3 weeks after the onset of symptoms, the mortality is 59%.

Hepatotoxicity occurs most frequently with the antimetabolites, L-asparaginase, and mithramycin. Any drugs incriminated in liver damage should not be used. Acetaminophen is not recommended as a postoperative analgesic.

Nephrotoxicity occurs most frequently with busulfan, methotrexate, mercaptopurine, mithramycin, streptozocin, and cisplatin. Balanced electrolyte solutions should be started the night before surgery to aid in maintenance of optimal renal blood flow and glomerular filtration. Perioperative monitoring of urinary output, central venous pressure, and fluids and electrolytes is mandatory [5].

Nausea and vomiting are common side effects with most chemotherapeutic agents, but are most severe with cisplatin, the alkylating agents, and mercaptopurine.

Stomatitis is a side effect of antibiotics, antimetabolites, alkylating agents, and plant alkaloids. Trauma can be avoided with intubation, throat packs, and oral airway [3].

Complications

The most common oral side effects of chemotherapeutic agents are stomatitis, ulcerations of the oral mucosa with secondary infections, and dental abscesses caused by immunosuppression.

Oral ulcerations can be managed locally by topical steroid, oral rinses, Kaopectate (Pfizer, Morris Plains, New Jersey), and local anesthetic rinses (eg, viscous lidocaine). Stomatitis is managed by local palliative therapy to relieve discomfort and permit a diet that will maintain an acceptable degree of nutritional intake.

Prevention is the best method of providing dental care to the patient who is a candidate for undergoing chemotherapy. Before the start of therapy, a dental team should evaluate the patient, perform a meticulous dental examination, and decide on a treatment plan that will include removal of questionable teeth, finalization of restorations, a dental cleaning, and topical fluoride application. Eliminating the possibility of any oral surgical or periodontal procedures is crucial in minimizing complications during treatment.

ONJ has recently been reported with the use of bisphosphonates [23–25]. This condition has attracted significant interest from the press [26] and oral and maxillofacial surgeons.

The US Food and Drug Administration approved bisphosphonates for the treatment of patients who have multiple myeloma and for use with standard cancer therapy in patients who have documented bone metastasis from solid tumors. These agents are used for bone metastasis to slow the resorption and reduce or delay the complications of bone metastasis.

Most cases of ONJ reported in patients undergoing treatment with bisphosphonates have been associated with dental procedures, mostly tooth extraction. Two theories regarding the cause of this condition are mentioned in the package insert of these medications [27]. One theory postulates that the osteoclastic-inhibiting properties of these drugs results in necrosis of bone with no turnover. The second theory suggests that inhibition of endothelial proliferation disrupts the new formation of capillaries in the haversian system of bone and causes an avascular condition. Surgical intervention in this avascular bone leads to osteomyelitis, bone necrosis, and sloughing of the overlying soft tissues. The exposed bone is usually permanent, and local surgical procedures, including debridement, resection, and attempted covering with vascular flaps, have all failed and often made the condition worse. The Marx hyperbaric oxygen protocol [28] was reported to have no benefit in treating ONJ caused by bisphosphonates.

The recommended management of ONJ is chlorhexidine oral rinse, twice daily. Acute exacerbation of the infection will be manifested as pain in the exposed bone. Penicillin is the antibiotic of choice and is potentially a life-long therapy. If the pain subsides, the penicillin should be gradually withdrawn but the twice-daily chlorhexidine rinses should continue (RE Marx, personal communication, 2005).

Because most of the instances (77%) of ONJ were precipitated by dental interventions, such as extracts or periodontal scaling [23], a dental examination with appropriate preventive dentistry must be considered before treatment with bisphosphonates. While on treatment, these patients should avoid invasive dental procedures if possible. No data are available as to whether discontinuation of bisphosphonate therapy reduces the risk for ONJ in patients who require dental procedures [29], but these agents seem to have permanent effects on the bone and always put the individual at risk for developing ONJ.

Despite multiple distressing side effects, chemotherapy remains an important and beneficial component of cancer therapy. Most of these drugs affect DNA synthesis and exploit kinetic differences between normal and malignant cells by acting preferentially on the cells that are dividing at a faster rate. Normal cells that have a turnover rate rivaling malignant cells (eg, bone marrow, GI mucosa, oral mucosa, skin, hair follicles) will also be severely affected, and the side effects of chemotherapeutic agents will therefore include myelosuppression, GI disturbance, and mucosal ulcerations. The perioperative considerations of patients undergoing cancer chemotherapy are related primarily to the multiplicity of noxious side effects presented by the various drugs. This article discusses the suggested management of the side effects most important to oral and maxillofacial surgeons.

References

[1] Andreoli TE, Carpenter CC, Plum F, et al. Cecil essentials of medicine. Philadelphia: W.B. Saunders (Elsevier B.V.); 2004.

[2] Chung F. Cancer, chemotherapy, and anesthesia. Can Anaesth Soc J 1982;29:364–71.

[3] Stoelting RK. Pharmacology and physiology in anesthetic practice. 3rd edition. Philadelphia: Lippincott Williams & Wilkins; 1999.

[4] Du XL, Osborne C, Goodwin JS. Population-based assessment of hospitalizations for toxicity from chemotherapy in older women with breast cancer. J Clin Oncol 2002;20(24):4636–42.

[5] Selvin BF. Cancer chemotherapy, implications for the anesthesiologist. Anesth Anal 1981;60:425–34.

[6] Boxer LA, Blackwood RA. Leukocyte disorders: quantitative and qualitative disorders of the neutrophil, part 1. Pediatr Rev 1996;17(1):19–28.

[7] Bain BJ. Ethnic and sex differences in the total and differential white cell count and platelet count. J Clin Pathol 1996;49:664–6.

[8] Wintrobe MM, Lee GR. Wintrobe's clinical hematology. 10th edition. Baltimore (MD): Williams & Wilkins; 1999.

[9] Hughes WT, Armstrong D, Bodey GP, et al. 2002 guidelines for the use of antimicrobial agents in neutropenic patients with cancer. Clin Infect Dis 2002; 34:730–51.

[10] Vial T, Gallant C, Choquet-Kastylevsky G. Treatment of drug-induced agranulocytosis with haematopoietic growth factors—a review of clinical experience. BioDrugs 1999;11(3):185–200.

[11] Armitage JO. Emerging applications of recombinant human granulocyte-macrophage colony-stimulating factor. Blood 1998;92(12):4491–508.

[12] Available at: http://www.neupogen.com. Accessed January 2005.

[13] McCullough J. Current issues with platelet transfusion in patients with cancer. Semin Hematol 2000; 37(2 Suppl 4):3–10.

[14] Platelet transfusion therapy. Natl Inst Health Consens Dev Conf Consens Statement 1986;6(7):1–6.

[15] Petz DP. Platelet transfusions. In: Petz LD, Swisher SN, Kleinman S, et al, editors. Clinical practice of transfusion medicine. 3rd edition. New York: Churchill Livingston; 1995. p. 359–412.

[16] Bishop JF, Schiffer CA, Aisner J, et al. Surgery in acute leukemia: a review of 167 operations in thrombocytopenic patients. Am J Hematol 1987;26: 147–55.

[17] Practice guidelines for blood component therapy. A report by the American Society of Anesthesiologists Task Force on Blood Component Therapy. Anesthesiology 1996;84(3):732–47.

[18] Schiffer CA, Anderson KC, Bennett CL, et al. Platelet transfusion for patients with cancer: clinical practice guidelines of the American Society of Clinical Oncology. J Clin Oncol 2001;19(5):1519–38.

[19] Lyons V, Triulzi DJ. Platelet transfusion therapy. Transfusion medicine update. The Institute of Transfusion Medicine. Available at: http://www.itxmdiagnostics.com/tmu1998/tmu9-99.htm. Accessed January 2005.

[20] Lee R, Purday J. Haematological disorders. In: Nichols A, Wilson I, editors. Perioperative medicine. Oxford: Oxford University Press; 2000. p. 206–20.

[21] Du X, Williams D. Interleukin 11: review of molecular, cell biology and clinical use. Blood 1997;89(11): 3897–908.

[22] Tepler I, Elias L, Smith JW, et al. A randomized placebo-controlled trial of recombinant human interleukin-11 in cancer patients with severe thrombocytopenia due to chemotherapy. Blood 1996;87: 3607–14.

[23] Marx RE. Pamidronate (Aredia) and zoledronate (Zometa) induced avascular necrosis of the jaws: a growing epidemic. J Oral Maxillofac Surg 2003; 61:1115–8.

[24] Ruggiero SL, Mehrotra B, Rosenberg TJ, et al. Osteonecrosis of the jaws associated with the use of bisphosphonates: a review of 63 cases. J Oral Maxillofac Surg 2004;62:527–34.

[25] Estilo CL, Van Poznak CH, Williams T, et al. Osteonecrosis of the maxilla and mandible in patients treated with bisphosphonates: a retrospective study [abstract]. J Clin Onc 2004;23:747 [Abstract 8088].

[26] Rubin R. Drug linked to death of jawbone. USA Today March 14, 2005:9D.

[27] Novartis Pharmaceutical Corporation: Oncology Drug Advisory Committee. Appendix 11: Expert Panel Recommendation for the Prevention, Diagnosis and Treatment of Osteonecrosis of the Jaw. Available at: http://www.fda.gov/OHRMS/DOCKETS/ac/05/briefing/2005-4095B2_02_12-Novartis-Zometa. Accessed November 2005.

[28] Lieutenant Commander Aaron P. Sarathy, DC, USN, and Commander Sidney L. Bourgeois Jr, DC, USN. Bisphosphonate-associated osteonecrosis of the jaws. Clinical Update. Vol. 27, No. 1, Jan. 2005. National Naval Medical Center, Bethesda, Maryland.

[29] Available at: http://www.us.zometa.com/info/patientsafetyinfo.jsp. Accessed January 2005.

Exam E-BOOKS!

These titles and other electronic and print collections are all searchable at http://www.swims.nhs.uk/ our library catalogue.

Add the limit PLYMOUTH to see our holdings and E-BOOK to refine your search.

Title	Author
100 Medical Emergencies for Finals	Sooriakumaran, Prasanna; Jayasena, Channa; Sharman, Anjla
Anaesthesia Science Viva Book, The	Bricker, Simon
Concise Notes in Oncology for MRCP and MRCS	
Emergency Radiology: Case Studies	Schwartz, David T.
EMQs for the MRCGP Paper 2! with answers discussed	Dawson, Hayley
EMQs in Obstetrics and Gynaecology	Akkad, Andrea; Habiba, Marwan; Konje, Justin
Essential OSCE Topics for Medical and Surgical Finals	Sritharan, Kaji; Elwell, Vivian A.; Sivananthan, Sachi
Extended Matching Items for the MRCPsych Part 1	Reilly, Michael; Raju, Bangaru
MCQs for the Final FRCA	Effurti, Khaled; Arthurs, Graham
MCQs for the MRCS	Mokbel, K.
MCQs for the Primary FRCA	Effurti, Khaled; Arthurs, Graham; Gemmell, Les; Shillito, Richard; Bailey, Tony
Medical Histories for the MRCP and Final MB	Khan, Iqbal
Memorizing Medicine: A Revision Guide	Bentley, Paul
MRCOG 2 Short Essay Questions	Abedin, Parveen; Sharif, Khaldoun
MRCOG Part 2: Essential EMQs	Habiba, Marwan; Akkad, Andrea; Konje, Justin C.
MRCP PACES Ethics and Communication Skills	Khan, Iqbal
nMRCGP Applied Knowledge Test Study Guide: Sample Questions and Explanatory Answers	Khan, Aalia; Jabbour, Ramsey; Rehman, Almas
Operative Surgery Vivas for the MRCS	Abbassian, Ali; Krishnanandan, Sarah; James, Christopher
Operative Surgery: Viva Practice for the MRCS/AFRCS	Mokbel, K.M; Jeswani, T. A.
Physics, Pharmacology and Physiology for Anaesthetists: Key Concepts for the FRCA	Cross, Matthew E.; Plunkett, Emma V. E.
Practice Examination Papers for the MRCPsych Part 1	Burza, Sabina; Mougey, Beata; Perecherla, Srinivas; Talwar, Nakul
Practice Questions in Trauma and Orthopaedics for the FRCS	Sharma, Pankaj
Rapid Revision in Endocrinology	Greenstein, Ben
Short Answer Questions for the MRCOphth Part 1	Cartwright, Nathaniel Know; Carvounis, Petros
Viva Tutorials for Surgeons in Training	Adams, Wendy; Bull, Jonathan; Epstein, Jonathan; Krishnan, Anant; Menezes, Leon; Modarai, Bijan; Patterson, Paul; Sahai, Arun; Schizas, Alexis

An Athens account is required to access these electronic titles.

To register for an Athens account, please visit www.library.nhs.uk and click 'Register Here'

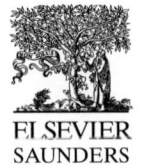
ELSEVIER
SAUNDERS

Oral Maxillofacial Surg Clin N Am 18 (2006) 195–202

ORAL AND
MAXILLOFACIAL
SURGERY CLINICS
of North America

Perioperative Management of the Female and Gravid Patient

Brett A. Ueeck, DMD, MD*, Leon A. Assael, DMD

*Department of Oral and Maxillofacial Surgery, Oregon Health and Sciences University, 611 SW Campus Drive,
Portland, OR 97239, USA*

Care of the female patient requires a detailed understanding of the unique issues inherent to quality treatment. Increasingly important data continue to accumulate about significant differences in the physiology of men and women and the way they express disease. Females react differently to treatment from physiologic and behavioral standpoints. With a new discipline and several journals devoted to the topic, staying current may seem intimidating in today's health care climate. However, from an oral and maxillofacial surgical standpoint, certain aspects of care are more relevant; this article attempts to focus on these.

The female patient

Until recently, practitioners made no conscious efforts to define differences between male and female patients. However, experts now understand that clinically significant differences exist. Possibly one of the most relevant differences is in communication.

Communication

For various conditions, women are more likely than men to seek health care and visit the doctor more frequently. These conditions include arthritis and dental care, but not cardiopulmonary conditions, partly because gender stereotypes may cause women to exclude these conditions from self-diagnosis. This exclusion prevents them from seeking care for con-

ditions for which they believe they are not at risk. These gender stereotypes have resulted in excess morbidity and mortality from delayed care.

Overall, women are less resistant to seeking help for medical conditions. Once treatment is decided, women also tend to be more agreeable to care. Therefore, more surgical procedures are performed each year on women than on men.

Several important points must be remembered regarding the clinical visit. Depending on the gender of the surgeon, the history and physical examination can yield different results for female patients. When dealing with a male surgeon, women are less likely to interrupt the interview process and volunteer information, and are generally less likely to identify and relate symptoms during their visit. When symptoms are described, they tend to be less specific and less directed than when discussed with a female surgeon [1–3].

These differences may occur for several reasons. Research has shown that female providers tend to smile more and create a more receptive and friendly environment than male providers. This finding does not imply that women should seek female surgeons, it simply means the male provider should consider this important difference in communication. In fact, several studies have shown that although women usually seek the care of a female gynecologist, the male gynecologist shows more patient-centeredness and higher levels of emotionally focused talk [4–6].

Physiology

Communication is not the only factor that causes differences in how women relate symptoms; physi-

* Corresponding author.
E-mail address: ueeckb@ohsu.edu (B.A. Ueeck).

ology also plays a large role. The most well-known difference is in cardiac angina and acute coronary syndrome. Men tend to give the classical description of angina, whereas women tend to be vague and may mention indigestion, belly pain, or nothing at all. Women are more likely to suffer a fatal infarction as the first event perhaps because the earlier symptoms were not recognized. Health professionals now have a greater understanding of this altered physiologic response to cardiac ischemia, which has stimulated more formal workup of vague cardiac symptoms in women.

More obvious differences in physiology are also important, especially the ability to become pregnant. Pregnancy status should be ascertained at every patient visit for every woman of childbearing years. This status can be determined verbally if the patient assures the treating doctor that they are not and could not be pregnant. If pregnancy is a possibility, a pregnancy test should be performed before surgical treatment. Lead shielding during radiographs should be used routinely on all women regardless of pregnancy status. Pregnancy status alters every decision for invasive procedures and choice of anesthetics. The impact not only applies to the patient, but also the fetus. The medical–legal aspects of failing to document or appropriately recommend treatment are equally important [7].

Oral contraceptive use is an essential factor to consider for female patients undergoing antibiotic therapy. Patients should be advised that antibiotics can impact the efficacy of contraceptives. Women taking contraceptives who will undergo antibiotic therapy should be informed of the risk for pregnancy. For female patients undergoing antibiotic therapy, alternative birth control methods should be used during the menstrual cycle. Oral contraceptives can also increase a woman's chance of experiencing a venous thrombosis or cerebrovascular accident perioperatively, and may increase blood pressure.

Women are more prone to osteoporosis than men, which has led to the wide use of bisphosphonates in women, usually those who are in the fourth decade of life and older. Because breast cancer is the most common female malignancy, it exposes women to bisphosphonates because these are a mainstay of metastatic breast cancer therapy. Bisphosphonates are shown to be important factors in the development of spontaneous osteonecrosis of the jaws and abnormal healing after oral surgery. Female patients are increasingly likely to experience and present with osteonecrosis of the jaws as a result of these drugs.

The gravid patient

Many aspects of the evaluation and treatment of gravid patients differ substantially from those who are nongravid. Although many elective procedures may be delayed until the baby has been delivered, several circumstances exist in which care cannot be postponed, including those involving trauma, acute infections of the head and neck, erupting or impacted teeth that are causing problems, and benign and malignant tumors.

An estimated 50,000 pregnant women each year undergo surgery related to conditions other than pregnancy, and therefore surgeons must understand the changes related to pregnancy, including those listed in Box 1, and the important impact these changes have on treatment. The change in maternal physiology is amazing when considering that such drastic changes seldom if ever take place in any other nonpathophysiologic process. From conception, a woman's body begins a remarkable transformation to allow another human to develop, grow, and be delivered. Each physiologic system is affected in ways that may or may not have clinical significance for the oral and maxillofacial surgeon. This article attempts to outline these effects based on each system.

Box 1. Normal hemodynamic and renal changes associated with pregnancy

Cardiovascular

Increased cardiac output
Decreased vascular resistance
Modest decrease in blood pressure
Increased blood volume with
     relative anemia

Renal and electrolyte

Increase in glomerular filtration
     rate (GFR)
Chronic partially compensated
     respiratory alkalosis
Hyponatremia
Decreased plasma concentration of
     blood urea nitrogen (BUN)
     and creatinine

Cardiovascular

Important hemodynamic changes that occur during pregnancy include increased cardiac output, reduced systemic vascular resistance, and decreased systemic blood pressure. Also, expansion of intravascular volume occurs with resulting anemia (hematocrit, 31%; hemoglobin, 10.5 g/dL). These changes begin early in pregnancy, peak during the second trimester, then plateau and remain until delivery. These changes contribute to the normal growth and devolvement of the fetus and help protect the mother from complications at delivery (Fig. 1) [8–11].

During the first 8 weeks the pregnant woman will be halfway to increasing her cardiac output by 30% to 50% above her baseline. By the first part of the second trimester, her cardiac output could be increased by 1.8 L/min. These changes remain constant until delivery. The surgeon must understand that the position of the patient and administration of drugs can greatly affect cardiac output during pregnancy [12].

This increase in cardiac output becomes very sensitive to postural changes. A woman in her third trimester must lie in the left lateral decubitus position, or at least at a 30° left lateral tilt, rather than supine (Fig. 2). Supine positioning leads to compression of the inferior vena cava with substantial reduction in venous return, accounting for a drop in cardiac output of up to 25% within 3 to 10 minutes. Furthermore, this position has been shown to compress the aorta, with a drop in blood flow in the common iliac arteries. Signs and symptoms of supine hypotensive syndrome in pregnancy are listed in Box 2. Both the mother and the fetal uteroplacental blood flow are affected by these phenomena (Fig. 3); however, the fetus is more susceptible to these changes and does not show warning signs [13–15].

Preload, afterload, and heart rate are important factors accounting for the increase in cardiac output. The preload is increased as total blood volume increases during pregnancy. Afterload is decreased because of a reduction in systemic vascular resistance. Finally, the maternal heart rate increases by 15 to 20 beats per minute. Early in pregnancy, stroke volume is the major factor accounting for the increased cardiac output, whereas heart rate accounts for it late in pregnancy and the ejection fraction remains at nonpregnant values [16].

A drop in systemic vascular resistance and blood pressure occurs early in pregnancy. A mean pressure of 105/60 by the second trimester is not abnormal. In the later part of pregnancy, pressures slowly return to pregravid levels. Several mechanisms may cause these decreases in resistance and pressures. Most experts believe that the vasculature loses responsiveness to effects of angiotensin II. Other theories involve circulating levels of vasoactive substances, such as endothelial prostacyclin, nitric oxide, and the female hormones estrogen, progesterone, and prolactin. Blood pressures that increase past normal levels should be followed-up because they could signal pregnancy-induced hypertension. Experts must understand the normal variation in blood pressures so they do not react to a presumed hypotensive situation, or worse yet, miss signs of a more serious condition.

Another clinically important change occurs in the coagulation pathway. Pregnancy produces a hyper-

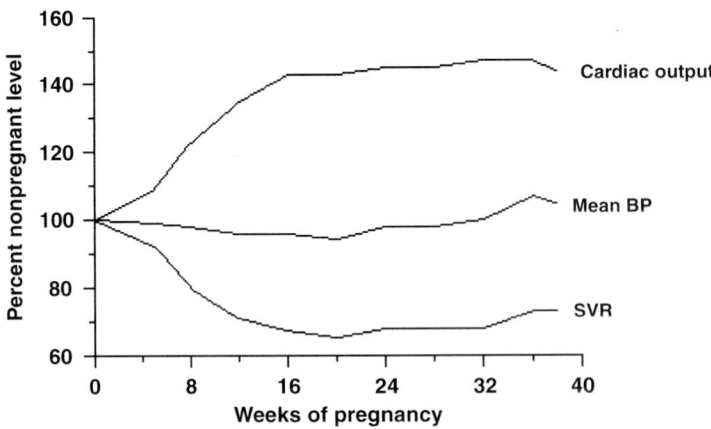

Fig. 1. Hemodynamic changes in normal pregnancy.

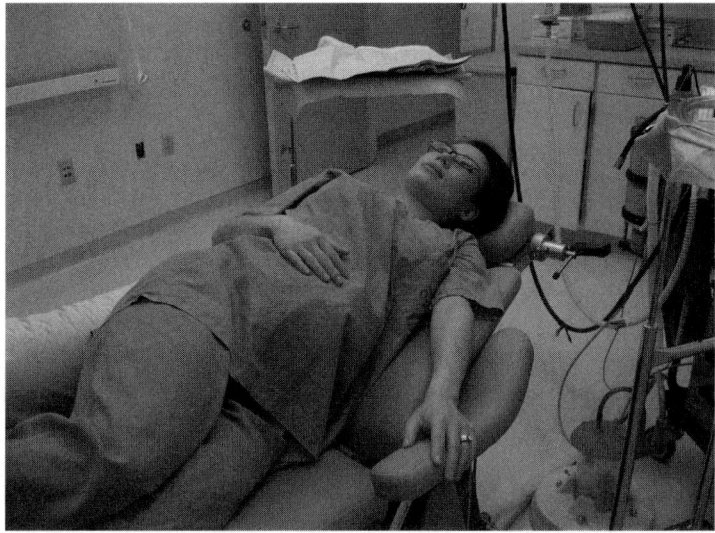

Fig. 2. Gravid patient in left lateral decubitus position.

coagulable state and causes a resistance to activated protein C in the second and third trimester. Protein S levels decrease. The levels of factors I, II, VII, VIII, X, and XII all increase. Finally, the activity of fibrinolytic inhibitors PAI-1 and PAI-2 increase. As a result, approximately 1 of 1000 women develop a venous thrombosis during pregnancy [17–19].

Respiratory

Changes in the respiratory system can be classified by functional and anatomic changes. The anatomic changes are related to the gravid uterus. The diaphragm is displaced upward by as much as 3 to 4 cm and the ribs flare out, creating a barrel-chest appearance. The overall excursion of the diaphragm remains the same, but may be impaired when the patient is in the supine position. Therefore, the total lung and vital capacities change very little. Functional residual capacity drops by 15% to 20%. Combined with the 20% increase in oxygen consumption, an overall decrease in the oxygen reserve occurs, which is important to remember during induction and maintenance of anesthesia [9,20–23].

The rise in progesterone from 25 to 150 ng/mL over the course of pregnancy is responsible for an increase in respiratory drive and rate leading to a 50% increase in minute ventilation. The increase in respiratory rate and tidal volume alter the blood gases of a pregnant patient, corresponding to a PCO_2 of 30 mmHg and a PO_2 of 105 mmHg. The kidney helps offset this respiratory alkalosis by increasing bicarbonate excretion. Even with the compensation, the normal pH rises slightly to 7.44. Furthermore, these changes also leave the patient feeling dyspneic. Up to 70% of pregnant women complain of dyspnea, and therefore physicians must differentiate between normal pregnancy hyperventilation and a more worrisome underlying cause, such as heart failure or pulmonary embolism, during the perioperative period [20–23].

Lastly, an increase in the blood flow and glandular activity of the mucosa occurs in the upper respiratory tract. The secretions also increase in amount and

---

Box 2. Signs and symptoms of supine hypotensive syndrome in pregnancy

Dizziness
Faintness
Nausea
Vomiting
Dyspnea
Pallor
Cyanosis
Hypotension
Headache
Tingling/numbness
Chest/abdominal pain

Systemic Hemodynamics During Normal Pregnancy †

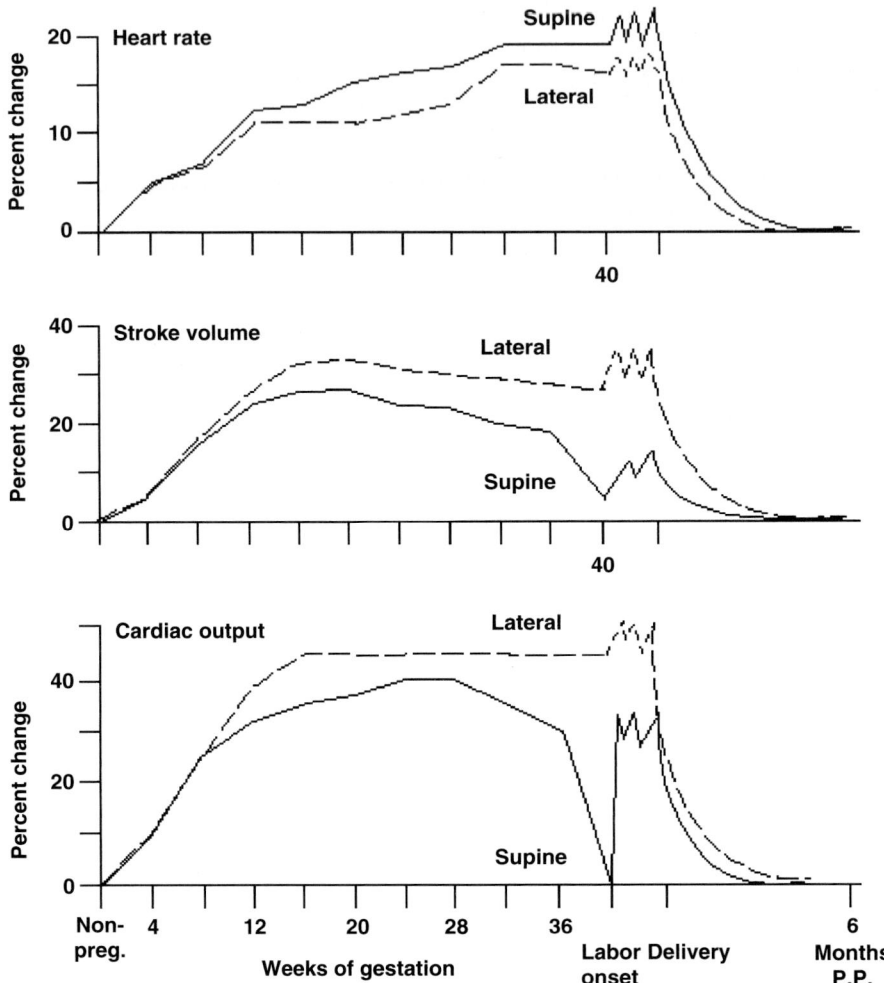

Fig. 3. Effects of position on maternal hemodynamics: systemic hemodynamics during normal pregnancy. (*Data from* Bonica JJ, McDonald JS. Principles and practice of obstetric analgesia and anesthesia. 2nd edition. Baltimore (MD): Williams & Wilkins; 1994. p. 60.)

viscosity. These changes often cause women to complain of nasal stuffiness and epistaxis [24].

Gastrointestinal

Of the changes that occur in the gastrointestinal tract during pregnancy, the most well-known to oral and maxillofacial surgeons is undoubtedly pregnancy gingivitis and the epulis. Gingivitis is multifactorial and is present in 50% to 100% of patients. The relationship between the hormonal effects and the increase in plasminogen activators, along with the

stable or reduced PAI 1 and 2 levels, create an environment where local tissue inflammation blossoms. Therefore, meticulous oral hygiene is warranted to reduce the causes of inflammation. The epulis is consistent with a pyogenic granuloma and can be treated with local hygiene measures. The gingivitis and epulis usually resolve past delivery. The epulis rarely must be removed surgically [25–27].

Gastric motility decreases and emptying times increase during pregnancy. The lower esophageal sphincter tone decreases and pressure on the stomach increases during pregnancy. These changes combine to increase the likelihood of gastroesophageal reflux and dyspepsia.

Positioning and anesthesia are important to consider during management. Sequence of induction, method of airway protection, and other means to eliminate or reduce the chance for aspiration of gastric contents in the perioperative period must be considered [28].

Lastly, nausea, vomiting, and constipation are problems for many women during pregnancy and must be considered when prescribing medications. Care should also be taken when prescribing laxatives because they can impact sodium retention and stimulate uterine contractions, and some are associated with teratogenic risk.

Renal

Plasma volume increases during pregnancy. This increase is partly caused by sodium and water retention. As much as 900 to 1000 mEq of sodium and 6 to 8 L of water are retained. The kidneys carefully regulate the sodium retention, and further sodium retention seldom produces further volume expansion. Even with this close regulation, pregnancy is associated with a chronic hyponatremia. A downward resetting of the osmostat is believed to be responsible for this. This change requires no intervention in a perioperative setting [9].

The renal plasma flow and GFR rise dramatically during pregnancy. The GFR can increase by as much as 50%. This increase, combined with the fact that neither creatinine nor urea nitrogen production changes, results in decreased plasma levels of creatinine and BUN. During pregnancy, normal creatinine and BUN levels are closer to 0.4 mg/dL and 8 mg/dL, respectively, compared with nonpregnancy levels of 0.8 mg/dL and 12 mg/dL. These levels slowly reverse to pregravid levels during the end of the third trimester, but do not fully restore until about 3 months postdelivery. Nevertheless, this change can impact the interpretation of laboratory values and the excretion and efficacy of various medications [29–31].

Changes in the urinary collecting system include dilation of the renal calyces, pelves, and ureters. These changes are poorly understood, but urinary stasis may develop, which explains why asymptomatic bacteriuria often leads to pyelonephritis during pregnancy. Therefore, perioperative catheterization should be used prudently [9].

Endocrine/metabolic

Maternal endocrine adaptations during pregnancy involve the hypothalamus and the pituitary, para-

thyroid, thyroid, and adrenal glands. These alterations affect the circulating levels and actions of the associated hormones. Also, glucose and lipid metabolism are altered. Although these changes have little direct clinical impact on patients during the perioperative period, the surgeon must be aware of them [9].

Fetal considerations

When dealing with pregnant women, surgeons must consider how treatment may impact the fetus. Interventions such as delivery of anesthesia, administration of medications, irradiation, and surgery and maternal disease must be carefully managed to decrease the hazards to the developing child. Benefits, risks, and alternatives for the mother and fetus must be considered. Surgeons must have full knowledge of the teratogenic or other possible harmful effects of medication (eg, induction of labor) before prescribing or administering medication. Surgeons are recommended to obtain approval from the patient's obstetrician for all medications administered during pregnancy [7].

Anesthesia

Preservation of maternal safety; avoidance of intrauterine fetal hypoxia and acidosis caused by decreased uterine blood flow; avoidance of teratogenic drugs; and prevention of preterm labor are objectives when anesthesia is administered to gravid patients undergoing nonobstetrical procedures. The maternal physiologic changes and important elements requiring attention and intervention were discussed previously.

Avoidance of maternal hypotension is the key to preventing fetal hypoxia and acidosis because uterine vessels are already somewhat dilated and cannot autoregulate to compensate. Furthermore, preventing arterial hypoxemia and excessive changes in the $PaCO_2$ preserves uterine blood flow and fetal oxygenation. The fetus depends on a steady rate of oxygen delivery and cannot increase the delivery or the extraction of oxygen. Compensation occurs through distributing blood flow to vital organs while limiting flow to others. Measures effective in returning uteroplacental blood flow include administering fluids, elevating the patient's legs, and placing the patient in the left lateral position. Administration of

Box 3. Food and Drug Administration drug classification

Category A: No known risk in the first trimester or later in pregnancy

Category B: Animal reproduction studies have not shown fetal risk; no controlled studies in pregnant women or animal reproduction studies have shown an adverse effect; human studies have not confirmed adverse effect

Category C: Adverse effects are shown in animal studies but no controlled human studies are available.

Category D: Evidence exists of human fetal risk but some use may be acceptable to preserve the health of the mother despite the risk to the fetus

Category X: Evidence exists of human fetal risk and the risk clearly outweighs any benefit in the pregnant mother

supplemental oxygen can increase maternal and fetal arterial oxygen supply [32,33].

Medications

Discussion of the many different medications and their effects on the pregnant patient and fetus is beyond the scope of this article. Any over-the-counter or prescription medication should be investigated before administration, and the patient's obstetrician usually participates in any medication decisions. Whenever possible, category A drugs (based on the FDA drugs classification system, presented in Box 3) should be prescribed.

Diagnostic radiation

The use of diagnostic radiation for maxillofacial imaging has some safety advantages: it occurs outside the realm of the abdomen and lead shields can be used for protection. Despite these advantages, the risk/benefit ratio should always be carefully calculated before studies are ordered. Increased risk for leukemia and other malignancies have been reported in children whose mothers underwent abdominal radiographs [34]. Of more related significance, the use of dental radiography has been associated with low birth weight and term low birth weight infants.

This finding challenges the assumption that only direct radiation to the fetus and reproductive organs is harmful [35].

Summary

To ensure successful treatment outcome of female and gravid patients, surgeons have certain responsibilities for appropriate management. The female patient has several obvious differences from the male patient, but subtle ones are often overlooked and result in poor patient-doctor communication and less than ideal outcomes. Care of the gravid patient may seem daunting, but use of resources helps focus the key issues of care.

References

[1] Dindia K, Allen M. Sex differences in self-disclosure: a meta-analysis. Psychol Bull 1992;112(1):106–24.

[2] Torpy JM, Lynm C, Glass RM. JAMA patient page. Men and women are different. JAMA 2003; 289(4):510.

[3] Roter DL, Hall JA, Aoki Y. Physician gender effects in medical communication: a meta-analytic review. JAMA 2002;288(6):756–64.

[4] LaFrance M, Hecht MA, Paluck EL. The contingent smile: a meta-analysis of sex differences in smiling. Psychol Bull 2003;129(2):305–34.

[5] van Dulmen AM, Bensing JM. Gender differences in gynecologist communication. Women Health 2000; 30(3):49–61.

[6] Roter DL, Geller G, Bernhardt BA, et al. Effects of obstetrician gender on communication and patient satisfaction. Obstet Gynecol 1999;93(5 Pt 1):635–41.

[7] Assael L. The pregnant patient. In: Bennett J, Rosenberg M, editors. Medical emergencies in dentistry. WB Saunders; 2002. p. 493–501.

[8] Metcalfe J, Ueland K. Maternal cardiovascular adjustments to pregnancy. Prog Cardiovasc Dis 1974;16: 363–74.

[9] Barron WM. The pregnant surgical patient: medical evaluation and management. Ann Intern Med 1984; 101:683–91.

[10] Ueland K. Maternal cardiovascular dynamics. VII. Intrapartum blood volume changes. Am J Obstet Gynecol 1976;126:671–3.

[11] Stephansson O, Dickman PW, Johansson A, et al. Maternal hemoglobin concentration during pregnancy and risk of stillbirth. JAMA 2000;284:2611–7.

[12] van Oppen AC, Stigter RH, Bruinse HW. Cardiac output in normal pregnancy: a critical review. Obstet Gynecol 1996;87:310–8.

[13] Kinsella SM, Lohmann G. Supine hypotensive syndrome. Obstet Gynecol 1994;83:774–88.

[14] Howard BK, Goodson JH, Mengert WF. Supine hypotension syndrome in late pregnancy. Obstet Gynecol 1953;1:371–7.

[15] Marx GF. Aortocaval compression: incidence and prevention. Bull N Y Acad Med 1974;50:443–6.

[16] Duvekot JJ, Cheriex EC, Pieters FA, et al. Early pregnancy changes in hemodynamics and volume homeostasis are consecutive adjustments triggered by a primary fall in systemic vascular tone. Am J Obstet Gynecol 1993;169:1382–92.

[17] Toglia M, Weg J. Venous thromboembolism during pregnancy. N Engl J Med 1996;335:108–14.

[18] McColl MD, Ramsay JE, Tait RC, et al. Risk factors for pregnancy associated venous thromboembolism. Thromb Haemost 1997;78:1183–8.

[19] Friederich PW, Sanson B-J, Simioni P, et al. Frequency of pregnancy related venous thromboembolism in anticoagulant factor-deficient women: implications for prophylaxis. Ann Intern Med 1996;125:955–60.

[20] Liberatore SM, Pistelli R, Patalano F, et al. Respiratory function during pregnancy. Respiration 1984; 46:145–50.

[21] Milne JA. The respiratory response to pregnancy. Postgrad Med J 1979;55:318–24.

[22] Prowse C, Gaensler E. Respiratory and acid-base changes during pregnancy. Anesthesiology 1965; 26:381–92.

[23] McAuliffe F, Kametas N, Costello J, et al. Respiratory function in singleton and twin pregnancy. BJOG 2002;109:765–9.

[24] Bende M, Hallgarde M, Sjogren U, et al. Nasal congestion during pregnancy. Clin Otolaryngol 1989;14:385–7.

[25] Kinnby B, Matsson L, Astedt B. Aggravation of gingival inflammatory symptoms during pregnancy associated with the concentration of plasminogen activator inhibitor type 2 (PAI-2) in gingival fluid. J Periodontal Res 1996;31:271–7.

[26] Kinnby B, Astedt B, Casslen B. Reduction of PAI-2 production in cultured human peripheral blood monocytes by estradiol and progesterone on effect on t-PA, a-PA, and PAI-1. Fibrinolysis 1995;9:152–6.

[27] Kinnby B, Lecander I, Martinsson G, et al. Tissue plasminogen activator and placental plasminogen activator inhibitor in human gingival fluid. Fibrinolysis 1991;5:239–44.

[28] Katz PO, Castell DO. Gastroesophageal reflux disease during pregnancy. Gastroenterol Clin North Am 1998; 27:153–67.

[29] Chapman AB, Abraham WT, Zamudio S, et al. Temporal relationships between hormonal and hemodynamic changes in early human pregnancy. Kidney Int 1998;54:2056–63.

[30] Lim VS, Katz AI, Lindheimer MD. Acid-base regulation in pregnancy. Am J Physiol 1976;231:1764–9.

[31] Iwasaki Y, Oiso Y, Kondo K, et al. Aggravation of subclinical diabetes insipidus during pregnancy. N Engl J Med 1991;324:522–6.

[32] Stoelting Robert K, Dierdorf Stephen F. Anesthesia and coexisting disease. 4th edition. Churchill Livingstone, Inc; 2002.

[33] Rosen MA. Management of anesthesia for the pregnant surgical patient. Anesthesiology 1999;91:1159–63.

[34] Stewart A, Kneale GW. Radiation dose effects in relation to obstetric x-rays and childhood cancers. Lancet 1970;1:1185–8.

[35] Hujoel PP, Bollen A, Noonan CJ, et al. Antepartum dental radiography and infant low birth weight. JAMA 2004;291(16):1987–93.

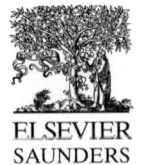

ELSEVIER
SAUNDERS

Oral Maxillofacial Surg Clin N Am 18 (2006) 203 – 212

ORAL AND
MAXILLOFACIAL
SURGERY CLINICS
of North America

Perioperative Management of Patients with Renal Disease

Lee R. Carrasco, DDS, MD[a,b,*], Joli C. Chou, DMD, MD[b]

[a]*Department of Oral and Maxillofacial Surgery, Hospital of University of Pennsylvania, 3400 Spruce Street, 5 White,
Philadelphia, PA 19104, USA*
[b]*University of Pennsylvania School of Dental Medicine, 240 South 40th Street, Philadelphia, PA 19104, USA*

Treating patients who have kidney disease can be a difficult and complex process. Understanding how to care for patients who have kidney disease is essential for lowering perioperative morbidity and mortality. The renal system eliminates metabolic waste; regulates fluid and electrolyte homeostasis; and maintains acid and base levels. In addition, the kidneys have endocrine functions that affect the cardiovascular and hematologic systems. The higher perioperative morbidity and mortality rates in patients who have renal disease, especially those who have end-stage renal disease (ESRD), reflects the importance of a properly functioning renal system [1–4].

Renal function is evaluated by measuring glomerular filtration rate (GFR). GFR is expressed per 1.73 m^2 surface area because it is affected by age, sex, and body size. The average value of GFR for an adult man is 130 mL/min per 1.73 m^2 and is 120 mL/min per 1.73 m^2 for an adult woman [5]. Chronic kidney disease occurs when the GFR is reduced by at least 50 mL/min [6].

Chronic kidney disease is becoming more prevalent in the United States. According to The Third National Health and Nutrition Examination Survey, 1988–1994, 8 million people in the United States experienced moderate to severe chronic kidney disease. Chronic renal disease (CRD) is characterized by a GFR lower than 60 mL/min per 1.73 m^2 [7].

These figures include patients who have chronic renal disease not yet on dialysis, patients who have end-stage renal disease who are undergoing dialysis, and patients who have undergone renal transplant but continue to have impaired renal function [8].

Acute renal failure (ARF) is also frequently encountered in the postoperative period. It can be seen either in patients who previously experienced impaired renal function or those who previously experienced normal renal function [9]. This article reviews the prevention of postoperative ARF and the perioperative management of patients who have ESRD who are undergoing surgery.

Acute renal failure

ARF is the rapid loss of renal function over the course of days to weeks, resulting in the patient's inability to clear nitrogenous waste, including creatinine and urea, from the body [10]. Renal failure is diagnosed through multiple clinical indicators. Urine output has been used to evaluate renal function in ARF, but depending on the cause of renal failure, the patient may or may not be oliguric (<400 mL/d) or anuric (<50 mL/d) [11].

Serum creatinine level has also been used by many investigators to define ARF because it grossly approximates the GFR. However, serum creatinine level may be elevated without change in GFR in patients taking drugs such as cimetidine and trimethoprim, or in those who have rhabdomyolysis. Cimetidine and trimethoprim compete with creatinine for secretion into the proximal tubule. This inhibition reduces the amount of creatinine cleared by the kidneys. In rhabdomyolysis, creatinine released from damaged muscle tissue increases. When the GFR is less than 20% of normal in patients who have

* Corresponding author. Department of Oral and Maxillofacial Surgery, Hospital of University of Pennsylvania, 3400 Spruce Street, 5 White, Philadelphia, PA 19104.
E-mail address: Carrasco11@comcast.net (L.R. Carrasco).

ARF, the serum creatinine level may overestimate the GFR [11]. In such cases, as the GFR declines, the 24-hour urine collection used to compare differences in plasma and urine creatinine and nitrogen levels may more accurately estimate renal function [12]. Nevertheless, many researchers agree that a 25% to 50% increase in the serum concentration of creatinine from baseline indicates ARF [13–15].

Etiology

ARF is categorized into three groups: prerenal, renal (intrinsic), and postrenal (obstructive) failure (Table 1) [11]. Prerenal ARF is caused by factors that result in diminished renal perfusion. Preoperative volume depletion or hypotension as seen in hemorrhage, diarrhea, or diuretics may decrease renal perfusion. Intraoperatively, stimulation of the sympathetic nervous system and the renin–angiotensin–aldosterone axis compromises GFR by inducing afferent arteriolar renal vasoconstriction. At the same time, angiotensin II causes renal vasoconstriction by stimulating renal release of prostaglandins. In the postoperative period, decreased GFR may be caused by relative intravascular volume depletion associated with redistribution of extracellular fluid, congestive heart failure (CHF), myocardial infarction, or vascular obstruction [3,16]. Pharmacologic agents such as nonsteroidal anti-inflammatory drugs (NSAIDs) and angiotensin-converting enzyme (ACE) inhibitors can also cause prerenal failure by changing the prostaglandin and angiotensin II levels that maintain renal perfusion (Table 1) [17].

Intrinsic ARF may be caused by acute tubular necrosis, interstitial nephritis, or renal parenchymal

Table 1
Causes and management of acute renal failure

Causes	Management
Prerenal	
Hypovolemia	Stop diuretics. Administer blood, crystalloid,
Reduced effective arterial blood volume	colloid infusions
Cardiac failure	Inotropes, diuretics, afterload reduction
Sepsis	Pressor agents, crystalloids, antibiotics
Drug-impaired autoregulation	Stop nonsteroidal anti-inflammatory agents, angiotensin-converting enzyme inhibitors, cyclosporine
Renal	
Renal artery occlusion	Anticoagulation, thrombolysis, angioplasty/stent/surgery
Renal parenchyma	
Lesions of the intrarenal vasculature	
Vasculitis	Immunosuppression
Hemolytic uremic syndrome/TTP	Plasma exchange/plasma infusion
Accelerated hypertension	Lower blood pressure: sodium nitroprusside, labetalol, etc
Glomerular disease	Consider immunosuppression, antibiotics if endocarditis, supportive care if postinfective
Ischemic ATN	Supportive care, treat cause of circulatory failure
Toxic ATN	Supportive care, discontinue toxin
Interstitial disease	
Allergic interstitial nephritis	Discontinue offending drug, consider steroids
Bilateral acute pyelonephritis	Antibiotics
Malignant infiltration	Chemotherapy
Intrarenal obstruction	
Myeloma casts	Consider plasma exchange and chemotherapy
Exogenous crystals	Stop offending drug
Endogenous crystals	Alkaline diuresis for rhabdomyolysis or acute urate nephropathy
Postrenal	
Renal vein occlusion	Anticoagulation. Treat glomerular disease if nephrotic
Urinary tract obstruction	Bladder catheter/nephrostomy
	Radiologic/surgical treatment of obstructing lesion

Abbreviation: ATN, acute tubular necrosis; TTP, thrombotic thrombocytopenic purpura.
From Lennon A, Colman PL, Brady HR. Management and outcome of acute renal failure. In: Johnson RJ, Feehally J, editors. Comprehensive clinical nephrology. Philadelphia: Mosby; 2000. p. 19.1–19.4; with permission.

infarcts secondary to renal vascular disease. Patients who have diabetes, hypertension, or vascular disease usually have a diminished baseline GFR that predisposes them to intrinsic types of ARF. Sustained hypotension or volume depletion, occurring in hemorrhage or sepsis, results in ischemia to the kidneys. This decrease in renal blood flow may lead to acute tubular necrosis (ATN). Nephrotoxin, such as aminoglycosides, radiocontrast materials, myoglobin, hemoglobin, and amphotericin B, can also lead to ATN. Penicillin, diuretics, cimetidine, and NSAIDs can lead to ARF by causing interstitial nephritis (Table 1) [18–21].

Obstructions of the urinary system causes postrenal ARF. These obstructions can be intrarenal, such as tubular obstruction caused by sulfonamide and acyclovir crystal deposits, or extrarenal, such as bladder dysfunction, obstructed urinary catheters, or pelvic or ureteral obstruction caused by blood clots, sloughed papillae, and retroperitoneal hematoma or masses [22]. However, in pelvic or ureteral obstruction, ARF only occurs when the obstruction is bilateral or in patients who have only one functioning kidney (Table 1) [17,23].

Evaluation

A thorough history and physical examination in combination with key laboratory measurements, such as complete blood count with leukocyte differential, metabolic panel, coagulation profile, microscopic urinalysis, and urine electrolytes, identify the etiology of acute renal failure. A detailed focused history may reveal important information about intravascular depletion, hypotension, heart failure, or exposure to endogenous and exogenous nephrotoxins.

Signs such as orthostatic hypotension, tachycardia, and dry mucous membranes noted on physical examination indicate volume depletion. Presence of rash, purpura, livedo reticularis, gangrene, or digital cyanosis may indicate acute interstitial nephritis or renal artery or atheromatous embolism. Cardiac failure is associated with third heart sounds, jugular venous distention and peripheral and pulmonary edema. Upper quadrant tenderness in abdominal palpation may indicate ureteral obstruction or renal infarction. Abdominal examination could identify palpable bladder caused by a blocked bladder catheter or enlarged prostate.

Assessment of serum and urinary electrolytes and a urinalysis may differentiate ARF into prerenal, intrinsic, or obstructive. Usually in prerenal ARF the urinalysis is normal, the ratio of blood urea nitrogen (BUN) to serum creatinine is elevated above 20:1,

urinary sodium concentration is less than 20 mEq/L, urine osmolality is higher than 500 mOsm/kg, and the fractional excretion of sodium (FENa) is less than 1%. FENa is defined as: [U Na/P Na]/[U Cr/P Cr] × 100%. It compares the differences of sodium and creatinine in the plasma (P) and urine (U).

Intrinsic ARF usually presents with a normal ratio of BUN and serum creatinine, urinary sodium concentration higher than 40 mEq/L, urine osmolality less than 350 mOsm/kg, and an abnormal urinalysis. The presence of many brown granular casts and renal tubular epithelial cells are commonly seen in ischemia or nephrotoxic ARF. A strongly positive dipstick reading for heme pigment in the absence of large amounts of red blood cells suggests rhabdomyolysis or intravascular hemolysis. Eosinophils in the urinalysis associated with fever, rash, and peripheral eosinophilia are typical of acute interstitial nephritis. Red cell casts, protein, and red blood cells in the urinalysis suggest acute glomerulonephritis.

Postrenal ARF typically presents with elevated ratio of BUN to serum creatinine, an FENa greater than 1%, and a normal urinalysis. Obstructive ARF could also be evaluated with renal ultrasound, which usually shows dilation of the urinary system. A renal ultrasound can also identify the location of the obstruction. Postvoiding residual of more than 100 cm^3 of urine suggests bladder obstruction and should be evaluated by cystoscopy. Further tests may be necessary, such as renal biopsy to identify the disease process causing acute glomerulonephritis, or radionucleotide tests if perfusion defects are suspected [23,24].

Management

Prevention is the most effective management of ARF. Before surgery, the potential risk factors such as volume depletion, hypotension, sepsis, nephrotoxin exposure, and preexisting chronic kidney disease should be identified (Table 2). To prevent ARF, elective surgery should be postponed until those abnormalities are improved.

Table 2
Risk factors for ARF

Risk factors for ARF
Surgery
Trauma (muscle injury, hemorrhage)
Administration of nephrotoxic drugs
Bladder catheterization
Sepsis
Shock

Preoperative hypotension and volume depletion must be corrected in a timely fashion to prevent perioperative renal ischemia. Renal ischemia can induce ATN and cause sloughing of the papillae, leading to tubular obstruction [25]. Infections should be treated with non-nephrotoxic antibiotics. Hypotension, renal vasoconstriction, and release of cytokines can result from sepsis and lead to ARF [25,26].

NSAIDs, including ketorolac and selective cyclooxygenase inhibitors, should be used cautiously or avoided. They can cause hemodynamically mediated ARF by inhibiting the synthesis of prostaglandins. Prostaglandins are important mediators in the maintenance of renal blood flow and GFR in volume depletion, cardiac failure, preexisting renal insufficiency, and liver cirrhosis [27–29]. ACE inhibitors (ACE-I) and angiotensin receptor blockers (ARB) should also be stopped because their inhibitory actions on the efferent arterioles worsen ARF.

Radiocontrast material may cause ARF through direct toxic effects or altering the production of nitric oxide [30,31]. Radiocontrast should be avoided whenever possible in patients who have chronic renal insufficiency. When the use of radiocontrast is indicated, contrast loads should be minimized and postprocedure hydration used [30,32]. Pretreatment with N-acetylcysteine or sodium bicarbonate should be considered because these have shown protective effects against radiocontrast-induced nephropathy [30,33,34].

When ARF is diagnosed in the postoperative period, causative agents should be eliminated efficiently. Volume repletion in patients who experience prerenal failure, and optimization of cardiac output in those experiencing hypotension ensure adequate renal perfusion. In patients who experience intrinsic failure, nephrotoxins should be eliminated. In addition, aggressive hydration should be used to ensure optimal renal perfusion and maintain extracellular fluid level and urine output to enhance the reparative phase. Finally, obstructive uropathy is treated with relief of obstruction [17]. Although diuretics such as furosemide, low-dose dopamine, and atrial natriuretic peptide have been used to prevent or improve ARF and avoid dialysis, no conclusive data currently show their efficacy [35–37]. Dialysis should be used if a patient experiences fluid overload, electrolyte abnormalities such as hyperkalemia, or acid–base imbalances.

Chronic renal disease

CRF is permanent renal insufficiency that develops over months or years caused by the structural and intrinsic damage of the glomerulus or tubulointerstitial system. The decrease in renal function causes damaging complications. This decrease usually occurs when GFR is reduced by 50 mL/min. In most cases, the progression of CRF leads to ESRD. ESRD causes death if renal replacement therapy such as dialysis or transplant is not provided [6].

The many different causes of CRF include hypertension; diabetes; adult polycystic kidney disease; reflux nephropathy and obstruction; glomerulonephritis; lupus; amyloidosis; and myeloma. The most common causes of CRF in North America, as listed in the 2001 report of the United States renal data system, are diabetes and hypertension [38]. Patients who have hypertension or diabetes often have other comorbidities, such as myocardial dysfunction, coronary artery disease (CAD), and peripheral vascular disease. In addition to loss of renal function, these patients are less able to handle fluids, sodium, and acid load and to metabolize or excrete medications. These medications include antibiotics, analgesics, and anesthetics. Patients who have ESRD are also immunocompromised and more susceptible to infections, and often have bleeding diathesis secondary to platelet dysfunction. Hence, those who have ESRD have increased surgical morbidity and mortality rates, requiring additional perioperative attention. Modification of the pre- and postoperative management depends on the severity of renal failure [3]. Conditions leading to ESRD are diabetes, primary hypertension, glomerulonephritis, interstitial nephritis, and polycystic kidney disease.

Clinical and laboratory evaluation

Perioperative evaluation of patients who have known CRF must include a detailed history; physical examination; ECG; complete blood count; metabolic panel; serum magnesium and phosphorus levels; and coagulation profile. Results of these screening tests may identify comorbidities associated with CRF that affect perioperative morbidity and mortality. Patients who have CRF experience increased atherosclerosis predisposing them to CAD and myocardial dysfunction. The decrease in renal function may result in fluid and electrolyte abnormalities, hypotension, hypertension, anemia, or bleeding diathesis. Correction or improvement of these abnormalities by avoidance of nephrotoxic medications and tight glycemic control decreases the risk for perioperative complications and may prevent infection.

Cardiac evaluation

Cardiac disease causes 50% of the mortality in patients who have ESRD [38,39]. CAD, an important contributory factor in the pathogenesis of cardiac disease, is found in 40% of all patients who have ESRD. In fact, 40% of all patients on dialysis have CHF. Left ventricular hypertrophy, a risk factor for CHF, is found in 75% of all patients who have ESRD. Patients who have renal failure have increased risk for developing cardiac disease, which may complicate the perioperative course. Preoperative evaluation of cardiac risk in patients who have chronic renal disease is difficult because clinical signs and symptoms of cardiac disease may present atypically in patients who have CRF. Patients undergoing dialysis often may complain of chest pain or exertional dyspnea but have no angiographic evidence of CAD [40]. Several studies have also found that 75% of patients who have diabetes and show significant CAD on angiography are asymptomatic [41,42].

Furthermore, functional capacity assessment is unreliable in patients who have ESRD because they may have anemia, dialysis-induced weakness, peripheral vascular disease with claudication, diabetic neuropathy, renal osteodystrophy causing joint or bone pain, or amyloidosis. Because of ultrafiltration at dialysis, patients who comply with their dialysis regimen do not experience the common symptoms of CHF [39]. Noninvasive tests such as echocardiography, thallium stress test, dipyridamole thallium imaging, or dobutamine stress ECG have been used with limited sensitivity and specificity to screen for cardiac disease in patients who have ESRD [43,44]. Targeting these tests toward patients who have risk factors may increase the positive predictive value of an abnormal test [45]. Cardiac risk factors include age older than 50 years; history of angina; diabetes or CHF; and an abnormal ECG. In patients who have high cardiac risk, coronary angiography may be required to detect CAD and allow for revascularization [46,47].

Fluid and electrolyte management

Euvolemia should be maintained perioperatively in patients who have ESRD. For patients not undergoing dialysis, euvolemia can be achieved with appropriate hydration or diuresis. Patients undergoing dialysis should be dialyzed before surgery to prevent fluid overload. Patients who have stable dry weight with minimal fluid gain between dialysis may undergo emergency surgery without dialysis if no other indications exist for dialysis. Postoperative dialysis may be required to remove extra volume if large amounts of fluids were given during surgery [48].

Hyperkalemia may be present before or after surgery. Although no guidelines exist for safe preoperative potassium level, one study suggests general anesthesia should be avoided in patients who have a potassium level more than 5.5 mEq/L [49]. If the ECG shows signs of arrhythmia, 10 mL of calcium gluconate should be infused with ECG monitoring to provide membrane stabilization and cardioprotection. Medical management of hyperkalemia includes use of polystyrene-binding resins, insulin in combination with intravenously administered dextrose, β_2-adrenergic agonist, and intravenously administered bicarbonate. A standard oral dosage is 40 g of polystyrene resin dissolved in 80 mL of sorbitol. If oral intake is not possible perioperatively then 50 to 100 g of polystyrene resin in 200 mL of water can be given as a retention enema. The resin should be given every 2 to 4 hours, although the surgeon must remember that the resin may cause intestinal necrosis especially when given with sorbitol within the first week after surgery.

Insulin administration decreases intravascular potassium by driving potassium intracellularly. This process occurs through the stimulation of Na-K-ATPase. Insulin should be given with glucose, and patients should be closely monitored for hypoglycemia. The administration of a β_2 agonist also stimulates the Na-K-ATPase to shift potassium into the cells. However, this technique is not typically used in patients who have ESRD because of the risk for tachycardia and arrhythmias. Sodium bicarbonate only reduces the serum potassium level by a small amount unless moderate or severe metabolic acidosis is present. Sodium bicarbonate, insulin, and β_2 agonist only decrease the serum potassium temporarily by shifting potassium from one compartment to another and levels may rebound with time. Only polystyrene-binding resins and dialysis remove excess potassium from the body. If the potassium level in a patient who has ESRD exceeds 6 mEq/L, either before or after surgery, dialysis is the treatment of choice [25].

Anemia

Anemia develops as renal function declines because of the decreased production of erythropoietin. No ideal hemoglobin level has been established for patients who have ESRD. The Anemia Work Group of the National Kidney Foundation—Kidney Disease Outcome Quality Initiative recommends that

hemoglobin be maintained between 11 and 12 g/dL [7]. Because of the formation of antibodies, transfusion may decrease a patient's future chances of successful renal transplantation and may also cause hyperkalemia from cellular lysis [1,50]. Nevertheless, transfusion is appropriate to help avoid complications from perioperative blood loss when hemoglobin levels fall below 8 to 10 g/dL in patients who have ESRD and are undergoing surgery. For elective surgery, erythropoietin should be initiated several weeks before surgery with iron supplementation to raise hemoglobin the desired level.

Bleeding

Patients who have ESRD may be susceptible to more intraoperative and postoperative bleeding for multiple reasons. Uremia can cause platelet dysfunction. Patients who have prolonged bleeding time or previous uremic bleeding must be treated before surgery (Table 3) [51]. Undergoing dialysis on the day before surgery may minimize uremic complications. Administering desmopressin intravenously or intranasally at a dose of 0.3 μg/kg 1 hour before surgery, cryoprecipitate at 10 units over 30 minutes intravenously 1 hour before surgery, and conjugated estrogens at 0.6 mg/kg/d intravenously or 2.5 to 25 mg orally for 5 days before surgery, and raising the hematocrit to 30% will decrease uremic bleeding [51]. Antiplatelet agents such as aspirin and dipyridamole should not be given within 72 hours before surgery to patients who have ESRD. Theoretically diphenhydramine, NSAIDs, chlordiazepoxide, and cimetidine can also increase the risk for intraoperative bleeding in patients who have ESRD and should be avoided preoperatively [52]. Heparin-induced bleeding is unusual. The anticoagulant effects of heparin last only 2.5 hours. If dialysis is performed on the day of surgery, heparin is withheld. During the postoperative period, patients should undergo heparin-free dialysis for at least 24 hours.

Hypertension

Fluid retention, augmented sympathoadrenal discharge, endothelin increase, and nitric oxide reduction all contribute to the hypertension of renal failure. Perioperative anxiety, withholding of antihypertensive drugs, and a catecholamine response related to the stress of the surgery worsen hypertension in patients who have ESRD. Antihypertensive medication should be continued perioperatively in most patients who have kidney disease. Oral agents should be replaced with intravenously administered agents. Oral agents that cannot be given intravenously may be replaced with transdermal clonidine 2 to 3 days before surgery. Unless diuretics are being used for volume management, these should be discontinued 2 to 3 days before surgery to avoid intraoperative hypotension and volume depletion [47].

Abrupt withdrawal of NSAIDs, antihistamines, and decongestants may cause rebound hypertension. Sudden discontinuation of these agent should be avoided immediately before surgery [53].

Glycemic control

Surgical stress and anesthetic-induced release of glucagon, growth hormone, cortisol, epinephrine, and norepinephrine can worsen insulin deficiency and resistance, resulting in hyperglycemia or even ketogenesis during surgery in patients who have kidney disease and type 1 diabetes mellitus. Patients who have kidney disease and diabetes may become hypoglycemic after surgery because of preoperative fasting. The goal for patients who have diabetes and uremia is to maintain glucose level between 150 and 200 mg/dL during surgery to prevent hypoglycemia. Postoperative ideal glucose level is between 120 and 180 mg/dL to reduce fluid and electrolyte imbalance, decrease the risk for infection, and promote wound healing. For patients who have diabetes who experience acceptable glycemic control (80–200 mg/dL) through diet alone or diet and oral hypoglycemic agents, no intraoperative intervention is generally necessary. For the patient who has insulin-dependant diabetes, perioperative insulin is used with frequent finger-stick glucose measurements. After outpatient surgery, the patient's preoperative regimen should be restarted when oral intake is resumed [54].

Drug therapy and anesthetic considerations

Patients experiencing renal failure have abnormalities in drug metabolism that inherently predispose them to adverse drug responses. Drugs and active metabolites excreted by the kidneys have a prolonged half-life in these patients. Changes in bioavailability, volume of distribution, and protein binding are also seen [55,56]. Some reports suggest that residual renal function is associated with a lower mortality in patients undergoing dialysis. Hence, avoidance of nephrotoxic drugs such as aminoglycosides, radiographic contrast media, and NSAIDs is

Table 3
Prevention and treatment of uremic bleeding

Treatment	Mechanism	Prescription	Dose	Onset of action	Maximum effect	Duration of effect after cessation
Dialysis	Remove uremic platelet receptors Allows re-expression of platelet vWF and fibrinogen receptors	—	—	Bleeding time may not improve immediately	Unknown	>48 h
Correct anemia to a hematocrit >30%	Enhances platelet level interaction	Transfusion of packed red blood cells Intravenous or subcutaneous epoetin	—	Immediate	—	NA
Estrogen	Vasoconstriction; enhances platelet-vessel interaction	Intravenous, conjugated Oral, conjugated Topical (patch) estradiol	0.6 mg/kg/d 50 mg/d 50–100 μg patch q 3.5 d	6 h 3–5 d 24–48 h	6 d 7 d 5–7 d	14 d 5–7 d unknown
DDAVP	Enhance platelet adhesion by increasing vWF serum levels and vWF platelet receptors	Intravenous Intranasal Subcutaneous	0.3 μg/kg in 50 mL normal saline over 30 min 3 μg/ kg 0.3 μg/kg	1 h 2 h 2 h	Unknown Unknown Unknown	4–8 h Unknown Unknown
Cryoprecipitate	Enhances platelet adhesions by increasing vWF levels	Intravenous	10 U/30 min	1 h	4–8 h	24 h

Abbreviation: DDAVP, Desmopressin; vWF, von Willebrand factor.
From Sloand JA. Platelet dysfunction and coagulation defects. In: Johnson RJ, Feehally J, editors. Comprehensive clinical nephrology. Philadelphia: Mosby; 2000; with permission.

essential for preservation of residual renal function [57]. In general, physicians should determine if dosage reduction is required or if the medication should be avoided before administering any drug to patients who have kidney disease.

Many patients who have ESRD require antibiotics in the perioperative period for treatment or prophylaxis of infection. Vancomycin has been used commonly for this purpose, resulting in an increase in vancomycin-resistant organisms. Use of a first-generation cephalosporin dosed according to the degree of renal failure is now advocated for empiric therapy. Antibiotic prophylaxis against endocarditis before surgery is recommended for the first several months after placement of synthetic vascular access grafts to avoid bacterial seeding of the graft before epithelialization occurs [58].

Sedative medication such as benzodiazepines should only be used in reduced doses. Patients receiving alprazolam who are undergoing dialysis may develop psychomotor and memory abnormalities [59]. In addition, meperidine should be avoided because its metabolite normeperidine can cause seizures [60]. Morphine should be used with caution because its conjugation with glucuronic acid–producing morphine-6-glucuronide, which also has opioid activity, is excreted by the kidney [61]. Fentanyl is metabolized in the liver, and only 7% is excreted unchanged in the urine. Fentanyl is moderately bound to plasma protein and its volume of distribution is large, and therefore it is safe for patients who have ESRD [62].

Inhaled anesthetics are eliminated primarily through the lung and not the kidney. However, most inhaled anesthetics have been shown to cause a transient reversible depression in renal function. Data suggest that halothane, desflurane, and nitrous oxide can be administered safely to patients experiencing kidney failure [62].

Propofol is a suitable induction agent for patients experiencing renal failure because no significant change occurs in protein binding and clinical effects of its liver metabolites. Also, propofol does not adversely affect renal function [63,64]. Barbiturates such as thiopental must be used in reduced dosages because their free fraction is markedly increased in patients who have CRF.

Succinylcholine is used cautiously in patients who have CRD because it can cause hyperkalemia, especially in patients who have experienced trauma, burns, or neurologic injuries. Large doses of succinylcholine should be avoided because of its weak active metabolite, succinylmonocholine, which is excreted by the kidney. Nondepolarizing agents have prolonged action in patients who have renal failure. This effect occurs because the drug or its metabolite or active metabolites have decreased elimination. A decreased activity of the enzyme that metabolizes the nondepolarizing agents is also seen. The action of atracurium is not prolonged in patients who have ESRD and is the muscle relaxant of choice in these patients [62].

Hemodialysis access sites are commonly occluded during the perioperative period because of thrombosis, hypotension, or pressure on the area during surgery. When patients who have ESRD are positioned for surgery involving general anesthesia, the hemodialysis access site must be protected. Pressure on the access site should be avoided. Frequent observation of the site to monitor for decreased function perioperatively is mandatory [23,24].

Summary

The patient who has renal disease is prone to many potential complications during the perioperative period. The prevention of postoperative ARF, especially in patients who have existing chronic kidney disease, and management of patients undergoing surgery who have ESRD are challenging. The treatment of these patients may require a team of specialists, including primary care physicians, nephrologists, cardiologists, anesthesiologists, endocrinologists, nutritionists, and surgeons. Elimination of risk factors for ARF and early diagnosis of ARF should improve patient outcomes. For patients who have ESRD, a thorough and comprehensive evaluation is necessary to decrease morbidity and mortality associated with the end-organ damage.

References

[1] Brenowitz JB, Williams CD, Edwards WS. Major surgery in patients with chronic renal failure. Am J Surg 1977;134:765–9.

[2] Horst M, Mehlhorn U, Hoerstrup SP, et al. Cardiac surgery in patients with end stage renal disease: 10-year experience. Ann Thorac Surg 2000;69:96–101.

[3] Kellerman PS. Perioperative care of the renal patient. Arch Intern Med 1994;154:1674–88.

[4] Schreiber S, Korzets A, Powsner E, et al. Surgery in chronic dialysis patients. Isr J Med Sci 1995;31: 479–83.

[5] Horio M, Orita Y, Fukunaga M. Assessment of renal function. In: Johnson RJ, Feehally J, editors. Comprehensive clinical nephrology. Philadelphia: Mosby; 2000. p. 3.1–3.6.

[6] Winearls CG. Clinical evaluation and manifestations of chronic renal failure. In: Johnson RJ, Feehally J, editors. Comprehensive clinical nephrology. Philadelphia: Mosby; 2000. p. 38.1–38.14.

[7] NKF-K/DOQI Clinical Practice Guidelines for Chronic Kidney Disease. Evaluation, classification, and stratification. Am J Kidney Dis 2000;37(Suppl 1):S1–266.

[8] Tilney NL, Lazarus JM. Surgical care of the patient with renal failure. Philadelphia: WB Saunders; 1982.

[9] Liano F, Pascual J. Epidemiology of acute renal failure: a prospective, multicenter community-based study. Kidney Int 1996;50(3):811–8.

[10] Anderson RJ, Schrier RW. Clinical spectrum of oliguric and non-oliguric acute renal failure. In: Brenner BM, Stein JH, editors. Acute renal failure (Contemporary issues in nephrology, volume 6). New York: Churchill Livingstone; 1980. p. 1–16.

[11] Iglesias J, Lieberthal W. Clinical evaluation of acute renal failure. In: Johnson RJ, Feehally J, editors. Comprehensive clinical nephrology. Philadelphia: Mosby; 2000. p. 15.1–15.16.

[12] Gehr T. Chronic kidney disease. In: Rakel RD, editor. Conn's current therapy. Philadelphia: WB Saunders; 2005. p. 831–7.

[13] Brady H, Brenner B, Lieberthal W. Acute renal failure. In: Brenner B, editor. The kidney. Philadelphia: WB Saunders; 1996. p. 1200–52.

[14] Faber MD, Kupin WL, Krishna GG, et al. The differential diagnosis of acute renal failure. In: Lazarus JM, Brenner BM, editors. Acute renal failure. 3rd edition. New York: Churchill Livingstone; 1993. p. 133–92.

[15] Nolan CR, Anderson RJ. Hospital-acquired acute renal failure. J Am Soc Nephrol 1998;9:710–8.

[16] Rudnick MR, Bastl CP, Elfinbein IB, et al. The differential diagnosis of acute renal failure. In: Lazarus JM, Brenner BM, editors. Acute renal failure. New York: Churchill Livingstone; 1988.

[17] Alam MG, Shaver-Lewis MJ, Shaw SV. Acute renal failure. In: Rakel RD, editor. Conn's current therapy. Philadelphia: WB Saunders; 2005. p. 822–31.

[18] Chertow GM, Lazarus JM, Christiansen CL, et al. Preoperative renal risk stratification. Circulation 1997; 95(4):878–84.

[19] Choundry D, Ahmed Z. Drug-induced nephrotoxicity. Med Clin North Am 1997;81:705–11.

[20] Humes HD. Aminoglycoside nephrotoxicity. Kidney Int 1988;33(4):900–11.

[21] Rudnick MR, Goldfarb S, Wexler L, et al. Nephrotoxicity of ionic and nonionic contrast media in 1196 patients: a randomized trial. Kidney Int 1995;47(1): 254–61.

[22] Perazella MA. Crystal-induced acute renal failure. Am J Med 1999;106(4):459–65.

[23] Kikeri D. Surgery in the patient with renal disease. In: Lubin MF, Walker HK, Smith RB, editors. Medical management of the surgical patient. Philadelphia: JB Lippincott; 1995. p. 291–304.

[24] Murray TG. The surgical patient with chronic renal failure. In: Goldmann DR, Brown FH, Levy WK, et al,

editors. Medical Care of the Surgical Patient. Philadelphia: JB Lippincott; 1982. p. 218–29.

[25] Rose BD. Pathogenesis and prevention of postischemic acute tubular necrosis. In: Rose BD, editor. UpToDate. Release 10.1, 2002.

[26] Beaufils M, Morel-Maroger L, Sraer JD, et al. Acute renal failure of glomerular origin during visceral abscesses. N Engl J Med 1976;295(4):185–9.

[27] Feldman HI, Kinman JL, Berlin JA, et al. Parenteral ketorolac: the risk for acute renal failure. Ann Intern Med 1997;127(6):493–4.

[28] Oates JA, Fitzgerald GA, Branch RA, et al. Clinical implication of prostaglandin and thromboxane A2 formation. N Engl J Med 1988;319(12):761–7.

[29] Perazella MA, Eras J. Are selective COX-2 inhibitors nephrotoxic. Am J Kidney Dis 2000;35(5):937–40.

[30] Solomon R, Werner C, Mann D, et al. Effects of saline, mannitol, and furosemide on acute decreases in renal function induced by radiocontrast agents. N Engl J Med 1994;331(21):1416–20.

[31] Yoshioka T, Fogo A, Beckman JK. Reduced activity of antioxidant enzymes underlies contrast media-induced renal injury in volume depletion. Kidney Int 1992; 41(4):1008–15.

[32] Solomon R. Radiocontrast-induced nephropathy. Seminar Nephrol 1998;18(5):551–7.

[33] Merten GJ, Burgess WP, Gray LV, et al. Prevention of contrast-induced nephropathy with sodium bicarbonate: a randomized controlled trial. JAMA 2004;291: 2328–34.

[34] Tepel M, van der Giet M, Schwarzfeld C, et al. Prevention of radiographic-contrast-agent-induced reductions in renal function by acetylcysteine. N Engl J Med 2000;343(3):180–4.

[35] Brown CB, Ogg CS, Cameron JS. High dose furosemide in acute renal failure: a controlled trial. Clin Nephrol 1981;15(2):90–6.

[36] Lassnigg A, Donner E, Grubhofer G, et al. Lack of renoprotective effects of dopamine and furosemide during cardiac surgery. J Am Soc Nephrol 2000;11(1): 97–104.

[37] Lewis J, Salem MM, Chertow GM, et al. Atrial natriuretic factor in oligouric acute renal failure. Anaritide Acute Renal Failure Study Group. Am J Kidney Dis 2000;34(4):767–74.

[38] United States Renal Data System. USRDS 2001 Annual data report: atlas of end-stage renal disease in the United States. Bethesda, MD: National Institute of Health, National Institute of Diabetes and Kidney Disease; 2001.

[39] Foley RN, Parfrey PS, Sarnack MJ. Clinical epidemiology of cardiovascular disease in chronic renal disease. Am J Kidney Dis 1998;32(5 Suppl 3):S112–9.

[40] Rostand SG, Kirk KA, Rutsky EA. Dialysis-associated ischemic heart disease: insights from coronary angiography. Kidney Int 1984;25(4):653–9.

[41] Braun WE, Phillips DF, Vidt DG. Coronary artery disease in 100 diabetic with end-stage renal failure. Transplant Proc 1984;16(3):603–7.

[42] Koch M, Gradaus F, Schoebel DC, et al. Relevance of conventional cardiovascular risk factors for the prediction of coronary artery disease in diabetic patients on renal replacement therapy. Nephrol Dial Transplant 1997;12(6):1187–91.

[43] Elsner D. How to diagnose and treat coronary artery disease in the uraemic patient: an update. Nephrol Dial Transplant 2001;16(6):1103–8.

[44] Marwick TH, Steinmüller DR, Underwood DA, et al. Ineffectiveness of dipyridamole stress in the diagnosis of coronary artery disease. J Nucl Med 1990;31(12): 1906–8.

[45] Reis G, Marcovitz PA, Leichtman AB, et al. Usefulness of dobutamine stress echocardiography in detecting coronary artery disease in end-stage renal disease. Am J Cardiol 1995;75:707–10.

[46] Eagle KA, Berger PB, Calkins H, et al. ACC/AHA guideline update for perioperative cardiovascular evaluation for noncardiac surgery-executive summary. A report of the American College of Cardiology/ American Heart Association Task Force on Practice Guidelines (Committee to Update the 1996 Guidelines on Perioperative Cardiovascular Evaluation for Noncardiac Surgery). Circulation 2002;105:1257–67.

[47] Palda VA, Detsky AS. Perioperative assessment and management of risk from coronary artery disease. Ann Intern Med 1997;127:313–28.

[48] Yee J, Parasuraman R, Narins RG. Selective review of key preoperative renal-electrolyte disturbances in chronic renal failure patients. Chest 1999;115(5 Suppl): S149–57.

[49] Haimov M, Glabman S, Schupak E, et al. General surgery in patients on maintenance hemodialysis. Ann Surg 1974;179:863–7.

[50] Poli F, Scalamogna M, Cardillo M, et al. An algorithm for cadaver kidney allocation based on a multivariate analysis of factors impacting on cadaver kidney graft survival and function. Transpl Int 2000;13(Suppl 1): S259–62.

[51] Sloand JA. Platelet dysfunction and coagulation defects. In: Johnson RJ, Feehally J, editors. Comprehensive clinical nephrology. Philadelphia: Mosby; 2000. p. 72.1–72.6.

[52] Steiner RW, Coggins C, Carbalho AC. Bleeding time in uremia: a useful test to asses clinical bleeding. Am J Hematol 1979;7:107–17.

[53] Krishnan M. Preoperative care of patients with kidney disease. Am Fam Phys 2002;66(8):1471–6.

[54] Jacober SJ, Sowers JR. An update on perioperative management of diabetes. Arch Intern Med 1999; 159(20):2405–11.

[55] Benett WM, Aronoff GR, Golper TA, et al. Drug prescribing in renal failure: dosing guidelines for adults. 4th edition. Philadelphia: American College of Physicians; 2000.

[56] Smith JW, Seidl LG, Cluff LE. Studies on the epidemiology of adverse drug reactions. V. Clinical factors influencing susceptibility. Ann Intern Med 1966;65(4):629–40.

[57] Shemin D, Bostom AG, Laliberty P, et al. Residual renal function and mortality risk in hemodialysis patients. Am J Kidney Dis 2001;38(1):85–90.

[58] Little JW, Falace DA, Miller CS, et al. Chronic renal failure and dialysis. In: Little JW, Falace DA, Miller CS, et al, editors. Dental management of the medically compromised patient. 6th edition. Philadelphia: Mosby; 2002. p. 147–60.

[59] Schmith VD, Piraino B, Smith RB, et al. Alprazolam in end-stage renal disease. II. Pharmacodynamics. Clin Pharmacol Ther 1992;51(5):533–40.

[60] Szeto HH, Inturissi CE, Houde R, et al. Accumulation of normeperidine, an active metabolite of meperidine, in patients with renal failure of cancer. Ann Intern Med 1977;86(6):738–41.

[61] Peterson GM, Randall CT, Paterson J. Plasma levels of morphine and morphine glucuronides in the treatment of cancer pain: relationship to renal function and route of administration. Eur J Clin Pharmacol 1990;38(2): 121–4.

[62] Malhotra V, Diwam S. Anesthesia and the renal and genitourinary systems. In: Miller R, editor. Anesthesia. 5th edition. New York: Churchill Livingstone; 2000. p. 1934–59.

[63] Ickx B, Cockshott ID, Varvais L. Propofol infusion for induction and maintenance of anaesthesia in patients with end-stage renal disease. Br J Anaesth 1998;81(6): 854–60.

[64] Kirvela M, Olkkola KT, Rosenberg PH, et al. Pharmacokinetics of propofol and haemodynamic changes during induction of anaesthesia in uraemic patients. Br J Anaesth 1992;68(2):178–82.

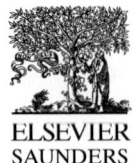

ELSEVIER
SAUNDERS

Oral Maxillofacial Surg Clin N Am 18 (2006) 213 – 225

ORAL AND
MAXILLOFACIAL
SURGERY CLINICS
of North America

Perioperative Management of the Patient with Liver Disease and Management of the Chronic Alcoholic

Earl Clarkson, DDS*, Sanjeev Raj Bhatia, MDS, FDS RCS (Eng), DDS

Oral & Maxillofacial Surgery, The Brooklyn Hospital Center, 121 DeKalb Avenue, Brooklyn, NY 11201, USA

Each year millions of Americans undergo surgical procedures requiring local, general, or spinal epidural anesthesia. A disproportionate number of the patients are older than age 65, and up to 10% of the patients have end-stage liver disease. Most patients do not suffer complications as a result of the surgical procedure or the anesthetic. However, about 3% to 10% of patients experience significant morbidity, often caused by infections or cardiac or pulmonary complications. Patients who have serious liver disease are generally believed to be at increased risk for perioperative morbidity and mortality. Appropriate preoperative evaluation is the cornerstone of successful intra- and postoperative management of the effects of anesthesia and surgery and is necessary for combating complications that may result from preexisting liver disease.

The presence of decompensated liver disease increases the risk for postoperative complications. Acute liver disease (eg, viral hepatitis, alcoholic hepatitis) is associated with more ongoing hepatocytic damage than chronic liver disease. Patients who have hepatitis generally have higher morbidity rates than those who have cholestatic disease. Patients who have chronic liver disease, including conditions such as chronic hepatitis C, whose liver function is preserved may not have an increased operative risk but are susceptible to hypoxic injuries. A comprehensive understanding of the pathophysiology of liver diseases, how the diseases impact liver physiology, and the effects of anesthesia is required for perioperative management of patients who have liver diseases. This article discusses each factor with emphasis on intricate management.

Pathophysiology

Liver disease is typically categorized as parenchymal or cholestatic in nature. Parenchymal diseases could be acute or chronic viral hepatitis and chronic alcoholic cirrhotic process, whereas cholestatic disease indicates obstruction of extrahepatic biliary system.

Parenchymal disease remains asymptomatic until liver damage reaches an advanced level. Nevertheless, the disease process is deeply embedded in the cellular level and ongoing injury occurs at a slow and steady pace; therefore, the injury is profound and extensive. Multiple organ system dysfunction is the hallmark of advanced parenchymal liver disease. Most of the parenchymal disease processes result in cirrhosis of liver.

In cirrhosis, hyperdynamic cardiovascular state becomes rampant with portal hypertension; high cardiac output; low peripheral vascular resistance and congestive heart failure; and impending cardiomyopathy. Portal hypertension results in decreased hepatic blood flow, decreased hepatocytic perfusion, formation of arteriovenous collaterals in splanchnic organs presenting as gastroesophageal varices, and precipitation of ascites. Ascites further interferes with alveolar ventilation and venous return. This process forms a whole array of complex cycle of events that become self-perpetuating, compromising the patient's homeostasis.

* Corresponding author.
E-mail address: eicddsoms@yahoo.com (E. Clarkson).

1042-3699/06/$ – see front matter © 2006 Elsevier Inc. All rights reserved.
doi:10.1016/j.coms.2005.12.007

Cholestatic disease is characterized by obstruction of biliary system and accumulation of bilirubin, cholesterol, and bile acids that are normally excreted with the bile. These patients have cardiovascular dysfunction similar to cirrhosis of the liver with decreased responsiveness to catecholamines. Therefore, these patients cannot tolerate hypotensive episodes or a hypovolemic state and are susceptible to cardiovascular collapse.

Altered physiologic functions

Patient response during the perioperative period may be influenced by disease-induced alterations of important functions of liver, including

- Glucose homeostasis
- Protein synthesis
- Drug metabolism
- Coagulation
- Bilirubin formation and excretion
- Phagocytizing bacteria absorbed from the gastrointestinal tract into the portal vein

Glucose homeostasis

The liver is responsible for the storage and release of glucose. Glucose enters hepatocytes where it is stored as glycogen. Glycogenolysis releases glucose back into the systemic circulation to maintain normal blood glucose concentration. The liver can store only about 75 g of glycogen, which can be depleted by 24 to 48 hours of starvation. Glucose homeostasis depends primarily on conversion of lactate, glycerol, and amino acids to glucose when liver glycogen stores are depleted. Exogenous sources of glucose during the fasting period associated with surgery become important when glycogen stores are depleted by poor preoperative nutrition and when gluconeogenesis is inhibited by anesthesia. Patients who have cirrhosis may develop hypoglycemia in the perioperative period.

Protein synthesis

All proteins except gamma globulins and antihemophiliac factor are synthesized in the rough endoplasmic reticulum of hepatocytes. Approximately 10 to 15 g of albumin is produced daily to maintain plasma concentrations of this protein in the normal range of 3.5 to 5.5 g/dL. Plasma albumin concentrations lower than 3.5 g/dL may reflect significant liver disease. The half-life of albumin, however, is about 23 days, emphasizing that decreased plasma concentrations of this protein will not reflect acute liver dysfunction. Protein synthesis in the liver is important for drug binding, coagulation, and production of enzymes necessary for hydrolysis of ester linkages.

Drug metabolism

Altered protein quantity and quality

When liver disease results in decreased albumin production, fewer sites will be available for drug binding. As a result, the unbound pharmacologically active fraction of drugs (eg, thiopental) increases. Increased drug sensitivities caused by decreased protein binding are most likely to manifest when plasma albumin concentrations are less than 2.5 g/dL.

Hydrolysis of ester linkages

Severe liver disease may decrease the production of pseudocholinesterase necessary for hydrolysis of drugs such as succinylcholine and mivacurium and ester local anesthetics. As a result, the duration of apnea after the administration of succinylcholine could be prolonged in the presence of liver disease. Prolonged effects of these drugs, however, are unlikely to be caused by liver disease alone, and atypical plasma cholinesterase enzyme must be suspected.

Metabolism

Drug metabolism characterized by the conversion of lipid-soluble drugs to more water-soluble and pharmacologically less active substances is controlled by microsomal enzymes, which are present in the smooth endoplasmic reticulum of hepatocytes. Chronic liver disease may interfere with metabolism of drugs because of decreased numbers of enzyme-containing hepatocytes or decreased hepatic blood flow seen with cirrhosis of the liver. Prolonged elimination half-times for morphine alfentanil, diazepam lidocaine, and pancuronium have been shown in these patents.

Repeated injections of these drugs are likely to produce cumulative effects in patients who have severe liver disease. Volatile anesthetics may interfere with clearance of drugs from the plasma because of decreases in hepatic blood flow or inhibition of drug-metabolizing enzymes. Accelerated drug metabolism could accompany cirrhosis of liver. For example, in the presence of decreased numbers of hepatocytes, the amount of drug presented to each cell increases. This effect stimulates microsomal enzyme activity. Enzyme induction may also be a response to chronic drug therapy or alcohol abuse.

Coagulation

Coagulation abnormalities must be suspected in patients who have liver disease because hepatocytes are responsible for the synthesis of most procoagulants. The adequacy of clotting factor levels is evaluated by measuring prothrombin time, partial thromboplastin time, and bleeding time. Liver function must be dramatically depressed before impaired coagulation manifests because many coagulation factors require only 20% to 30% of their normal levels to prevent bleeding. Nevertheless, the plasma half-time of hepatic clotting factors such as prothrombin and fibrinogen is short, and acute liver dysfunction is likely to be associated with clotting abnormalities.

Liver disease associated with splenomegaly can alter the normal coagulation mechanism independent of procoagulant synthesis by trapping platelets in the spleen, precipitating thrombocytopenia. Another predisposing factor to bleeding diathesis is the failure of a diseased liver to clear plasma activators of the fibrinolytic system.

Bilirubin formation and excretion

Bilirubin is the end product of hemoglobin metabolism in the reticuloendothelial system. It is transported to the liver in protein-bound or unconjugated form where it is conjugated with glucuronic acid to become water-soluble and is thus excreted into biliary canaliculi to reach the intestines. The conjugation process is controlled by glucosyltransferase, which is regulated by the microsomal enzyme–induction system of the liver.

The liver is involved in pharmacokinetics by eliminating exogenous and endogenous compounds through metabolism and excreting unchanged compounds in the bile. The hepatic elimination of drugs is influenced by hepatic blood flow and hepatocytes function.

The concept of hepatic blood flow

The liver receives 25% of the cardiac output, but 70% of its hepatic blood flow occurs through the portal vein and less than 30% comes from the hepatic artery, indicating that its oxygen supply is very minimal. In normal conditions the liver receives 50% of its oxygen through the unsaturated blood in the portal vein and 50% from oxygenated blood in the hepatic artery. A reciprocal relationship exists between these vascular systems; when portal venous supply decreases, the hepatic artery supply increases, and vice versa.

This relationship could be altered perioperatively for several reasons, making the liver susceptible to decreased blood flow and ischemia. Volatile anesthetic agents cause peripheral vasodilatation, hypotension, and decreased cardiac output, which decrease not only the hepatic artery flow but also the portal venous flow. Hepatic blood flow is decreased by 20% to 30% with volatile anesthetic agents. Isoflurane does not cause as much decrease in blood flow compared with halothane. Arterial hypoxemia, hypercarbia, or increased circulating catecholamines cause an increase in splanchnic vascular resistance and decreased hepatic blood flow. Hepatic circulation is also supplied by beta receptors, and use of β-blockers could decrease the hepatic blood flow if used for cardiac conditions. Positive pressure ventilation, cirrhosis, or presence of CHF increases the central venous pressure causing backpressure or increase in hepatic venous pressure, thereby decreasing the perfusion of hepatocytes. And lastly, closeness of the liver during surgery, such as laparotomy, or undue pressure during iliac crest harvest could decrease the hepatic flow as well.

Liver function tests

Liver function tests are rarely specific and only indicate change in the homeostasis of liver (Table 1). Moreover, liver has an abundant reserve of structure and function and the tests are not altered until the hepatic damage is advanced.

Researchers have suggested that existing liver disease makes the hepatocytes more vulnerable to intraoperative insults such as hypoxia and hypercarbia. These conditions could lead to postoperative hepatic dysfunction. Nevertheless, hepatic injury

Table 1
Live function tests

Test	Normal range
Albumin	3.5–5.5 g/dL
Bilirubin	0.3–1.1 mg/dL
Unconjugated B (indirect)	0.2–0.7 mg/dL
Conjugated B (direct)	0.1–0.4 mg/dL
SGOT	10–40 U/mL
SGPT	5–35 U/mL
Alkaline phosphatase	10–30 U/mL
Prothrombin time	12–14 s

Abbreviations: SGOT, serum glutamic-oxaloacetic transaminase; SGPT, serum glutamine pyruvate transaminase.

Table 2
Modified Child-Pugh scores

	Points*		
	1	2	3
Albumin (g/dL)	>3.5	2.8–3.5	<2.8
Bilirubin (mg/dL)	<2	2–3	>3
Prothrombin (seconds prolonged)	<4	4–6	>6
International Normalized Ratio	<1.7	1.7–2.3	>2.3
Ascites	Absent	Slight-moderate	severe
Encephalopathy	None	Grade 1–11	Grade 111–IV

Class A = 5–6 points.
Class B = 7–9 points.
Class C = 10–15 points.
  * Points indicate the scoring system for cirrhosis.

could be related to prehepatic, perioperative, or post-operative causes.

*Prehepatic causes of hepatic injury
(bilirubin overload)*

Prehepatic causes of hepatic injury, which reflect bilirubin overload, include hemolysis (decrease in hematocrit or increase in reticulocyte count), hematoma resorption, whole blood transfusion (shows increase in unconjugated bilirubin; one unit contains 250 mg of bilirubin), intrahepatic events (direct hepatocyte injury), drug toxicity, septicemia, hypoxemia, and hypercarbia. Serum aminotransferase increases as injured hepatocytes release their stored enzymes, and conjugated bilirubin increases more than unconjugated bilirubin.

Posthepatic causes (bile duct obstruction)

Posthepatic causes reflect bile duct obstruction and show increased conjugated bilirubin and alkaline phosphatase, which is a characteristic finding. Benign postoperative intrahepatic cholestasis may occur in elderly patients who experience complications related to intraoperative events of hypoxemia and massive blood transfusions.

Risk factor assessment for surgery

The extent of surgery and the type and severity of liver disease play key roles in determining the specific risk. Other factors, such as cardiac disease, pulmonary gas exchange abnormalities, and malnutrition, compound the risks for surgery in patients who have liver disease. Laparotomy in patients who have viral hepatitis has a 10% mortality and 12%

morbidity rate and correlates with the extent of surgery. Patients who have mild chronic hepatitis and well-preserved liver function tolerate surgery well, unlike patients who have decompensated disease.

In patients who have alcoholic hepatitis, elective surgery is associated with a high mortality rate unless surgery is deferred until prolonged abstinence and biochemical and clinical progress is noted. Patients who have stable cirrhosis without signs of liver failure, encephalopathy, poor nutritional status, albumin more than 3.5, and bilirubin less than 3.0 can usually tolerate surgery [1].

Elective surgery is tolerated in Child-Pugh's class A cirrhosis; permissible in class B cirrhosis (with preoperative preparation); and contraindicated in class C cirrhosis (Table 2). Table 3 defines the surgical risk based on preoperative evaluation of liver functions.

The liver diseases must be well understood to fully comprehend the perioperative or postoperative management of patients who have underlying liver

Table 3
Surgical risk based on preoperative evaluation of liver functions

Test	Risk		
	Minimal	Modest	Marked
Bilirubin mg/dL	<2	2–3	>3
Albumin g/dL	>3.5	3.0–3.5	<3
Prothrombin time increase	None	Moderate	Severe
Nutrition	Excellent	Good	Poor
Ascites	None	Moderate	Marked

Prothrombin time and bilirubin are probably the best measures of hepatic function.
Data from Strunin L. Preoperative assessment of the patient with liver dysfunction. Br J Anaesth 1978;50:25–34.

pathology. The most common diseases are discussed with a wider perspective regarding management.

Hepatitis A

Hepatitis A virus (HAV) has a worldwide distribution. The highest seropositivity (antibody to HAV) is observed in adults in urban Africa, Asia, and South America. The United States has low endemicity. HAV has recently been considered one of the more common causes of acute hepatitis. A shift in the pattern of infection from a younger to an older patient population has occurred, which may lay the framework for potential epidemics in the future. In the United States, most cases are symptomatic, with an 80% frequency of icteric cases. HAV commonly has four phases:

> Prodromal phase: flu-like symptoms, anorexia, nausea, vomiting, fatigue, malaise, low-grade fever, myalgia (1–14 days)
> Icteric phase: bilirubinuria, pale stool, jaundice (adults more than children), abdominal pain, pruritus, arthralgia, vasculitic rash (14–21 days)
> Post-icteric phase: gradual recovery (10–14 days)
> Relapse: protracted course of symptoms or relapse of acute symptoms after apparent resolution (adults more than children)

The various laboratory studies used to determine HAV include:

- Anti-HAV IgM: sensitive and specific, positive for 3 to 6 months, rises with acute phase, usually accompanies first rise in ALT
- Anti-HAV IgG: appears soon after IgM, persists for years; absence of IgM indicates past infection or vaccination; provides protective immunity
- Alanine aminotransferase (ALT) and aspartate aminotransferase (AST): sensitive for disease of levels more than 10,000 U/mL; levels return to normal in 20 weeks
- Alkaline phosphatase: rises during acute phase and after rise in ALT during cholestatic phase
- Bilirubin: follows rise in ALT and AST, remains high for up to 3 months; rise lasting more than 3 months indicates cholestatic HAV infection. Older patients have higher levels; direct and indirect fractions increase because of hemolysis
- Albumin levels: modest fall
- Prothrombin time: usually normal range but could rise with protracted disease process
- Complete blood count: mild lymphocytosis

Pathophysiology

HAV is a single-stranded, linear RNA enterovirus and a member of the Picornaviridae family. It is resistant to denaturation by ether, acid (pH 3.0), drying, and temperatures as high as 56°C and as low as −20°C. HAV can remain viable for many years. In humans, viral replication depends on hepatocyte uptake and synthesis, and assembly occurs exclusively in liver cells. No antibody cross-reactivity with other viruses causing acute hepatitis has been identified. Acquisition results almost exclusively from ingestion (ie, fecal–oral transmission), although isolated cases of parenteral transmission have been reported.

Complications

Generally, HAV infection elicits no lasting sequel. Death is rare, occurring in less than 0.2% of cases. Death is more frequent in elderly patients and those who have underlying liver disease. Acute renal failure, interstitial nephritis, pancreatitis, red blood cell aplasia, agranulocytosis, bone marrow aplasia, transient heart block, Guillain-Barré syndrome, acute arthritis, Still's disease, lupus-like syndrome, and Sjögren syndrome have been shown to be associated with HAV infection.

Hepatitis B

Hepatitis B virus (HBV) is a worldwide health care problem, especially in developing areas. An estimated one third of the global population has been infected with this virus. Approximately 350 million people are lifelong carriers, and only 2% spontaneously seroconvert annually. In the United States, an estimated 200,000 new cases of HBV occur annually, and 1 to 1.25 million people are carriers [2]. The prevalence of the disease is higher among African Americans and persons of Hispanic or Asian origin. HBV is transmitted hematogenously and sexually. Antiviral treatment may be effective in approximately one third of patients, and liver transplantation currently seems to be the only viable treatment for the latest stages of this disease for select candidates. The immunology of HBV is as follows:

> Hepatitis B surface antigen (HBsAg): the S gene encodes the viral envelope
> Hepatitis B core antigen (HBcAg): encloses viral DNA, initiates cellular immune response

Hepatitis B early antigen (HBeAg): part of core gene, marker of active viral replication, can be detected in patients who have circulating serum HBV DNA

Anti-HBsAg: confers immunity, detected in patients who had HBV infection and were vaccinated

Anti-HBcAg: detected in every patient who had previous exposure to HBV

Anti-HBeAg: indicates antigen has been cleared and suggests nonreplicative stage

IgM: indicates acute infection or reactivation

IgG: indicates chronic infection

Pathophysiology

HBV is a Hepadnavirus. It is an extremely resistant strain capable of withstanding extreme temperatures and humidity. It can survive when stored for 15 years at $-20°C$, for 24 months at $-80°C$, for 6 months at room temperatures, and for 7 days at $44°C$. The pathogenesis and clinical manifestations are caused by the interaction of the virus and the host immune system. The latter attacks the HBV and causes liver injury. Activated $CD4^+$ and $CD8^+$ lymphocytes recognize various HBV-derived peptides located on the surface of the hepatocytes, and an immunologic reaction occurs. Impaired immune reactions (eg, cytokine release, antibody production) or tolerant immune status result in chronic hepatitis. In particular, a restricted T-cell–mediated lymphocytic response occurs against the HBV-infected hepatocytes. The outcome of this infection is a complicated viral–host interaction resulting in either an acute symptomatic or asymptomatic disease. Patients may become immune to HBV or may develop a chronic carrier state. Later consequences are cirrhosis and the development of hepatocellular carcinoma (HCC).

Stages in the viral life cycle

Four stages have been identified in the viral life cycle. The first stage is immune tolerance. The duration of this stage for healthy adults is approximately 2 to 4 weeks and represents the incubation period. For newborns, the duration of this period is often decades. Active viral replication is known to continue despite little or no elevation in the aminotransferase levels and no symptoms of illness.

In the second stage, an inflammatory reaction with a cytopathic effect occurs. HBeAg can be identified in the sera and a decline of HBV DNA levels is seen. The duration of this stage for patients who have acute infection is approximately 3 to 4 weeks (symp-

tomatic period). For patients who have chronic infection, 10 years or more may elapse before cirrhosis develops.

In the third stage, the host can target the infected hepatocytes and the HBV. Viral replication no longer occurs, and HBeAb can be detected. The HBV DNA levels are lower or undetectable, and aminotransferase levels are within the reference range. In this stage, the viral genome is integrated into the host's hepatocyte genome. HBsAg is still present.

In the fourth stage, the virus cannot be detected and antibodies to various viral antigens have been produced.

Acute phase

Anicteric hepatitis

Anicteric hepatitis is the predominant form of expression for this disease. Most patients are asymptomatic. Patients who experience symptomatology have the same symptoms as patients who develop icteric hepatitis. Patients who have anicteric hepatitis have a greater tendency to develop chronic hepatitis.

Icteric hepatitis

Icteric hepatitis is associated with the prodromal period, during which a serum sickness–like syndrome can occur. The symptomatology is more constitutional and includes anorexia; nausea; vomiting; low-grade fever; myalgia; fatigability; disordered gustatory acuity and smell sensations (eg, aversion to food and cigarettes); and right upper-quadrant and epigastric pain.

Hyperacute, acute, and subacute hepatitis

Hyperacute, acute, and subacute hepatitis present as advanced stages that may be characterized by hepatic encephalopathy, somnolence, disturbances in sleep pattern, mental confusion, and coma. Physical examination shows low-grade fever, jaundice (10 days after the appearance of constitutional symptomatology and lasting for 1 to 3 months), hepatomegaly (mildly enlarged soft liver), splenomegaly (5%–15%), palmar erythema (rarely), and spider nevi (rarely).

Chronic phase

Patients who have chronic hepatitis can be healthy carriers without any evidence of active disease, and are also asymptomatic.

In the replicative stage these patients may complain of symptoms similar to those of acute hepatitis, including fatigue, anorexia, nausea, mild upper-quadrant pain, or discomfort, or hepatic decompen-

sation. Hepatomegaly, palmar erythema, or spider angioma would be indicative signs. The chronic phase could end in an asymptomatic carrier state, chronic hepatitis, chronic cirrhosis, or hepatocellular carcinoma.

Hepatitis C

The World Health Organization [3] estimates that 170 million individuals worldwide are infected with hepatitis C virus (HCV). According to the Centers for Disease Control and Prevention, an estimated 1.8% of the United States population is positive for HCV antibodies. Three of four persons who are seropositive are also viremic, corresponding with an estimated 2.7 million people who have active HCV infection nationwide. Infection caused by HCV accounts for 20% of all cases of acute hepatitis, an estimated 30,000 new acute infections, and 8,000 to 10,000 deaths each year in the United States. The various laboratory studies used to determine HCV include:

- Anti-HCV (enzyme immunoassay): 97% specific but cannot differentiate acute versus chronic. False-positive results in patients infected with HIV, those who are immunocompromised, those who have renal failure, blood donors, and even health care workers
- ALT: increases or decreases with course of infection
- Recombinant immunoblot assay: used to confirm HCV infection when detection of antibodies against two or more antigens found a positive result followed by two negative results suggest resolution
- Qualitative assay: polymerase chain reaction—an amplified qualitative test for HCV
- Quantitative assay: polymerase chain reaction or transcription-medicated amplification to monitor response
- HCV genotyping: helpful in predicting the likelihood of response and duration of treatment. Patients who have genotype 1 and 4 are treated for 12 months, whereas 6 months is sufficient for other genotypes

Pathophysiology

HCV is a spherical, enveloped, single-stranded RNA virus belonging to the Flaviviridae family. The natural targets of HCV are hepatocytes and, possibly, B lymphocytes. More than 50% of hepatocytes are infected with the virus. Moreover, it generates several mutant viruses known as *quasispecies*. Quasispecies pose a major challenge to immune-mediated control of HCV and may explain the variable clinical course and the difficulties in vaccine development.

Currently, HCV is predominantly transmitted by means of percutaneous exposure to infected blood. In the past, blood products were a major source of HCV, but in 2004 Stramer and colleagues [4] estimated the risk for acquiring HCV from blood transfusions to be 1 in 230,000 donations. HCV may also be transmitted through acupuncture, tattooing, and sharing razors. Needle stick injuries in the health care setting result in a 3% risk for HCV transmission, but HCV prevalence among health care workers has been found to be similar to that of the general population. Nosocomial patient-to-patient transmission may occur through a contaminated colonoscope, through dialysis, or during surgery. In 2001, Yeung and colleagues [5] reported that uncommon routes of HCV transmission, which affect less than 5% of the individuals at risk, include high-risk sexual activity and maternal–fetal transmission. Coinfection with HIV type 1 seems to increase the risk for sexual and maternal–fetal HCV transmission.

Severe progression of hepatitis C to cirrhosis was shown to occur in approximately 20% of patients who have chronic infection, and is largely responsible for the recent increase in the incidence of HCC in the United States. This number is expected to increase because of the current large pool of patients who have chronic infections.

Course of disease

Most patients with chronic HCV are asymptomatic or may experience nonspecific symptoms such as fatigue or malaise in the absence of hepatic synthetic dysfunction. In these patients, abnormal physical examination findings are not shown until portal hypertension or decompensated liver disease develops. A patient who has chronic HCV infection could present with features such as palmar erythema, spider nevi, Dupuytren's contracture, clubbing, icteric sclera, temporal muscle wasting, enlarged parotid, gynecomastia, ascites, and ankle edema.

The treatment goals for chronic HCV infection are sustained eradication of HCV and prevention of progression to cirrhosis, HCC, and decompensated liver disease requiring liver transplantation. Physicians should remember that HCV is prevalent in patients who have end-stage renal disease and can also be an important cause of renal failure, and that 30% to 50% of HIV patients are coinfected with HCV. Coinfection with HIV accelerates the clinical progression of HCV

and increases the risk for perinatal HCV transmission. These patients could be taking multiple antiviral medications, such as interferon, ribavirin, and polyethylene glycol therapy.

Hepatitis D

Approximately 15 million people are reported to be infected worldwide with hepatitis D virus (HDV). HDV is observed more commonly among patients who have a history of intravenous drug use and in persons from the Mediterranean basin.

Pathophysiology

HDV was discovered in 1977 and is an RNA virus that is structurally unrelated to HAV, HBV, or HCV. HDV causes a unique infection that requires the assistance of viral particles from HBV (HBsAg) to replicate and infect other hepatocytes. Its clinical course is varied and ranges from acute self-limited infection to acute fulminant liver failure. Chronic liver infection can lead to end-stage liver disease and associated complications.

Course of disease

HDV infection is clinically indistinguishable from other forms of viral hepatitis. As many as 90% of patients are asymptomatic. Simultaneous infection with HBV and HDV is known as *coinfection* and results in fulminant liver failure in 1% of patients. Complete clinical recovery and clearance of HBV and HDV coinfection are the most common outcomes except in 5% of patients who become chronic carriers. Infection with HDV in a patient who is already HBsAg-positive is known as *superinfection* and results in fulminant liver failure in 5% of patients. Approximately 80% to 90% develop chronic HDV infection. In these patients, disease progresses more rapidly to cirrhosis and they may develop HCC. The various laboratory studies used to determine HDV include:

- HDV Ag: positive in 20%
- HDV RNA: positive in 90% by reverse transcriptase polymerase chain reaction
- Anti-HDV IgM: positive initially
- Anti-HDV IgG: positive later in the course of disease
- Anti-HDV IgA: exclusively associated with chronic HDV infections
- Anti-HBc IgM: positive except with superinfection in which it is absent

- HBsAg: required for HDV replication but may be suppressed to undetectable levels with active HDV replication
- ALT: increased more than 500 IU/L
- Prothrombin: international normalized ratio may be raised in fulminant or chronic conditions

Hepatitis E

Hepatitis E virus (HEV) has worldwide distribution, but is predominantly seen in tropical climates, areas with inadequate sanitation, and in people who have poor personal hygiene. The reservoir of HEV is unknown, but it may be transmitted through animals. The prevalence rate of anti-HEV antibodies is less than 2% [6].

Pathophysiology

HEV is a icosahedral and nonenveloped virus. HEV is an enterically transmitted self-limited infection. It is spread by water contaminated with fecal matter within endemic areas. Outbreaks can be epidemic and individual. HEV has similar features with HAV. The incubation period ranges from 15 days to 60 days and the course of infection has two phases, termed *prodromal* and *icteric*, which are similar in signs and symptoms to HAV and do not develop into a chronic state. The various laboratory studies used to determine HEV include:

- Anti-HEV IgM: nonsensitive and nonspecific, positive for 3 to 6 months, rises with acute phase, usually accompanies first rise in ALT
- Anti-HEV IgG: appears soon after IgM, persists for years; absence of IgM indicates past infection or vaccination; provides protective immunity; indicates chronic phase
- AST ALT: sensitive for disease of levels more than 10,000 U/mL; levels return to normal in 20 weeks
- Alkaline phosphatase: rise during acute phase and after rise in ALT during cholestatic phase
- Bilirubin: follows rise in ALT and AST, remain high for up to 3 months. Older patients have higher levels; both direct and indirect fractions increase
- Albumin levels: modest fall
- Prothrombin time: usually normal range but could rise with protracted disease
- Complete blood count: mild lymphocytosis or sometimes leukopenia

Alcoholic hepatitis

Alcohol abuse is the most common cause of serious liver disease in Western societies. In the United States alone, alcoholic liver disease affects more than 2 million people (approximately 1% of the population). Although no genetic predilection is noted for any particular race, alcoholism and alcoholic liver disease are more common in minority groups, particularly among Native Americans. Likewise, since the 1960s, death rates of alcoholic hepatitis and cirrhosis have consistently been far greater for the nonwhite population than for the white population. The nonwhite male rate of alcoholic hepatitis is 1.7 times the white male rate, 1.9 times the nonwhite female rate, and almost 4 times the white female rate. Women are more susceptible than men to the adverse effects of alcohol. Women develop alcoholic hepatitis after a shorter period and smaller amounts of alcohol abuse than men, and alcoholic hepatitis progresses more rapidly in women than in men.

Alcoholic hepatitis is a syndrome of progressive inflammatory liver injury associated with long-term heavy intake of ethanol. Patients who are severely affected present with subacute onset of fever, hepatomegaly, leukocytosis, marked impairment of liver function (eg, jaundice, coagulopathy), and manifestations of portal hypertension (eg, ascites, hepatic encephalopathy, variceal hemorrhage). The true prevalence of alcoholic hepatitis, especially its milder forms, is unknown because patients may be asymptomatic and never seek medical attention, presenting a challenge for operative management.

Pathophysiology

Genetic, environmental, nutritional, metabolic, and, more recently, immunologic factors have been implicated as various causes of alcoholic hepatitis, principally affecting ethanol metabolism. The major site of ethanol metabolism is the liver, although most tissues can perform enzymatic oxidative or nonoxidative metabolism of ethanol. In the liver, alcohol dehydrogenase, the microsomal ethanol oxidizing system, and peroxisomal catalase oxidize the ethanol to acetaldehyde, which is then further metabolized to acetate by acetaldehyde dehydrogenase. Acetaldehyde is a hepatotoxic reactive metabolite.

The estimated minimum daily ethanol intake required for the development of cirrhosis is 40 g for men and 20 g for women older than 15 to 20 years. Furthermore, in patients who continue to drink after a diagnosis of alcoholic liver disease, the 5-year survival rate is approximately 30% for women compared with 70% for men [7].

Course of disease

Heavy alcohol use is a prerequisite for the development of alcoholic hepatitis. The history is usually apparent; however, some patients' alcohol use may be covert and therefore should be suspected during preoperative stage.

Clues to the presence of alcoholism include a history of multiple motor vehicle accidents, convictions for driving while intoxicated, and poor interpersonal relationships. Alcoholism exhibits a genetic predisposition, and a history of alcoholism in a close relative may also indicate that a patient is at risk.

Patients who have clinically symptomatic alcoholic hepatitis typically present with nonspecific symptoms of nausea, malaise, and low-grade fever.

Mild tachypnea with primary respiratory alkalosis may be observed. The liver is usually enlarged, often with mild hepatic tenderness. Hepatomegaly results from steatosis and swelling of injured hepatocytes.

In milder cases of alcoholic hepatitis, a slight elevation of the aspartate aminotransferase level may be the only diagnostic clue [8]. The clinical presentation may be precipitated through complications of impaired liver function or portal hypertension, such as upper gastrointestinal hemorrhage from esophageal varices; confusion and lethargy from hepatic encephalopathy; or increased abdominal girth from ascites.

Spider angiomata, proximal muscle wasting, altered hair distribution, and gynecomastia may be observed, although these findings most commonly reflect coexistent cirrhosis.

A person who uses alcohol heavily may seek medical attention with complaints of a medical illness that produces altered mental status or persistent vomiting, which in turn triggers alcohol withdrawal symptoms. In such instances, the physician must be alert to the presence of a precipitating illness (eg, subdural hematoma, acute pancreatitis, gastrointestinal hemorrhage), the likelihood of alcohol withdrawal symptoms (eg, seizures, delirium tremens), and the problems associated with alcoholic hepatitis.

Complications

Coagulopathy and thrombocytopenia

Hypoprothrombinemia ensues in the course of severe alcoholic hepatitis. Administering fresh-frozen plasma temporarily restores the depleted hepatic prothrombin stores. The value of parenteral ad-

ministration of vitamin K is dubious because the hepatocytes are incapable of synthesizing new pro-thrombin. Platelet transfusions are indicated to correct thrombocytopenia before or during the surgery.

Hemochromatosis
Iron overload.   Several histopathologic studies have shown that as many as 50% of patients who have alcoholic liver disease have increased hepatic iron content compared with healthy controls. This excess deposition of iron may play a significant role in the progression of the alcoholic liver damage.

Altered drug metabolism
Acetaminophen toxicity.   Increased levels of toxic metabolites lead to hepatic necrosis.

Other common considerations include chronic pancreatitis with biliary strictures and pancreatico-biliary neoplasms. Patients who have alcoholic liver disease should be immunized against common infectious pathogens, including HAV, HBV, pneumo-cocci, and influenza A virus.

Alcohol withdrawal

Alcohol withdrawal occurs when illness or hospitalization interrupts alcohol intake, and is associated with significant mortality. Tremors, irritability, anorexia, and nausea characterize minor alcohol withdrawal. Symptoms usually appear within a few hours after reduction or cessation of alcohol consumption and resolve within 48 hours.

Treatment of alcoholic withdrawal includes (1) placing the patient in a well-lit room, offering them reassurance, and having family or friends present, (2) administering thiamine, 100 mg intramuscularly, followed by 100 mg administered orally every day, (3) administering multivitamins that contain folic acid and a balanced diet as tolerated, and (4) administering chlordiazepoxide, 25 to 100 mg orally every 6 hours, with dosage adjusted until the patient is calm.

Alcohol withdrawal seizures, which may be one or a few brief generalized convulsions, occur 12 to 48 hours after cessation of ethanol intake. Antiepileptic drugs are not indicated in such a situation. Other causes for seizures must be excluded. If hypoglycemia is present, thiamine should be administered before glucose.

Maintenance of fluid and electrolyte balance is important because these patients are susceptible to hypomagnesemia, hypokalemia, hypoglycemia, and fluid losses.

Anesthesia and liver disease

Decreased hepatic blood flow

Most inhaled anesthetics decrease hepatic blood flow because of their potential for peripheral vaso-dilatation [9]. This decease could lead to episodes of hepatic hypoxia and concomitant hepatocytic necrosis, as discussed in the context of hepatic blood flow. Isoflurane is a safer choice because the effect on hepatic blood flow and oxygenation is much less that that of halothane and is supposed to increase hepatic blood flow. Hypercarbia causes decreased portal blood flow and must be avoided. Hypotension resulting in shock liver injury is possible. Close monitoring of renal function is necessary, especially if fluid shifts have occurred. Meticulous hemostasis is very important in preventing a hypotensive crisis.

Halothane hepatitis

Halothane hepatitis is a life-threatening immune-mediated condition. On exposure to halothane, the proteins on the surface of hepatocytes are modified by trifluoroacetyl chloride (TFC), a metabolite of halo-thane. Thus, these surface proteins are converted from self-antigen to neoantigens or nonself antigens. The body forms IgG antibodies against these neo-antigens. Further exposure of halothane causes the antigen–antibody assault on the liver, precipitating halothane hepatitis. Risk factors include multiple exposures, obesity, female gender, and middle age.

Other fluorinated anesthetic agents, such as isoflurane, desflurane, and enflurane, may also have TFA as one of their metabolites and therefore could potentially cause similar liver injury, but this has been found to be much less likely than with halothane [10]. However, patients who are genetically susceptible to this condition who have become sensitized to halothane could experience clinical evidence of hepatitis later in life when exposed to isoflurane or similar anesthetic. Sevoflurane does not metabolize to TFA, and therefore has the least possibility of causing immune-mediated hepatotoxicity or even cross-sensitivity in patients previously exposed to halothane.

Altered metabolism of drugs

In liver disease, the metabolism of drugs is altered and results in delayed clearance of drugs such as midazolam, fentanyl, and morphine. The half-life of lidocaine is increased by 300%, and the half-life of benzodiazepines is increased by 100%. Succinylcho-

line or mivacurium may have prolonged actions. Atracurium and doxacurium may be safer to use as muscle relaxants. However, the drugs can be decreased by half and modified as needed. Modifying drug dosages based on liver function and titrating sedative and pain management prevent exacerbation of hepatic encephalopathy.

Perioperative management

The perioperative management of patients who have liver dysfunction is summarized in Box 1.

Box 1. Synopsis of perioperative management — a systematic approach

Consider differentials

- Hepatitis A, B, C, D, and E
- Alcoholic hepatitis
- Autoimmune hepatitis
- Biliary obstruction/stricture
- Budd-Chiari syndrome
- Cholangitis, cholecystitis
- Isoniazid hepatotoxicity/acetaminophen poisoning
- Drug-induced hepatitis/possibility of halothane hepatitis

Functional disturbances associated with liver disease

Bleeding problems
- Deficiency of fibrinogen, factors 11, V11, 1X, and X
- Portal hypertension
- Thrombocytopenia

Central nervous system dysfunction
- Hepatic encephalopathy

Fluid and electrolyte imbalance
- Edema, ascetic
- Sodium retention, hypokalemia, hypocalcaemia,
- Hypoalbuminemia

Immunocompromise
- Decreases host defense
- Increased risk for infections
- Malnutrition

Baseline investigations

- Complete blood cell count with differential and coagulation profile
- Basal metabolic panel
- Liver function tests, including an alanine aminotransferase level determination
- Cardiovascular assessment, stress testing may be necessary in appropriate patients
- Respiratory system assessment
- Renal function assessment
- Screen the patient for alcohol abuse, drug abuse, or depression
- Screen the patient for coinfection with HIV or HBV
- Anti-HCV antibody enzyme immunoassay, genotyping could be performed as an aid for guiding prognosis (HCV)

Manage coagulopathy

- Keep prothrombin time to within 3 seconds of normal
- Provide vitamin K (eg, 10 mg intramuscularly) if prothrombin time prolonged. If vitamin K does not improve prothrombin level, severe hepatocellular disease should be suspected
- Cryoprecipitate, deamino-8-D-arginine
- Platelet transfusion, platelet counts >50,000 for minor and >100,000 for major surgeries

Nutrition and water – electrolyte balance

- Consider the possibility of hypoglycemia (patient nothing by mouth)
- Check for ongoing gastrointestinal bleeding from portal gastropathy or varices, if concomitant anemia, hydrate and transfuse as needed
- Manage hypoalbuminemia (immunocompromised state, altered healing, drug toxicity, hyposmolarity). Restrict protein without compromising nutrition (30 g/d)
- Electrolyte replacement or management/ avoid excess sodium load in patients who have cirrhosis (sodium retention)/ check hypokalemia, hypocalcaemia

---

- Assure preoperative diuresis/check renal function (patients who have total serum bilirubin higher than 8 mg/dL are likely to develop acute renal failure and sepsis postoperatively)
- Monitor for hemochromatosis
- Management of encephalopathy/avoid sedatives that may precipitate the process

Steroid supplement
- In patients who have autoimmune hepatitis or patients who have other conditions who are on long-term prednisone, stress doses of hydrocortisone may be needed.

Perioperative considerations
- DVT prophylaxis: for moderate-risk patients (obese or elderly), heparin 5000 U should be given every 8 hours through subcutaneous injection. Initial dose must be given at least 2 hours before surgery. Use sequential pneumatic stockings and low molecular weight heparin before anesthetic induction and muscular relaxation. For high-risk patients (h/o DVT, PE), heparin infusion should be continued until the patient is ambulatory.
- The action of microsomal enzymes may be altered because of liver disease. For example, accelerated metabolism of drugs in the presence of alcohol-induced microsomal-enzyme stimulation might alter the amount of inhaled anesthetic needed to achieve a given partial pressure.
- Decreased responsiveness to catecholamines occurs manifesting an impaired tolerance to blood loss.
- In alcohol-induced cardiomyopathy, the myocardium's sensitivity to depressant effects of anesthetic agents is increased.
- Decreased serum proteins increase the pharmacodynamics and -kinetics of active drugs.
- Halothane hepatitis and possible decreased hepatic blood flow with halothane compared with isoflurane and desflurane should be considered. Con-

comitant use of nitrous oxide and narcotics is probably beneficial.
- Use of regional anesthesia should be preferred if possible.
- Alcohol abuse renders peripheral nerves vulnerable to ischemia, therefore use of positional padding should always be considered to avoid pressure necrosis.
- Use of succinylcholine and mivacurium may cause prolonged response. Elimination and metabolism of atracurium, cisatracurium, vecuronium, and rocuronium are not affected by compromised hepatic function and may be preferable.
- Blood gases, pH, coagulation status, and urine output should be monitored and exogenous glucose levels considered.
- When blood transfusion is indicated, transfusion should be slow to compensate for decreased clearance of citrate.
- Cardiac filing pressure should be monitored with central venous or pulmonary artery catheter for fluid administration.
- Unnecessary esophageal instrumentation (eg, gastric tube, esophageal stethoscope) should be avoided in patients who have esophageal varices.

Postoperative considerations
- Catecholamine response is impaired in patients who have liver disease; therefore, intraoperative or postoperative hypovolemia or hemorrhage may not trigger adequate compensatory mechanisms.
- Postoperative liver function is usually exaggerated because of detrimental nonspecific effects of anesthetic drugs on hepatic blood flow and hepatocytic oxygenation.
- Postoperative jaundice may be caused by increased bilirubin resulting from infection, hemolysis, hematomas, and blood transfusion.
- Cholestasis should be considered with postoperative jaundice. Cholestatic jaundice increases the risk for postoperative renal failure.

- Patients should be monitored for hypoglycemia and signs of hepatic decompensation, such as jaundice, ascites, and encephalopathy. These reactions could be triggered by post-operative constipation, bleeding, infection, or alkalosis.
- Sepsis is always an impending possibility, especially with postoperative liver dysfunction.

References

[1] Strunin L. Preoperative assessment of the patient with liver dysfunction. Br J Anaesth 1978;50:25–34.

[2] Chitturi S, George J. Predictors of liver-related complications in patients with chronic hepatitis C. Ann Med 2000;32(9):588–91.

[3] CDC. Guidelines for prevention of transmission of human immunodeficiency virus and hepatitis B virus to health-care and public-safety workers. MMWR Morb Mortal Wkly Rep 1989;38(Suppl 6):1–37.

[4] Stramer SL, Glynn SA, Kleinman SH, et al. Detection of HIV-1 and HCV infections among antibody-negative blood donors. Med 2004;351(8):760–8.

[5] Yeung LT, King SM, Roberts EA. Mother-to-infant transmission of hepatitis C virus. Hepatology 2001; 34(2):223–9.

[6] Fields HA, Favorov MO, Margolis HS. Hepatitis E virus: a review. J Clin Immunoassay 1993,16.215–23.

[7] French SW. Mechanisms of alcoholic liver injury. Can J Gastroenterol 2000;14(4):327–32.

[8] Spies CD, Rommelspacher H. Alcohol withdrawal in the surgical patient: prevention and treatment. Anesth Analg 1999;88:946–54.

[9] Ziser A, Plevak DJ, Wieser RH, et al. Morbidity and mortality in cirrhotic patients undergoing anesthesia and surgery. Anesthesiology 1999;90:42–53.

[10] Gelman S, Fowler KC, Smith LR. Liver circulation and function during Isoflurane and halothane anesthesia. Anesthesiology 1984;61:726–30.

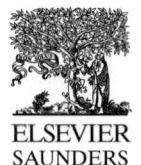

ELSEVIER
SAUNDERS

Oral Maxillofacial Surg Clin N Am 18 (2006) 227 – 239

ORAL AND
MAXILLOFACIAL
SURGERY CLINICS
of North America

Perioperative Management of Maxillofacial Tumor and Reconstruction Patients

Christopher M. Harris, MD, DMD[a], Bartlomiej L. Nierzwicki, MD, DMD, PhD[a],
Remy H. Blanchaert, Jr, MD, DDS[b],*

[a]Department of Oral and Maxillofacial Surgery, University of Missouri—Kansas City, Truman Medical Center,
2301 Holmes Street, Kansas City, MO 64108, USA
[b]Private Practice, Oral & Maxillofacial Surgery Associates, 1919 North Webb, Wichita, KS, 67206, USA

Perioperative management of patients who undergo maxillofacial surgery can be challenging. The Truman Medical Center is a regional referral center for the management of patients who undergo complex maxillofacial surgery. Over the last 3 years, the practice has treated more than 250 complex maxillofacial oncology and reconstructive cases, including many benign and malignant head and neck tumors, complex traumatic injuries (eg, avulsive gunshot wounds), and severe infections (eg, necrotizing fasciitis). Approximately 50% of all cases are disease-related, and most involve malignancies. Many of the patients are also significantly medically compromised and need intensive surgical care to maximize outcomes. These cases are not those of typical outpatient surgery and therefore management must be highly individualized.

The pathology presenting in these patients requires urgent, and in some cases, emergent management. Surgeons must be aware that patients may not see any other medical provider before undergoing operative intervention. Medical maximization of these patients in the preoperative period is frequently not an option. Any comorbid conditions must be recognized and factored into the treatment plan. Many patients have significant cardiovascular, pulmonary, and metabolic diseases, which can negatively impact recovery throughout the perioperative period. These patients undergo prolonged surgeries.

They may even require multiple staged surgeries. Frequently these patients require surgical airways, mechanical ventilation, prolonged hospitalization, and intense hemodynamic and metabolic support. The accepted complication rate associated with head and neck surgery is approximately 20% to 25%, with pulmonary, infectious, and cardiovascular complications the most common [1]. Surgeons can improve patient outcome by recognizing these risks and applying aggressive prophylactic management strategies. Preoperative assessment standardization is warranted to assure that all relevant measures are considered. Table 1 presents a useful memory tool for initial patient evaluation.

This article describes management, rationale for treatment, and the common complications that are encountered in the treatment of patients undergoing maxillofacial surgery. General considerations for patients undergoing complex surgery, suggestions for preventing infection in head and neck surgery, and comprehensive discussions of cardiovascular and pulmonary concerns are presented. Table 2 presents a clinical pathway developed to assist in managing these patients. Application of this pathway allows ongoing evaluation of inpatient progress towards discharge after head and neck surgery.

Preventative perioperative management—general considerations

The statement, "an ounce of prevention is worth a pound of cure," is particularly true for perioperative

* Corresponding author.
  E-mail address: rblanchaert@aol.com
(R.H. Blanchaert, Jr).

1042-3699/06/$ – see front matter © 2006 Elsevier Inc. All rights reserved.
doi:10.1016/j.coms.2005.12.001

oralmaxsurgery.theclinics.com

Table 1
Preoperative assessment and interventions

Preoperative assessment	Intervention
Cardiovascular evaluation	Rate control (start beta blockade, if indicated) EKG Cardiology consultation (perfusion study, if indicated)
Pulmonary evaluation	Pulmonary consultation Anesthesia evaluation
Nutritional evaluation	Physical examination Serum albumin, prealbumin Begin nutritional supplements PEG tube placement
Laboratory evaluation	Complete blood count Basic metabolic panel Coagulation profile Liver function studies
Oncology consultation	Adjuvant therapy evaluation
Surgical consultation	PEG tube placement (if needed) Venous access placement (if needed)
Social work referral	Financial, psychosocial, hospice needs

Abbreviation: PEG, percutaneous endoscopic gastrostomy.

prophylaxis. Early measures to identify and prevent common and potentially fatal postoperative problems are imperative. Gastrointestinal hemorrhage, pulmonary embolism, decubitus ulcer formation, and peripheral neurologic injuries are preventable. Avoiding these complications requires a proactive approach, especially in the patient undergoing maxillofacial tumor and reconstruction surgery who often experiences lengthy surgeries and prolonged convalescence. This section focuses on perioperative prophylaxis, which has become the standard of care.

Gastrointestinal bleeding is a well-recognized phenomenon in conditions of extreme stress. This risk has been documented in the surgical and critical care literature. Stress-related mucosal ulcerations, thought to be caused by mucosal ischemia, are more commonly seen in patients who are critically ill. Experts believe this ischemia, along with disuse of the gastrointestinal tract, increases the risk for gastrointestinal bleeding in patients in the surgical intensive care unit (ICU). The surgical and critical care literature supports perioperative suppression of acid formation and early enteral nutrition. This approach has been shown to reduce the morbidity associated with these episodes [2,3], and is therefore used in patients treated at the authors' institution.

Enteral nutrition is begun the on the evening of surgery at a very low (10 cm^3/h) rate. The nutrition supplied is rapidly titrated to the patient's goal rate within the first 36 hours. The patient undergoes careful observation for intolerance, which occurs rarely. H_2 receptor antagonists are started immediately after surgery and continued throughout the ICU stay until the goal rate of enteral nutrition is reached or adequate nutrition is obtained orally. Of course, patients chronically receiving these medications continue on their preoperative regimen without interruption. Patients who have a history of peptic ulcer or gastroesophageal reflux disease undergo proton pump inhibitor therapy because they are at even greater risk for gastrointestinal bleeding. Unexplained decreases in hemoglobin with no obvious surgical source should prompt immediate evaluation for upper (eg, gastritis) and lower (eg, hemorrhoids) gastrointestinal tract sources.

Pulmonary embolism can be a catastrophic event in any patient undergoing surgery. Particular types of surgery are associated with increased risk. Maxillofacial tumor and reconstructive surgery is generally considered a low-risk procedure in patients not otherwise predisposed (eg, previous deep venous thrombosis or pulmonary embolism). The increased risk for pulmonary embolism in patients undergoing surgery, particularly surgeries of long duration, is well recognized. Prophylaxis has become standard and the appropriate means of handling these risks has been documented. Intermittent sequential compression devices may increase venous blood movement and most importantly activate the fibrinolytic system. This simple, drug-free therapy should be used for all patients undergoing surgery that lasts more than 90 minutes. In addition, the devices should remain in place until the patient returns to normal ambulation (hospital discharge).

Low-dose heparins (low molecular weight and unfractionated) are also commonly used [4,5]. The addition of drug therapy is typically limited to patients who have a previous history of deep venous thrombosis or pulmonary embolism because they have an increased perioperative risk. Staff (eg, nurses, residents, physical therapists) participation is often needed to assist and support adequate early mobilization. Additional measures are often helpful in preventing thrombosis and can be required based on preexisting comorbid disease. Also, aspirin therapy is routinely administered immediately after surgery to patients who undergo free-flap reconstruction. This procedure is primarily used for flap maintenance, although antiplatelet therapy (although not a recommended prophylaxis when used alone) has also

shown some benefit in preventing deep venous thrombosis [6].

Decubitus ulcers and peripheral neuropathies injuries can prolong hospital stay and increase overall costs. These injuries should be preventable. Failure to attempt to prevent these injuries is considered medicolegal negligence. Meticulous perioperative management is essential in preventing positioning errors. The entire staff involved with patient care, from the operating room to the ICU to the surgical wards, must be concerned with these injuries. Pressure-distributing mattresses should be used for all patients. Early and frequent mobilization (eg, early ambulation, turns every 2 hours when bedridden) is required. Ensuring adequate nutrition is also critical to overall wound healing and prevention [7].

The authors have seen decubitus ulcers on the sacrum, heels, lips, nasal ala, and forehead of patients after surgery. These injuries resulted from positioning and padding issues that were overlooked in the operating theater and ICU. The surgeon must inspect the positioning and padding of the patient to ensure adequacy before proceeding with a lengthy operation. Forehead ulcerations have been noted with over-zealous attempts to secure head wraps and endotracheal tubes. Probes, sensors, and folds in towels or drapes underneath a taped head wrap can easily cause ulceration during a long surgery and should be eliminated. Common sense, attention to detail, and judicious amounts of force should minimize forehead wounds. Ulcers of the nasal ala are seen with prolonged nasal endotracheal tube tension and pressure on the ala. These wounds can occur after surgery when patients who have ventilator tubing secured to the bed rails slide down in the ICU bed. This sliding causes an increased pressure on the ala from the nasal tube which can quickly develop into a cosmetically deforming alar wound. Lip ulcers are often overlooked because they are obscured by the tape used to secure the endotracheal tube. Careful attention in taping and frequent inspection of the lips underneath the tape help prevent these ulcerations. Prefabricated, manufactured endotracheal tube holders can be used in prolonged oral intubations to secure the tube well and distribute the forces required for stabilization.

Prevention of wound infection in head and neck surgery

Surgical wound infection after head and neck tumor surgery can have a devastating impact on patient outcomes. Infection can lead to flap necrosis, fistula formation, and delay in definitive adjuvant therapies, resulting in increased tumor recurrence rates. Similar to findings in other areas of surgery, costs are closely and directly linked to perioperative wound infection because of increased hospital stay. Most head and neck surgeries are classified as clean-contaminated procedures because of the field's communication with the oral cavity, oral pharynx, or upper airway. Head and neck tumor extirpation results in complex three-dimensional defects that complicate reconstruction and predispose to salivary leakage, wound contamination, and subsequent wound sepsis. This section provides an evidence-based approach to wound infection prevention after head and neck surgery. The newest edition of *Oral and Maxillofacial Infections* provides an expanded discussion of this topic [8].

Microbiology of head and neck wound infections

To prevent surgical site wound infections, the microbiology present in established postoperative wound infections must first be understood. Clayman and colleagues [9] published a prospective study of 43 wound infections in 212 patients who underwent head and neck surgery. Standardized perioperative prophylactic antibiotics (ampicillin-sulbactam, 1.5 g, or clindamycin, 600 mg) were administered 1 hour before incision, followed by eight additional doses at 6-hour intervals. The investigators isolated 55 organisms from 34 of the infected wounds. Table 3 summarizes these isolates.

Anaerobic bacteria were more frequently isolated from postoperative wound infection when dental extractions were performed concurrently with tumor excision and reconstruction. These results show that extraction of teeth in poor condition should be considered at diagnostic endoscopy or biopsy rather then at definitive surgery. Additionally, when periodontally diseased teeth cannot be removed before definitive tumor surgery, use of ampicillin-sulbactam as antibiotic prophylaxis should be considered because of the high incidence of *Eikenella* sp reported in wound infections in these cases.

Recommended protocol for prevention of infection in head and neck surgery

A comprehensive protocol for the prevention of infection in head and neck surgery requires that surgeons consider a multifactorial approach. Decontamination of the surgical site, copious antibiotic impregnated irrigation before closure, elimination of dead space, and appropriate intravenous antibiotic administration should be evaluated for each patient

Table 2
Clinical pathway for the patient undergoing maxillofacial surgery

	Cardiovascular hemodynamics	Fluid electrolytes nutrition	Pulmonary	Prophylaxis	Infectious wound
POD 1 (ICU care)	Ensure adequate fluid status Invasive blood pressure monitoring Accurate I & Os IV antihypertensive therapy (eg, BBs, hydralazine) IV antihypotensive therapy (eg, fluid boluses, dopamine) Initiate alcohol withdrawal precautions Adequate analgesia and anxiolysis Supplemental oxygen Fluid and electrolyte management BBs for tachycardias and arrythmias CCBs for tachycardias and arrhythmias (diltiazem)	Daily electrolyte, complete blood count laboratory evaluation Fluid boluses as needed Accurate I & O Tube feedings initiated at 25 mL/h (Nutren 1.5), (low carb for COPD) Tight serum glucose control (<140 mg/dL), insulin infusion if needed	Aggressive ventilator management or weaning Postoperative arterial blood gas Postoperative chest radiograph (ET and feeding tube placement) Routine nebulizer therapy (albuterol-ipratropium) Hourly incentive spirometry post extubation Frequent suctioning Humidified oxygen	Sequential compression devices ASA (if flap reconstruction) H₂ blocker (Zantac 50 mg IV q8h) or PPI (Protonix 40 mg IV q d) initiated Initiate bowel regimen (eg, Colace 100 mg bid)	Antibiotic regimen (Unasyn 3.0 g q6h or Clindamycin 900 mg q8h) Initiate nutrition regimen Serial wound evaluations
POD 2 (ICU care or surgical ward)	Maintain adequate fluid status Invasive blood pressure monitoring, consider discontinuing if stable Initiate transition to oral antihypertensives IV antihypotensive therapy (eg, fluid boluses, dopamine) Continue alcohol withdrawal precautions Maintain analgesia and anxiolysis, transition to oral route Maintain supplemental oxygen BBs/CCBs for tachycardias and arrhythmias, transition to oral	Daily electrolyte, complete blood count laboratory evaluation Fluid boluses as needed Accurate I & O Enteral feedings near goal rate Maintain tight serum glucose control	Continue ventilator management, may wean if appropriate Routine nebulizer therapy (albuterol-ipratropium) Continue incentive spirometry Frequent suctioning Humidified oxygen OOB to chair tid (nonventilator pt)	Continue all measures	Continue all measures

POD 3 (ICU care or surgical ward)	Maintain adequate fluid status Discontinue invasive monitoring Oral agents for hypertension control Continue alcohol withdrawal precautions Analgesia and anxiolysis per oral medications Maintain supplemental oxygen if clinically indicated BBs/CCBs for tachycardias and arrhythmias, per oral medications	Electrolyte evaluation Accurate I & O Enteral feedings at goal rate Maintain tight glucose control	Wean off ventilator, if clinically appropriate Routine nebulizer therapy (albuterol-ipratropium) Continue incentive spirometry Frequent tracheostomy suctioning Humidified oxygen OOB to chair tid and ambulate with assistance	Discontinue GI prophylaxis when enteral feeding effective Continue all other measures	Continue all measures
POD 4–7 (Surgical ward)	Maintain adequate fluid status Continue all hypertensive medications Continue alcohol withdrawal precautions	Transition feedings to bolus Accurate I & O Maintain tight glucose control	Continue aggressive pulmonary toilet Continue oxygen (if clinically indicated) Downsize or decannulate tracheostomy (POD 5–7)	Continue all measures Physical therapy goals met (POD 5)	Remove suction drains (POD 4–5) D/C antibiotics Serial wound evaluations Remove bolster (POD 5) Remove STSG dressing (POD 5) Remove staples, sutures (POD 5)

This represents an ideal course for hypothetical patient undergoing complicated maxillofacial surgery (eg, tumor ablation, neck dissection, reconstruction). Use of this pathway by the treatment team assures consideration of all relevant interventions within the early postoperative period. The use of pathways has been shown to improve outcomes through decreasing length of hospital stay.

Abbreviations: ASA, acetylsalicylic acid; BB, β-blockers; Carb, carbohydrates; CCB, calcium channel blockers; COPD, chronic obstructive pulmonary disease; D/C, discontinue; ET, endotracheal tube; GI, gastrointestinal; ICU, intensive care unit; I & O, intake and output; IV, intravenously; OOB, out of bed; POD, postoperative day; PPI, proton pump inhibitor; Pt, patient; STSG, split thickness skin graft.

Table 3
Common isolates identified in postoperative wound infections

Organism	Incidence (%)
Aerobic	
Gram-positive	
Coagulase-negative	5
Staphylococcus spp	
Streptococcus (non-group A)	2
Gram-negative	
Eikenella corrodens	8
Escherichia coli	5
Pseudomonas aeruginosa	4
Klebsiella spp	3
Anaerobic	
Gram-negative	
Bacteroides	5
Fusobacterium	4
Haemophilus parainfluenza	2

Data from Clayman GL, Raad II, Hankins PD, et al. Bacteriologic profile of surgical infection after antibiotic prophylaxis. Head Neck 1993;15:526–31.

undergoing head and neck surgery. Hair should be removed from surgical sites only by clipper to avoid follicle inflammation and elaboration of additional organisms. Skin preparation using iodine, chlorhexidine, or alcohol products is acceptable. Mucosal surfaces should be appropriately treated with either clindamycin solution or chlorhexidine solution. Using antibiotic-impregnated saline solution to decontaminate surgical sites at the completion of surgery decreases the number of organisms within the surgical site and provides increased local antibiotic concentration. Before definitive closure, dead space should be eliminated through either suture closure or closed suction drainage. Drains should be removed as early as possible after surgery. Intravenous antibiotic administration should be completed before incision, and continuation of the regimen for three doses should be considered in patients when contamination occurs. _Oral and maxillofacial infections 4th Edition_ provides an expanded review of the literature and justifies the protocols outlined in the following paragraphs [8].

Clean case

A single dose of empiric antibiotic therapy should be considered within 30 minutes of skin incision in a clean head and neck case. These cases are at low risk for infection, and use of additional prophylactic antibiotics is not supported by the literature and may cause resistant organisms to develop. Appropriate site decontamination, attention to hemostasis,

elimination of dead space, and reduction of surgical time are measures that the surgeon may take to minimize perioperative surgical site infections.

Contaminated case

The measures outlined in the previous section are also relevant to contaminated cases. Further measures are often necessary in these cases to optimize patient outcome, such as administering additional antibiotics up to three doses. This intervention is well supported by the literature. Because increased risks for infection have been reported when extraction is performed at definitive surgery, surgeons should consider eliminating poor dentition before major surgery. This measure requires only some foresight and proper case planning. A final and perhaps most important additional measure surgeons should consider in contaminated head and neck surgical cases is flap transfer of well-vascularized tissue to the operative site of resection during reconstruction to avoid wound tension and subsequent breakdown. Wound margin breakdown results in salivary contamination of surgical sites with resultant infection. In most contaminated head and neck surgical cases, this problem is addressed with microvascular free-tissue transfer reconstruction of surgical resection defects.

Cardiovascular complications

Cardiovascular disease is a common comorbidity in patients who have head and neck cancer. The generally accepted risk for ischemic perioperative cardiovascular events in head and neck surgery is less than 5% [10]. Recognizing and initiating therapy for cardiovascular disease as early as possible during the preoperative evaluation is crucial to minimize these risks. Postoperative myocardial infarction and hemodynamic instability are potentially lethal events.

The preoperative interview should determine any serious cardiovascular disease history, such as angina, recent or old myocardial infarction, hypertension, congestive heart failure, valvular disease, and arrhythmias, and should provide some assessment of exercise tolerance. Findings of peripheral vascular disease, renal disease, chronic pulmonary disease, and diabetes may also indicate occult cardiac disease. The physical examination should determine signs of cardiovascular disease, such as peripheral edema, jugular venous distension, and heart murmurs. Preoperative cardiac testing in patients who have minor risk factors only consists of an EKG, chest radio-

graph, basic electrolyte panel, and complete blood count. Patients at greater risk require coordination of care with a cardiologist. For these patients, consultation often results in further evaluation, such as perfusion studies and echocardiogram. Preoperative consultation facilitates early involvement in patients who develop cardiac complications.

Patients who have ischemic cardiovascular disease should be rate-controlled with β-blockers. Researchers have consistently shown that β-blockers decrease the risk for postoperative myocardial infarctions and overall mortality [11]. These medications decrease sympathetic outflow and reduce myocardial oxygen demand [10,11]. Arterial lines are used commonly to closely monitor blood pressure during and after surgery, whereas central venous pressure monitoring is rarely used. An arterial line also allows serial laboratory testing. Bladder catheterization with urine output monitoring is a reliable estimate of adequate cardiac output and tissue perfusion. Hemodynamic status and oxygenation must be closely monitored and fluid management optimized throughout the perioperative course. The patient must recover from anesthesia and undergo extubation without dramatic changes in hemodynamic state or Valsalva. A rough emergence with coughing and blood pressure elevation may result in wound hematoma requiring evacuation. Patients who will remain sedated and undergo mechanical ventilation immediately after surgery require neuromuscular blockade and appropriate depth of anesthesia throughout transfer to the intensive care setting.

Strict management of hemodynamics and tissue oxygenation are required, particularly after surgery. Hypotension, hypertension, and tachycardia must be avoided. Appropriate administration of analgesia significantly improves the postoperative hemodynamic profile by minimizing the patient's sympathetic response to the stress of surgery and postoperative pain. Postoperative hypertension and tachycardia are commonly caused by inadequate analgesia. Intravenous beta blockade (ie, labetalol, esmolol hydrochloride) is used to treat hypertension and tachycardia when other factors, particularly pain, have been ruled out. Tachyarrhythmias seen in the postoperative course include sinus tachycardia, supraventricular tachycardia, and atrial fibrillation. When tachyarrhythmias occur, an EKG and extended serum electrolyte panel should be performed immediately. Any abnormality in potassium, magnesium, calcium (ionized), and phosphorous should be corrected. Adequate analgesia and oxygenation must be provided and the volume status should be optimized. Persistent arrhythmia requires prompt cardiology intervention.

Sedation is used throughout the first 18 to 36 hours after major surgeries, particularly in flap reconstructions, to minimize the challenges of hypertension and tachycardia. An additional benefit of sedation may be that decreased movement minimizes kinking, laxity, or tension of the microvascular flap vessel while a surrounding fibrin network develops that helps stabilize the vessel geometry.

Postoperative myocardial oxygen demand is increased because endogenous catecholamine is released as a natural stress response to surgery. Hypertension increases the myocardial oxygen demand because increased contractile force is required to offset the elevated pressures. Tachycardia decreases the duration allotted for diastolic coronary artery perfusion and therefore decreases oxygen delivery to the myocardium. This combination can precipitate myocardial insufficiency, especially in patients who have preexisting cardiovascular disease. Hypotension must also be avoided because insufficient coronary blood flow may result. Sustained hypotension, defined as a 30% decrease in mean blood pressure for 10 minutes, is associated with postoperative myocardial infarctions.

Myocardial infarctions are most common within the first 3 days after surgery and are also associated with tachycardia in the early postoperative period [12]. Postoperative myocardial infarctions, although rare compared with thoracic and abdominal surgery, occur after head and neck surgery. Data suggest that postoperative myocardial infarctions occur when catecholamine levels and myocardial oxygen demands are increased. Excess oxygen demand, rather than a sudden loss of tissue oxygenation, is the more likely key component in a postoperative myocardial infarction. This altered physiology also makes patients who have underlying cardiovascular disease more prone to plaque rupture. Plaque rupture, which is the final mechanism for occlusion, plays a lesser role in the cause of perioperative myocardial infarction compared with its primary role in spontaneous myocardial infarctions. Therefore, imbalances in postoperative myocardial oxygen demand are limited through assuring hemodynamic stability and providing supplemental oxygen, beta-blockade (in patients considered at risk), and adequate pain control.

The presentation and treatment of postoperative myocardial infarction differ somewhat from the commonly recognized myocardial infarction. Standard clinical, laboratory, and electrocardiographic testing are employed in the diagnosis. ST-segment depression and non−Q wave infarctions are common and up to 90% of patients have no anginal symptoms associated with these myocardial infarctions [12].

The most glaring difference in treatment is the inability to use systemic fibrinolytic agents (eg, tissue plasminogen activator, streptokinase). The use of antiplatelet agents, nitrates, β-blocker, analgesia, and oxygen is still recommended. With the contraindication of fibrinolytic therapy, interventional cardiology may have a more prominent role in therapy [13]. A cardiologist should be involved immediately when a postoperative myocardial infarction is suspected.

Pulmonary complications

Pulmonary complications contribute significantly to overall perioperative morbidity and mortality in maxillofacial tumor and reconstructive surgery. The incidence of postoperative pulmonary complications reported in the literature varies from 2% to 70%. The wide range is influenced partially by patient selection and procedure-related risk factors. The lack of uniform and standardized definitions for postoperative complications also accounts for much of the variability. The most commonly encountered definition is a pulmonary abnormality that produces identifiable disease or dysfunction that is clinically significant and adversely affects the clinical course [14]. This definition includes several major categories of complications, including atelectasis; tracheobronchitis and aspiration pneumonitis; nosocomial pneumonia; and hypoxemia and respiratory failure.

In upper abdominal and thoracic surgery, diaphragmatic dysfunction plays the most important role in the development of these complications through reduction of vital capacity and functional residual capacity. In head and neck surgery, local factors, including oropharyngeal edema; tongue obstruction; impaired cough and gag reflex; and difficulty clearing secretions, lead to colonization of the tracheobronchial tree with oral microflora. This colonization leads to clinically evident infection in susceptible hosts.

Risk factors for pulmonary complications can be categorized into patient-related and procedure-related risks. Potential patient-related factors include chronic lung disease, smoking, general health status, obesity, and age.

Known chronic lung disease is the most important patient-related risk factor for postoperative pulmonary complications. A prospective study of 272 patients who were referred for preoperative evaluation before undergoing nonthoracic surgery found that patients who had a history of chronic obstructive pulmonary disease (COPD) had an odds ratio (OR) of 4.2 for pulmonary complications [15,16]. Important predictors of complications were: age of 65 years or

older (OR 1.8), history of 40 or more pack-years of smoking (OR 1.9), and maximum laryngeal height of 4 cm or less (distance from the top of the thyroid cartilage to the suprasternal notch at end expiration). These findings complemented the previously published risk-prediction equations for respiratory failure and pneumonia [17].

Despite early reports indicating increased rates of postoperative pulmonary complications among patients who had asthma, subsequent studies did not confirm the correlation for patients who had well-controlled asthma [18]. Therefore, patients who have asthma who are well controlled and have a peak flow measurement more than 80% of predicted (or personal best) can be considered at average risk. Current cigarette smokers carry an increased risk for postoperative pulmonary complications even in the absence of chronic lung disease. A prospective cohort study of 410 patients undergoing elective, noncardiac surgery found that smoking had an OR of 5.5 for postoperative complications [19]. In a multivariate regression model, a prospective study of 272 patients referred for medical evaluation before undergoing nonthoracic surgery found that those who had 40 pack-years or more of smoking had an OR of 1.9 for pulmonary complications [16,17]. Patients undergoing elective surgery should be advised to stop smoking at least 8 weeks before surgery. A brief period of abstinence does not improve morbidity and seems to increase the risk for postoperative pulmonary complications.

General health status is an important determinant of pulmonary risk. The Goldman cardiac risk index predicts postoperative pulmonary and cardiac complications. The commonly used American Society of Anesthesiologists (ASA) classification also correlates with pulmonary risk.

Obesity induces reduction in lung volumes, ventilation/perfusion mismatch, and relative hypoxemia; accentuates similar changes seen with general anesthesia; and increases the risk for pulmonary complications. A prospective study of 272 patients referred for preoperative evaluation before undergoing nonthoracic surgery showed an OR of 4.1 for pulmonary complications in patients who had body mass index (BMI) of 30 kg/m² or more; however, a multivariate regression model deemed this correlation insignificant [16,17]. In a review of six studies comprising 4526 patients, the risk for pulmonary complications was identical for patients who were obese and those who were not [20].

When stratified by ASA class, the risk for surgical mortality is remarkably similar across all age groups [21]. A multivariate model for postoperative respira-

tory failure identified age older than 60 years as a minor risk factor [17]. The ORs for age 60 to 69 years and age older than 70 years were 1.51 and 1.91, respectively. Other studies reported similar ORs [15,16].

Procedure-related risk factors in the head and neck region that may potentially affect pulmonary risk include surgical site and duration. The incidence of pulmonary complications is inversely related to the distance of the surgical incision from the diaphragm. Thus, the complication rate in the cervical region is much lower than in the upper abdomen or thorax. Surgical procedures lasting more than 3 to 4 hours, however, correlate with higher risk for pulmonary complications [15,16]. Atelectasis, aspiration pneumonia, hospital-acquired pneumonia (HAP), and hypoxemia are common.

Atelectasis

Atelectasis is undoubtedly the most common pulmonary complication in the postoperative period. Its pathogenesis consists of altered compliance of lung tissue, impaired regional ventilation, and retained tracheobronchial secretions. Clinically significant atelectasis is characterized by increased work of breathing and hypoxemia. Atelectasis is best prevented by appropriate empiric intervention, including respiratory therapy, incentive spirometry, and rapid weaning from mechanical ventilation. In treating acute lobar atelectasis, removal of secretions through bronchoscopy has not shown superiority to respiratory therapy, although further evaluation is warranted based on stratification of the currently available studies.

Aspiration pneumonia

The prevalence of aspiration pneumonia was 0.8% in a large observational study of more than 300,000 adult patients undergoing surgery [22]. Prevalence varied among the 52 hospitals surveyed (from 0% to 1.9%) and by surgical procedure (from <0.1% to 19%). An increased risk for aspiration pneumonia was independently associated with male gender, nonwhite race, age older than 60 years, dementia, COPD, renal disease, malignancy, moderate-to-severe liver disease, and emergency department admission. The clinical features of chemical pneumonitis include abrupt onset of dyspnea and tachycardia. Patients may exhibit fever, bronchospasm, or cyanosis, with pink and frothy sputum. Radiographic evidence of infiltrates in one or both lower lobes usually appears in the first 24 hours. Treatment

should begin with prompt lateral head positioning (assuming integrity of the cervical spine), suctioning, and consideration of endotracheal intubation. Thereafter, treatment is supportive; supplemental oxygen or even mechanical ventilation may be necessary in the setting of hypoxemia. Administration of either corticosteroids or prophylactic antibiotics is controversial and currently not recommended. These therapies are commonly used, however, although their value in the treatment of aspiration pneumonia is not substantiated by scientific data.

Hospital-acquired pneumonia

HAP is pneumonia occurring 48 hours after admission in patients who have no evidence of infection at admission. Ventilator-associated pneumonia (VAP), a subset of nosocomial pneumonia, is a bacterial pneumonia that develops in patients who have acute respiratory failure and have been receiving mechanical ventilation for at least 48 hours. VAP is such a common event that the question clinicians should consider is not *if* pneumonia may develop, but *when*.

VAP requires bacterial colonization of the aerodigestive tract and concomitant aspiration of contaminated secretions into the lower airway [23]. These two processes lead to development of bronchiolitis, followed by bronchopneumonia. The prevalence of distal airway colonization relative to duration of mechanical ventilation has been estimated to be a 1% increase in colonization for each day of ICU stay. In one study, 275 patients undergoing mechanical ventilation were assessed through alternate-day bronchial lavage. Based on their findings, the investigators suggested particular vigilance between day 5 and 15 of ICU admission [24]. The microbiology of nosocomial pneumonia was evaluated in a large prospective consecutive case series of 837 patients who were suspected to have developed pneumonia in the first 14 days after surgery [25]. VAP occurred in 303 patients (36%). Microbiologic sampling was performed in 718 patients (86%). The pulmonary infection was polymicrobial in 94 patients (29%), and in 73 patients (22%) the infection resulted from a combination of two organisms: Enterobacteriaceae and *Staphylococcus aureus* or Enterobacteriaceae and streptococci (24% and 17%, respectively). Considering all isolates, 61% of cultured Enterobacteriaceae, 51% of *Pseudomonas*, and 57% of *S aureus* were isolated among patients who were diagnosed with pneumonia before the fifth postoperative day [25].

Gram stain of sputum, sputum culture, and blood cultures are routinely obtained. Although some

authors believe Gram stain is useful, culture results tend to be unreliable because of contamination with bacteria colonizing in the oropharynx (an exception may be the presence of *S aureus*). Blood cultures are extremely helpful only when results are positive. Sputum culture obtained through either expectorated sputum or suctioned secretions (in patients who are intubated endotracheally) is the optimal method for determining localized infection. A controversy exists as to whether invasive diagnostic techniques should be used on a routine basis or only in select cases. Multiple studies show that bronchoscopic and non-bronchoscopic bronchoalveolar lavages are superior in sensitivity and specificity to nonquantitative endotracheal aspirate cultures in the microbiologic diagnosis of VAP [23]. Initial empiric treatment of nosocomial pneumonia in patients who are immunocompetent after surgery consists of broad-spectrum systemic antibiotic therapy for gram-negative and gram-positive organisms with activity against *Pseudomonas* and *S aureus*, two of the most common causes of HAV and VAP.

Prevention strategies should be implemented routinely to reduce the incidence of VAP. Because duration of mechanical ventilation creates a linear risk for VAP, non–physician-directed ventilator-weaning protocols and guidelines must be followed in all ICUs to ensure timely discontinuation of mechanical ventilation [26]. Reduction of gastroesophageal reflux and resultant aspiration can be effectively reduced by placing patients in a semi-recumbent position. Continuous aspiration of subglottic secretions has shown potential benefit; however, its definitive effectiveness must be assessed in randomized prospective studies. Use of chlorhexidine gluconate oral rinses reduces bacterial colonization in the posterior oropharynx, contributing to lower nosocomial infection rate [27].

Hypoxemia

Postoperative hypoxemia has been defined either as an arterial oxygen saturation of less than 90% or a PaO_2 that is 75% or less of the preoperative value. In the early postoperative period, airway tissue edema, accumulation of oropharyngeal secretions, posterior tongue prolapse, and hypoventilation caused by residual anesthetic effects are common causes of hypoxemia. In the later postoperative period, atelectasis and a decline in the functional residual capacity contribute to hypoxemia. Treatment consists of supplemental oxygen and prompt correction of underlying pathology, such as chemical pneumonitis, pulmonary edema, or COPD exacerbation. Noninvasive positive-pressure ventilation may be helpful in improving gas exchange and pulmonary function in patients who experience respiratory distress or impending respiratory failure after surgery. Although high-flow oxygen can be provided through a face mask, more than approximately 70% oxygen is difficult to provide noninvasively because environmental air is entrained. By comparison, up to 100% oxygen is delivered easily when administered through an endotracheal tube. Almost all patients who have significant hypoxemia require intubation and mechanical ventilation. Specific abnormalities suggestive of the need for mechanical ventilation are presented in Table 4.

During the peri-intubation period, 100% oxygen should be given to ensure an adequate oxygen saturation (SaO_2). Because oxygen uptake may exceed replenishment in areas with low ventilation/perfusion (V/Q) ratios, some clinicians use slightly less than 100% oxygen (eg, 95%) in attempt to prevent absorptive atelectasis. Once it has been well established, absorptive atelectasis is not easily reversed by reduction of the fraction of inspired oxygen (FiO_2) to maintenance levels, emphasizing the desirability of rapid downward titration of FiO_2 to the lowest fraction necessary to maintain an SaO_2 of more than 90% [28]. Mechanical ventilation strategies designed to allow a decrease in the FiO_2 generally require the use of positive end-expiratory pressure. Airway access for mechanical ventilation can be provided either through endotracheal or tracheostomy tube. Initially, patients are generally ventilated through an endotracheal tube; changing to a tracheostomy tube is usually considered when a prolonged need for mechanical ventilation is expected. Early tracheostomy at 7 days of mechanical ventilation is appropriate for patients who are not likely to undergo weaning and extubation before day 14. Advantages of elective tracheostomy versus endotracheal intubation in patients undergoing max-

Table 4
Abnormalities suggestive of the need for mechanical ventilation

Parameter	Value
Respiratory rate	>35 breaths/min
Tidal volume	<5 mL/kg
Vital capacity	<10 mL/kg
Minute ventilation	<10 L/min
Rise in PCO_2	>10 mmHg
Alveolar-arterial gradient (FiO_2=1.0)	>450
PaO_2/PAO_2	<0.15
PaO_2 with supplemental O_2	<55 mmHg

Box 1. Advantages of tracheostomy versus endotracheal intubation

- Most optimal airway control
- Ease of performing sequential surgeries under general anesthesia
- Ease of suctioning
- Patient can be nursed outside of surgical ICU
- Ease of replacement (once tract has formed)
- Decreased work of breathing
- Ease of decannulation
- Patient comfort
- Enhancement of speech, mobility, and swallowing
- Radiation therapy access

---

illofacial tumor and reconstructive surgery are presented in Box 1.

Several factors contribute to the development of pulmonary complications in patients who undergo tracheostomy. First, patients lose the ability to contract expiratory muscles against a closed glottis, which prevents a sudden increase in intrathoracic pressure thereby decreasing the energy required to expectorate. Second, the loss of the natural positive end-expiratory pressure provided by the glottis may cause atelectatic collapse of small airways, predisposing the patient to pneumonia. Furthermore, smoking history plays a role in mucociliary clearance impairment.

For the high-volume, low-pressure endotracheal and tracheostomy tube cuffs currently in use, pressures should be maintained above 18 mmHg to reduce aspiration, but below 25 mmHg to minimize the risk for ischemic airway complications caused by pressure necrosis. The minimum cuff pressure required to prevent an air leak is correlated in a linear fashion with the peak inspiratory pressure measured on the ventilator. Thus, patients whose peak airway pressures exceed 48 cmH$_2$O will require cuff pressures greater than 25 mmHg to avoid a cuff leak, and are therefore presumably at increased risk for ischemic complications [29]. However, a properly inflated cuff does not provide complete protection from aspiration. Leakage around the cuff allows the penetration of secretions pooled above the larynx to enter trachea.

Mechanical ventilation has two beneficial effects: it improves gas exchange and decreases the work of

breathing. The application of positive pressure to the respiratory system can improve V/Q matching and decrease intrapulmonary shunting, thereby relieving hypoxemia and diminishing hypercapnia. Appropriate candidates for tracheal decannulation after weaning from mechanical ventilation include patients who fulfill the following criteria:

- No upper airway obstruction
- Ability to clear secretions
- Presence of an effective cough
- No aspiration with swallowing test
- No need for further surgeries
- No need for radiation therapy

Techniques for weaning patients from tracheostomy tubes include: progressive decrease of tracheostomy tube size, progressive capping of a fenestrated tracheostomy tube until tolerated for 12, 24, or 24 hours, and use of a tracheostomy plug (button). The tracheostomy plug is particularly useful in patients who have borderline clearance of secretions.

Pulmonary complications are a major cause of morbidity and mortality in the perioperative period. These complications range in clinical severity from asymptomatic hypoxemia to acute respiratory failure necessitating intubation and initiation of mechanical ventilation. A careful history and physical examination are the most useful tools for assessing preoperative risk in patients who are being evaluated for potential postoperative complications. Known chronic lung disease; current cigarette use; general health status according to Goldman cardiac risk index and ASA classification; and type and length of the procedure are among the most important determinants of pulmonary risk. Initial treatment should be supportive, including use of supplemental oxygen, inhaled bronchodilators, mechanical clearance of secretions, and possibly noninvasive mechanical ventilation. Bronchoscopy with pulmonary medicine consultation may be warranted in equivocal or refractory cases. Airway access for mechanical ventilation can be provided by either endotracheal or tracheostomy tube. Subsequent therapy is guided by the underlying condition or conditions responsible for acute decompensation. The risk for development of VAP increases 1% with each day of mechanical ventilation, and the clinician should consider not if, but when it will occur. Two strategies have been found to reduce the incidence of VAP, and an effort should be made to implement them in all ICUs: use of ventilator-weaning protocols and placement of the patient in the semirecumbent position.

Summary

Management of patients undergoing maxillofacial tumor and reconstruction surgery is complex. The clinician must consider many factors in surgical planning and perioperative management. This article reviews the impact of common comorbidities and the challenges related to the complexity and length of the surgical procedures. Strategies for dealing with these challenges are presented based primarily on the published literature, with added emphasis from clinical experience in a regional referral center. Many clinical tools are found within this article, including the Critical Pathway presented in Table 2. The hope is that application of these tools has a positive impact on clinical practice to the benefit of patients.

References

[1] Girod DA, McCulloch TM, Tsue TT, et al. Risk factors for complications in clean-contaminated head and neck surgical procedures. Head Neck 1995;17(1):7–13.

[2] Daley RJ, Rebuck JA, Welage LS, et al. Prevention of stress ulceration: current trends in critical care. Crit Care Med 2004;32(10):2008–13.

[3] Hiramoto JS, Terdiman JP, Norton JA. Evidence-based analysis: postoperative gastric bleeding: etiology and prevention. Surg Oncol 2003;12(1):9–19.

[4] Agnelli G. Prevention of venous thromboembolism in surgical patients. Circulation 2004;110(24, Supp 1): IV4–IV12.

[5] Geerts WH, Pineo GF, Heit JA, et al. Prevention of venous thromboembolism: The Seventh ACCP Conference on Antithrombotic and Thrombolytic Therapy. Chest 2004;126(3 Suppl):338S–400S.

[6] Group Participating in Pulmonary Embolism Prevention Trial. Prevention of pulmonary embolism and deep vein thrombosis with low dose aspirin. Pulmonary Embolism Prevention (PEP)Trial. Lancet 2000;15(355): 1295–302.

[7] Mechanick JI. Practical aspects of nutritional support for wound healing patients. Am J Surg 2004; 188(1A Suppl):52–6.

[8] Blanchaert RH. Identification, management, and prevention of infections after head and neck surgery. In: Topazian RG, Goldberg MH, Hupp JR, editors. Oral and maxillofacial infections. 4th edition. Philadelphia: W.B. Saunders; 2002. p. 399–409.

[9] Clayman GL, Raad II, Hankins PD, et al. Bacteriologic profile of surgical infection after antibiotic prophylaxis. Head Neck 1993;15:526–31.

[10] Eagle KA, Berger PB, Calkins H, et al. ACC/AHA guideline update for perioperative cardiovascular evaluation or noncardiac surgery: executive summary report of the American College of Cardiology/American Heart Association Task Force on Practice Guidelines (Committee to Update the 1996 Guidelines on Perioperative Cardiovascular Evaluation for Noncardiac Surgery). Circulation 2002;105(10):1257–67.

[11] Mangano DT, Layug EL, Wallace A, et al. Effect of atenolol on mortality and cardiovascular morbidity after noncardiac surgery. N Engl J Med 1996;335: 1713–20.

[12] Ashton CM, Petersen NJ, Wray NP, et al. The incidence of perioperative myocardial infarction in men undergoing noncardiac surgery. Ann Intern Med 1993;118(7):504–10.

[13] Berger PB, Bellot V, Bell MR, et al. An immediate invasive strategy for the treatment of acute myocardial infarction early after noncardiac surgery. Am J Cardiol 2001;87(9):1100–2.

[14] O'Donohue Jr WJ. Postoperative pulmonary complications. When are preventive and therapeutic measures necessary? Postgrad Med 1992;91:167–75.

[15] McAlister FA, Khan NA, Straus SE, et al. Accuracy of the preoperative assessment in predicting pulmonary risk after nonthoracic surgery. Am J Respir Crit Care Med 2003;167:741–4.

[16] Smetana GW, Cohn SL, Lawrence VA. Update in perioperative medicine. Ann Intern Med 2004;140: 452–61.

[17] Arozullah AM, Daley J, Henderson WG, et al. Multifactorial risk index for predicting postoperative respiratory failure in men after major noncardiac surgery. The National Veterans Administration Surgical Quality Improvement Program. Ann Surg 2000;232:242–53.

[18] Warner DO, Warner MA, Barnes RD, et al. Perioperative respiratory complications in patients with asthma. Anesthesiology 1996;85:460–7.

[19] Bluman LG, Mosca L, Newman N, et al. Preoperative smoking habits and postoperative pulmonary complications. Chest 1998;113:883–9.

[20] Smetana GW. Preoperative pulmonary evaluation. N Engl J Med 1999;340:937–44.

[21] Thomas DR, Ritchie CS. Preoperative assessment of older adults. J Am Geriatr Soc 1995;43:811–21.

[22] Kozlow JH, Berenholtz SM, Garrett E, et al. Epidemiology and impact of aspiration pneumonia in patients undergoing surgery in Maryland, 1999–2000. Crit Care Med 2003;31:1930–7.

[23] Napolitano LM. Hospital-acquired and ventilator-associated pneumonia: what's new in diagnosis and treatment? Am J Surg 2003;186:4S–14S [discussion 31S–4S].

[24] Garrard CS, A'Court CD. The diagnosis of pneumonia in the critically ill. Chest 1995;108:17S–25S.

[25] Montravers P, Veber B, Auboyer C, et al. Diagnostic and therapeutic management of nosocomial pneumonia in surgical patients: results of the Eole study. Crit Care Med 2002;30:368–75.

[26] Ely EW, Meade MO, Haponik EF, et al. Mechanical ventilator weaning protocols driven by nonphysician health-care professionals: evidence-based clinical practice guidelines. Chest 2001;120:454S–63S.

[27] DeRiso II AJ, Ladowski JS, Dillon TA, et al.

Chlorhexidine gluconate 0.12% oral rinse reduces the incidence of total nosocomial respiratory infection and nonprophylactic systemic antibiotic use in patients undergoing heart surgery. Chest 1996;109:1556–61.

[28] Santos C, Ferrer M, Roca J, et al. Pulmonary gas exchange response to oxygen breathing in acute lung injury. Am J Respir Crit Care Med 2000;161:26–31.

[29] Guyton DC, Barlow MR, Besselievre TR. Influence of airway pressure on minimum occlusive endotracheal tube cuff pressure. Crit Care Med 1997;25:91–4.

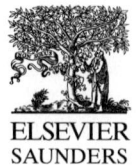
ELSEVIER
SAUNDERS

Oral Maxillofacial Surg Clin N Am 18 (2006) 241 – 254

ORAL AND
MAXILLOFACIAL
SURGERY CLINICS
of North America

Gastrointestinal Diseases and Considerations in the Perioperative Management of Oral Surgical Patients

Orrett E. Ogle, DDS[a,b,]*

[a]Department of Dentistry/Oral and Maxillofacial Surgery, Woodhull Medical and Mental Health Center, 760 Broadway,
Brooklyn, NY 11206-5317, USA
[b]School of Dental and Oral Surgery, Columbia University, 630 West 168th Street, New York, NY 10032, USA

The human gastrointestinal (GI) system is a long complex tract of varied components and related organs that are affected by an extensive array of diseases in the categories of malformations; nutritional and metabolic disorders; infections; inflammatory conditions; and malignancies. Its major function is to ingest food, digest it to extract energy and nutrients, and eliminate harmful waste. The human GI tract is approximately 25 feet (7.5 m) long and consists of the following components:

Mouth and pharynx
Esophagus
Stomach
Small intestine: duodenum, jejunum, and ileum
Large intestine: colon (ascending, transverse, and descending), cecum, rectum, and anus
Organs: liver and biliary system, pancreas, and spleen

So many diseases affect the above components of the GI system that even a fraction of them is impossible to address in this article. Commonly encountered and clinically significant problems are therefore selected and briefly discussed with emphasis on assisting the clinician in developing management strategies to reduce the risk associated with GI

diseases. The best strategy, of course, is always a good medical history, which allows identification of comorbid conditions of the GI system that may affect perioperative clinical decisions. An educated assessment of the type and magnitude of intraoperative risk can be made along with identification of potential postoperative complications, which may be reduced if considered preoperatively.

Mouth

Two significant oral conditions that are important to the oral surgeon are xerostomia and postradiation of the jaws.

Xerostomia

Xerostomia is not a disease, but a symptom. Surgical risks include compromised nutritional status, poor healing of the oral mucosa in intraoral cases, opportunistic infections, and increased postoperative pain and patient discomfort. Mucositis may contribute to fragile tissue and increased intraoperative bleeding. Causes of xerostomia include drugs, anticancer treatment, and conditions such as Sjögren' syndrome and diabetes.

Although more than 400 commonly used medications can cause dry mouth, the risks for significant surgical complications from most of these drugs are fortunately generally low. The main classes of medications that cause dry mouth are antihypertensives, antidepressants, tranquilizers, diuretics, anti-

* Department of Dentistry/Oral and Maxillofacial Surgery, Woodhull Medical and Mental Health Center, 760 Broadway, Brooklyn, NY 11206-5317.
    E-mail addresses: orrett.ogle@woodhullhc.nychhc.org, ogle-me@att.net

psychotics, anti-Parkinson's agents, and antihistamines. Specific perioperative problems are pain from tender mouth tissues; increased inflammation, particularly at suture locations; slow healing; and increased risk for infection.

Antineoplastic therapy produces the most severe cases of xerostomia, and increased risk for bacterial, fungal, and herpetic infections. Chemotherapeutic drugs can temporarily change the flow and composition of the saliva. The severity and type of symptoms are specifically related to the pharmacologic class of drug being used, the dosage, and the extent of the leukopenia (a characteristic of all chemotherapeutic drugs). Radiation treatment that is focused on or near the salivary glands can permanently damage salivary glands. Radiation-induced mucositis is dependent on absorbed radiation dose, fractionation, and delivery modality.

The two most common diseases that cause xerostomia are Sjögren' syndrome and diabetes. Other causes are bone marrow transplantation, systemic lupus erythematosus, and thyroid dysfunction.

Swallowed saliva provides a neutralizing effect, which when coupled with the esophageal motor body response (which involves the peristaltic action of the esophagus) clears the esophagus of acid-pepsin–containing refluxate. Investigations have shown that 90% of gastric refluxate is cleared by one or two peristaltic sequences, and the remainder is neutralized by swallowed saliva [1]. In this regard, xerostomia can predispose to or worsen damage from gastroesophageal reflux.

Management strategy

The magnitude of the xerostomia must be assessed, the sources identified, and steps taken to minimize the causes and ensure the patient's comfort. Because smoking is extremely deleterious to dry oral mucosa, smokers should use nicotine replacement therapy to assist with cessation [2]. The use of alcohol should also be discouraged. Pilocarpine, 5 mg, may be helpful to individuals who have residual functional salivary gland tissue [3]. Otherwise, taking frequent sips of cold (iced) water or sucking on ice cubes soothes the oral mucosa and helps keep sutures clean.

Postradiation

The patient who has undergone radiotherapy is at risk for osteoradionecrosis (ORN), a complication resulting from regional radiation-induced hypovascularity, hypoxia of the affected bone, hypocellularity, and cytotoxicity of bone-forming cells [4,5]. The risk

increases after completion of radiation treatment and is present throughout the patient's life span [5]. ORN is associated with large areas of nonvital bone and necrotic soft tissue; oral and cutaneous fistulas; and pathologic fractures. It usually occurs after oral trauma, with 84% of reported ORN associated with tooth extraction.

Management strategy

A careful assessment of the risk for ORN should be performed by determining the fields and total radiation dosage. ORN has not been reported to occur in patients undergoing less than 5000 cGy of radiation. ORN has been reported in patients undergoing between 5000 cGy and 6000 cGy of radiation, but these cases are extremely rare. In contrast, a radiation dose of 7000 cGy produces 10 times the relevant risk when compared with 5000 cGy [6]. Therefore, patients who have undergone more than 6000 cGy of radiation should be considered at risk for ORN and given hyperbaric oxygen (HBO) therapy using the Marx protocol. This regimen consists of 20 preoperative dives followed by 10 postoperative HBO exposures to 100% humidified oxygen at 2.4 atmospheres absolute pressure for 90 minutes per exposure [4,7]. The surgery should be performed as atraumatically as possible.

Esophagus and stomach

The esophagus, stomach, and duodenum form the upper GI tract. Comorbid concerns are associated with acid-related problems, infections, inflammatory disorders, hemorrhage, alterations of upper GI motility, and nutrition. Risk factors the oral and maxillofacial surgeon must consider include aspiration during anesthesia, ulcerations with possible gastric bleeds, postoperative nausea and vomiting, and poor nutritional status.

Aspiration

Aspiration occurs when material, either solid (food or a foreign body) or liquid (gastric contents, blood, or saliva), enters the trachea from the pharynx, usually during a general anesthesia when the patient's airway reflexes are depressed. Pulmonary aspiration of gastric contents during general anesthesia is a rare event in healthy patients undergoing elective surgery [8]. The incidence is 1 in 7000 to 9000 in patients who are American Society of Anesthesiologists

Box 1. Patient conditions that lead to an increased risk for aspiration

- Recent meal (< 4 – 6 hours)
- Morbid obesity (may have increased stomach acid contents or volumes)
- Intoxication or sedation (alcohol, heroine, or heavy sedation with other sedatives)
- Difficult airway access (eg, short fat neck or micrognathia; increased risk for regurgitation if gastric insufflation occurs)
- Head trauma
- Hiatal hernias or esophageal reflux disease
- Pregnancy (decreased lower esophageal sphincter tone)
- Diabetes (slow stomach emptying)
- Narcotics use or significant pain (delayed stomach emptying)
- Connective tissue disorders that affect the esophagus (eg, scleroderma)
- Coma or semiconsciousness
- Gastrointestinal motility disorders
- Dysphagia symptoms

pneumonitis will also make the patient susceptible to more serious bacterial pulmonary infections with a very high associated morbidity and mortality. Prevention of aspiration by identifying patients at risk, requiring preoperative fasting, and using conscious sedation techniques is part of the foundation of safe anesthesia practice in oral surgery offices. Conditions that put patients at increased risk for aspiration are listed in Box 1.

The most important principle in minimizing the risk for aspiration is to have the stomach empty at the time of the anesthesia. The best preventive strategy is to ensure solids are prohibited. Nothing by mouth (NPO) recommendations from the ASA [12] are listed in Table 1 The guidelines for clear liquid NPO status in patients undergoing surgery apply primarily to patients who are at low risk for pulmonary aspiration and who are outpatients. Children and adults undergoing ambulatory surgery can drink clear liquids up to 2 hours preoperatively and will still be at low risk for pulmonary aspiration during general anesthesia if they do not have conditions that are associated with increased volume of gastric contents [13]. Clear liquids are defined as noncoagulating, nonemulsion, or non – particulate-containing fluids, such as water, juices without pulp, punch, soft drinks, tea, or coffee. The type of liquid ingested is more significant than the volume. With solids, however, the type and quantity are important considerations [14]. For pediatric sedation performed in the oral and maxillofacial surgery (OMFS) office, the child should not have any solids or nonhuman milk for 4 hours before sedation. Small amounts of clear liquids or human milk are acceptable up to 2 hours before the procedure. Children at risk for regurgitation or aspiration (eg, those who have known gastroesophageal reflux, those who are extremely obese) should be

(ASA) class I and II, but increases to 1 in less than 400 in patients who are ASA class III to V [9]. However, the reported incidents are widely variable. In one report of patients undergoing general surgery, the rate was as high as 1 in 2000 and was only slightly higher in obstetric or pediatric patients [10]. In an older South African study, the rate was as low as 1 in 240,483 cases [11].

Other situations that predispose patients to aspiration include incision and drainage of pharyngeal abscesses, intranasal surgery, tracheotomy, prolonged endotracheal intubation, nasogastric tubation, deep sedation with loss of swallowing reflex, dysphagia, esophageal strictures, gastroesophageal reflux disease, Parkinson's disease, and myasthenia gravis. Patients experiencing altered mental status caused by conditions such as drug or alcohol ingestion, acute stroke, or head trauma are at extremely high risk for aspiration.

Aspiration of gastric contents is the most relevant and serious type of aspiration for the oral and maxillofacial surgeon. It can result in a spectrum of lung injuries ranging from a very mild subclinical pneumonia to more severe progressive diseases such as adult respiratory distress syndrome. Aspiration

Table 1
NPO recommendations (ASA guidelines)

Ingested material	Minimum fasting period
Clear liquids[a]	2 h
breast milk	4 h
Infant formula	6 h
Nonhuman milk	6 h
Light meal[b]	6 h
Fatty meal	≥8 h

[a] Water, artificial fruit juices, fruit juices without pulp, black coffee, clear tea, carbonated beverages (must not include alcohol).

[b] Toast, crackers, clear liquids in small portions. The meal must never include meat products or fried or fatty foods. The amount and type of food must be considered.

given a longer NPO period before sedation and analgesia [14].

Gastroesophageal reflux disease

Gastroesophageal reflux disease (GERD) is the most common GI disorder, affecting nearly 20 million Americans. It is a digestive disorder that affects the lower esophageal sphincter muscle (LES) connecting the esophagus to the stomach. GERD occurs when the LES is weak or relaxes inappropriately, permitting the stomach's contents to flow up into the esophagus. The most frequently reported symptom is a burning sensation in the chest, but other less common symptoms include chest pain, coughing, wheezing, and hoarseness.

Notably, the symptoms associated with the head and neck manifestation of GERD are different from those seen in individuals who have GI symptoms alone. Heartburn, the classic symptom of GERD, is common in patients who have GI symptoms but uncommon in those who have head and neck manifestations. One study reported only a 20% to 43% incidence of heartburn in patients who had head and neck symptoms [15]. The most common symptom is the sensation of a "lump in the throat" (globus sensation) and studies have shown that GERD is the etiologic factor in 23% to 60% of patients presenting with globus sensation [15,16]. Other symptoms include constant throat clearing (caused by increased secretions and irritation of the laryngeal mucosa), chronic sore throat, coughing, halitosis, and food sticking in the throat.

Two theories attempt to explain how GERD can precipitate an extraesophageal pathologic response. The first theory proposes that injury to the larynx and surrounding tissues is caused directly by refluxed acid–pepsin rising from the stomach [17,18]. The second theory suggests that acid in the distal esophagus stimulates vagally mediated reflexes that result in bronchoconstriction [19], chronic throat clearing, and coughing, eventually leading to mucosal lesions [20,21]. GERD-related airway problems include aspiration; apnea; recurrent pneumonia, bronchitis, and croup; asthma; tracheal stenosis; stridor; hiccups; and sudden infant death syndrome [22]. Direct complications of GERD are bleeding, ulcerations, narrowing of the esophagus, and development of esophageal cancer.

Patients who have GERD should be questioned so that extraesophageal pathologic conditions can be identified, particularly those that would affect the airway. The frequency and severity of symptoms of heartburn should be ascertained. Patients who experience severe symptoms of heartburn daily may be at higher risk for airway problems. Preoperative efforts should be taken to minimize the potential for aspiration. GERD is associated with an alteration in the rate of gastric emptying [23] and will require longer NPO times before surgery. In high-risk patients, prophylactic medications should be considered preoperatively. Ranitidine or cimetidine (the second choice because of its nondesirable side effects) can effectively decrease gastric acid secretion and increase gastric pH for up to 3 hours. Ranitidine is four to six times more potent than cimetidine and has fewer side effects. Famotidine and nizatidine are similar to ranitidine but have a longer duration (Table 2). Efforts should be made to protect the airway from GI secretions throughout surgery and during emergence from anesthesia. Insertion of a nasogastric tube for awake nasogastric suctioning is recommended for patients who are at high risk for aspiration. This tube may be attached to suction or left open to drain freely [24]. During the postoperative phase, nausea and vomiting must be aggressively managed in patients who have GERD. Box 2 describes the management of regurgitation/aspiration in the oral surgery office.

Table 2
Drugs used to treat gastroesophageal reflux disease and most common adverse effects

Drug/antacid	Side effects
H$_2$ receptor blocking agents	
Cimetidine	Headache, gynecomastia in men, depression, disorientation
Famotidine	Constipation, dizziness, fatigue, fever
Nizatidine	diarrhea, headaches, nausea and vomiting, abdominal pain, flatulence, dyspepsia, rhinitis, sore throat
Ranitidine	Headache, constipation, nausea, joint pain, rash, hepatitis
Proton pump inhibitors	
Esomeprazole	Headache, diarrhea, abdominal pain, constipation, nausea, flatulence, dry mouth
Lansoprazole	Abdominal pain, nausea, constipation/diarrhea
Omeprazole	Nausea and vomiting, headache, diarrhea, abdominal pain
Pantoprazole (oral)	Headache, flatulence, diarrhea, abdominal pain
Rabeprazole	Headache, diarrhea, pancreatitis

Proton pump inhibitors are more effective than H$_2$ receptor blockers. H$_2$ receptor blocking agents have several drug interactions.

Box 2. Management of vomiting/ regurgitation or aspiration in the oral and maxillofacial surgery office

1. Turn patient's head towards the shoulder as far as possible and slightly raise the chin to allow gastric contents to flow out of the side of the mouth
2. Use high-speed suction to evacuate fluids from the oral cavity.
3. When possible lower the back of the chair and position it so that the patient will be in a slight Trendelenburg position. If vomiting continues, position patient on the left side.
4. Be aware that entry of fluid into the larynx may produce a (vagal) reflex laryngospasm. Observe chest movement, monitor air flow with pretracheal stethoscope, and observe for laryngospasm.
5. Maintain continuous pulse oximetry and supplemental oxygen to maintain oxygen saturation near 100%. (Tracheal intubation may be necessary if patient has persistent hypoxia. In this case, activate 911 and transfer to a hospital.)
6. Place a stable intravenous catheter in a good vein if not already done. Replace "butterfly" or metal needle.
7. If aspiration occurs, the size of the inoculum will generally be small and the postoperative course will be insidious. Monitor patient for 2 to 4 weeks.
8. Perform a chest radiograph.
9. Depending on chest radiograph findings, consult pulmonologist and an infectious disease specialist.
10. Prophylactic use of antibiotic, steroid therapy, and pulmonary lavage have not been shown to be useful.

Ulcerations and gastric bleeds

Peptic ulcer disease is a common disorder that causes pain and severe discomfort and affects millions of Americans each year. The three most common causes of peptic ulcers are *Helicobacter pylori* infection of the gastric mucosa, ingestion of nonsteroidal anti-inflammatory drugs NSAIDs), and stress (eg, postoperative, shock).

Peptic ulcers are called *primary* when they occur without any predisposing factors, such as an acute medical illness, trauma, use of ulcerogenic medications (eg, salicylates, NSAIDs, steroids), smoking, or dietary intake of secretagogues (eg, alcohol). They occur most commonly in the duodenum or pyloric channel and are uncommon in the stomach. *H pylori*, described by Warren and Marshall [25] in 1983, is now recognized as an important factor in the pathogenesis of primary peptic ulcer disease [26].

Secondary peptic ulcers are usually associated with stress, systemic infection, head trauma, burns, chronic illness, and ulcerogenic medications. Secondary peptic ulcers are not associated with hyperacidity and usually occur in the stomach. Several conditions linked to increased prevalence of peptic ulcer disease in children include cystic fibrosis, type 1 diabetes mellitus, sickle cell disease, pseudo–Zollinger-Ellison syndrome, and Crohn's disease involving the stomach or duodenum.

Perioperative concerns for patients who have chronic peptic ulcers are focused on preventing or minimizing acute ulceration with or without bleeding after surgery. Inactive peptic ulcer disease may become active after surgery, causing persistent pain, and may even bleed and complicate the recuperation. Patients who have a history of ulcers, GI bleeding, or dyspepsia should therefore be considered for preventive therapy after surgery.

NSAID-related ulcers (Table 3) are more likely to bleed than those caused by *H Pylori*, perhaps because ulcers caused by NSAIDs are often diagnosed late and are therefore more difficult to treat. This late

Table 3
Ulcer risk by specific nonsteroidal anti-inflammatory drugs

| Lowest risk | Medium risk | | Highest risk |
	Lower	Higher	
COX-2–selective	Aspirin[a]	Naproxen	Flurbiprofen
Meloxicam	Ibuprofen	Tolmetin	Piroxicam
Nabumetone	Diclofenac	Aspirin	Fenoprofen
Etodolac			Indomethacin
COX-2–specific			Meclofenamate
Rofecoxib			Ketoprofen
Valdecoxib			Ketorolac
Nonacetylated salicylates			
Salsalate			
Nonselective			
Sulindac			

[a] Low-dose aspirin, 81 mg.

diagnosis occurs because usually no GI symptoms from NSAIDs appear until the ulcers are advanced and bleeding occurs.

When an active peptic process is present, surgery should not be performed and the GI disease should be treated before major surgical procedures. Some individuals may also become anemic and require treatment before major surgery. Patients at risk for developing GI bleeding should also undergo repeated postoperative stool testing for occult blood.

In primary peptic ulcers the object of therapy is to ameliorate the symptoms and prevent postoperative recurrence and complications. The most important goal of treatment is the eradication of *H pylori* because otherwise primary peptic ulcers are likely to recur. Several combinations of therapeutic agents are recommended. The first-line treatment is the combination of omeprazole with two antibiotics: clarithromycin and amoxicillin. Second-line treatment incorporates bismuth subcitrate with metronidazole and tetracycline [27].

Secondary ulcers, however, are treated by stopping the offending substances (eg, aspirin, NSAIDs, corticosteroids, alcohol) and using acid-suppressing medications such as H_2 blockers, proton pump inhibitors, and mucosal protectants. NSAIDs and aspirin-containing analgesics should be avoided in any patient who has a history of gastric ulcers.

Postoperative nausea and vomiting

Many oral and maxillofacial surgeons may not regard postoperative nausea as a serious complication, viewing it as a short-term annoyance that will eventually pass. To many patients, however, it is the worst aspect of their surgical experience. Despite years dedicated to improving anesthetic agents and developing shorter-acting agents and better techniques, one out of three patients still experiences nausea and vomiting after surgery. This condition not only influences patient satisfaction but also can prolong recovery, lengthen hospital stay, and negatively impact surgery. One study estimated that nausea affects up to 35% of patients after day surgery [28] and that about 1% of patients undergoing ambulatory surgery are admitted overnight because of uncontrolled postoperative nausea and vomiting [29]. According to Gan [30], four groups at high-risk for experiencing postoperative nausea and vomiting (PONV) are females, young patients, nonsmokers, and patients who have a history of PONV or motion sickness. Nausea, vomiting, and retching are defined in Box 3.

The use of postoperative opioids for pain is one of the most predictive risk factors for PONV. Some

---

Box 3. Definitions of nausea, vomiting, and retching

Nausea: a subjectively unpleasant sensation associated with flushing, tachycardia, and an awareness of the urge to vomit.

Vomiting: the contraction of the abdominal muscles, descent of the diaphragm, and opening of the gastric cardia, resulting in the expulsion of stomach contents from the mouth.

Retching: a spasmodic contraction of the diaphragm and thoracic and abdominal walls without expulsion of gastric contents.

---

surgical procedures are also associated with a higher incidence of PONV, including craniotomy; ear, nose, and throat procedures; major breast procedures; strabismus surgery; laparoscopy; and laparotomy. Agents used during anesthesia, including opioids, nitrous oxide, and volatile inhalational anesthetics, are emetogenic. Pain, anxiety, and dehydration may also increase the incidence of PONV [31]. Ulcers that form in the duodenum can swell and scar, resulting in a narrowing or closing of the intestinal opening. In such cases, gastric emptying is slowed and the patient may vomit.

The underlying physiology of emesis must be understood so the pharmaceutical strategies that are involved in the elimination of PONV can be appreciated. The emetic center is an ill-defined area located in the lateral reticular formation of the medulla that receives nerve signals from many areas of the body. During and after surgery, signals involving several neurotransmitters mediated through central and peripheral pathways arrive and activate the center, causing the nausea and vomiting. An important structure that affects the vomiting center is the chemoreceptor trigger zone (CTZ) located in the area postrema which lies outside the blood–brain barrier. The nucleus of the tractus solitarius (NTS) and the vagal nuclei receive afferent impulses through the vagus nerve and interconnect in the CTZ. Within the CTZ the signals are modulated and transferred to the vomiting center. Serotonin, dopamine, and acetylcholine are the active transmitters in this area. Peripheral structures that trigger the vomiting center include the mechanoreceptors in the muscular wall of the distal stomach and proximal duodenum, and the chemo-

Table 4

Drugs used to manage postoperative nausea and vomiting by class

Anticholinergic (antimuscarinic) drugs	Dopamine antagonists	Antihistamines	5-HT$_3$–receptor antagonists	Other
Scopolamine	Phenothiazines	Dimenhydrinate	Ondansetron	Dexamethasone
	Butyrophenones	Meclizine	Dolasetron	Trimethobenzamide
	Metoclopramide		Palonosetron[a]	Aprepitant[a]
	Domperidone		Granisetron[a]	

The receptor sites implicated in nausea and vomiting include acetylcholine (muscarine), dopamine, histamine, and serotonin.

[a] Chemotherapy-related.

receptors in the gut mucosa of the upper small intestine. Serotonin and cholinergic pathways are involved. Other connections to the vomiting center come from cranial nerves, the hypothalamus, the cortex, and the vestibular system [31]. Learned responses (from the cortex), such as a strong history of motion sickness, are also important and are mediated by histamine.

In summary, the receptor sites implicated in nausea and vomiting include dopamine, acetylcholine (muscarine), serotonin, and histamine. Pharmacologic agents acting as antagonists of these receptors are the agents used to manage PONV. Tables 4 and 5 list the agents that are used to treat PONV. The administration of an antiemetic acting on one receptor site typically reduces the incidence of PONV by about 30%. Using a combination of antiemetics acting at different receptor sites has been found to further reduce this incidence and many antiemetic combinations have been investigated. Ondansetron and

droperidol combined can achieve at least a 90% response rate (no nausea, vomiting, or need for rescue antiemetics) [30,32]. Speculating that the use of multiple (more than two) drug combinations will further enhance effectiveness is tempting, but published data have not been conclusive. Scuderi and colleagues [33] described one special combination involving more than two agents, showing that multimodal management incorporating combination antiemetics and propofol resulted in a 98% complete response rate. Evidence also suggests that intravenous anesthesia with propofol reduces the incidence of PONV [33] and may be beneficial for sedating patients in the OMFS office who are at high risk or have a previous history of PONV. Propofol's mechanism of action as an antiemetic has not been conclusively elucidated; however, some evidence suggests that it may act by reducing serotonin levels in the area postrema [34]. Recognizing that nausea, like pain, is more difficult to control once it becomes severe, some clinicians recommend using antiemetics before the nausea begins (preemptively). The timing of antiemetic administration is outlined in Box 4.

Table 5

Drugs commonly used to manage postoperative nausea and vomiting by name

Drug	Brand names	Dosage
Chlorpromazine	Ormazine, Thorazine	Oral/IM: 0.5–1 mg/kg/dose q6h
Prochlorperazine	Compazine	Oral: 5–10 mg qid; IM: 5–10 mg q4h prn
Granisetron	Kytril	1 mg IV over 30 sec
Promethazine	Phenergan	25 mg initially, then 12.5–25 mg q6h prn
Metoclopramide[a]	Reglan	10–20 mg IM near end of surgery
Ondansetron	Zofran	4 mg IV/IM immediately before anesthesia or at end of surgery. Oral: 16 mg 1 h before anesthesia with small sip of water

Abbreviations: IM, intramuscularly; IV, intravenously; prn, as needed.

[a] First drug of choice.

Box 4. Timing of antiemetics

- Drug should be administered at the end of the surgical procedure before extubation.
- If dexamethasone is to be used, it should be administered 1 hour before the end of the procedure.
- If an NSAID (ketorolac) will be used for postoperative pain management, it should be given at the end of anesthesia before the patient leaves the operating room.
- For high-risk surgery with two or more patient-specific risk factors, the drug should be administered at the start of anesthesia.

Lower intestinal tract

The small and large intestines constitute the lower GI tract. The small intestine is where 90% of digestion and absorption occurs, whereas the large intestine is involved with the absorption of water and elimination of solid waste. Dietary fibers and other solid products that are not digested by the stomach or small intestine and reach the large intestine are broken down by microorganisms in the colon. This microflora is also important in the development of the intestinal immune system. Diseases of the lower GI tract involve motility issues; infections; inflammatory and malabsorption problems; malfunctions in the secretion of digestive enzymes; malformations and deformities; and malignancies. The major symptoms of lower GI disorders are diarrhea, constipation, pain, rectal bleeding, and fecal incontinence.

Motility problems

Disruptions of normal gut motility can lead to diarrhea, constipation, or paralysis. Peristalsis is used to propel chyme from the proximal (duodenum) to distal (rectum) intestinal tract. It consists of coordinated contractions that end in relaxation and move as a wave pushing the chyme along the intestinal tract. Normal peristalsis is controlled by the action of stimulatory and inhibitory effectors on muscle-wave activity. These effectors are initiated by stomach wall distention and transmitted through the myenteric plexus. Several factors can disrupt this normal process, resulting in motility changes ranging from increased motility to total paralysis.

Diarrhea

Diarrhea consists of loose, watery stools occurring more than three times in one day (people who have diarrhea may pass more than 2 liters of stool per day). The most significant perioperative diarrhea is antibiotic-associated diarrhea and colitis. The term *antibiotic-associated diarrhea* (AAD), which may affect up to 20% of people undergoing antibiotic therapy, refers to a benign, self-limited diarrhea that occurs during antimicrobial use. The risk for developing AAD more than doubles when patients undergo more than 3 days of antibiotic therapy (risk ratio, 2.28) [35], but cases of colitis involving administration of a single perioperative dose for surgical prophylaxis have been reported [36]. When antibiotics (especially broad-spectrum agents with poor intestinal absorption or high biliary excretion) are used over an extended period, they induce a change in the composition and function of the intestinal flora

that results in AAD. The degree of alteration is influenced by the ability of the normal flora to resist colonization and the type of antibiotic used [31].

A decrease in the colonic anaerobic flora interferes with carbohydrate and bile acid metabolism, which can cause an osmotic or secretory diarrhea. The colon is unable to absorb carbohydrates, and as much as 70 g of undigested carbohydrate reaches the colon each day. Colonic bacteria, especially certain anaerobes, metabolize these carbohydrates as an energy source, producing lactic acid and short-chain fatty acids that are then readily absorbed by the colon [37]. Loss of these bacteria from antibiotic treatment can lead to increased amounts of carbohydrate in the colonic lumen, resulting in an osmotic diarrhea. Overgrowth of opportunistic pathogens occurs as a result of microbiologic and metabolic alterations in the normal gut flora. However, in general, no pathogens are identified in AAD and the diarrhea is caused only by the changes in the composition and function of the intestinal flora, and is osmotic in nature. Removing the offending antibiotic will often resolve the diarrhea.

All groups of antibiotics may cause AAD, but those with broad-spectrum coverage, in particular cephalosporins, extended-coverage penicillins, and clindamycin, are the most common causative agents (Tables 6 and 7). The aminoglycosides (amikacin sulfate, gentamicin sulfate, tobramycin), erythromycin, trimethoprim-sulfamethoxazole, and the newer fluoroquinolones seem less likely to cause AAD. The risk also increases with how often and how long the antibiotics are taken. However, any antibiotics, even

Table 6
Frequency of antibiotic-associated diarrhea (AAD) when treated with one antibiotic only

Common	Less common	Rare
Ampicillin (6.7%)	Penicillin (3.3%)	Chloramphenicol
Clindamycin (5.0%)	Erythromycin (3.4%)	Metronidazole
Cephalosporins (6.1%)		Tetracycline (2.0%)
Ciprofloxacin (10.3%)		Aminoglycosides
		Vancomycin

Note: Other studies have shown higher incidents, up to as much as 20%. Numbers used in this table are closer to those consistently seen by the author.
Data from Epocrates.com. Available at: http://www2.epocrates.com/index.html/palm. Accessed January 2005; and Wiström J, Ragnar Norrby SR, Myhre EB, et al. Frequency of antibiotic-associated diarrhoea in 2462 antibiotic-treated hospitalized patients: a prospective study. J Antimicrob Chemother 2001; 47:43–50.

Table 7
Frequency of antibiotic-associated diarrhea according to duration of antibiotic treatment when taking one antibiotic only

Number of treatment (days)	Percentage developing AAD (%)
1–3 d	2.4
4–7 d	5.2 (>100% increase)
8–10 d	4.5
10–21 d	4.9
>3 weeks	6.7

A significant increase in risk (more than double) for AAD occurs when antibiotics is taken for >3 d.
Abbreviation: AAD, antibiotic-associated diarrhea.
Data from Wiström J, Ragnar Norrby SR, Myhre EB, et al. Frequency of antibiotic-associated diarrhoea in 2462 antibiotic-treated hospitalized patients: a prospective study. J Antimicrob Chemother 2001;47:43–50.

when given for a short time, can occasionally lead to this problem [38]. Most patients will experience response when antibiotics are discontinued and supportive measures are undertaken.

Pseudomembranous colitis

Pseudomembranous colitis is a much less common but more serious form of AAD that can lead to serious morbidity, such as toxic megacolon which may require surgical resection. Although rare, it may even be fatal. A severe inflammation of the inner lining of the colon (irritation and swelling with presence of excess immune cells) occurs in pseudomembranous colitis, characterized by pus and blood in the stool. For years the cause of pseudomembranous colitis was uncertain and experts widely believed staphylococci to be the source. In the late 1970s, however, studies of clindamycin-associated pseudomembranous colitis and the demonstration of the potent cytopathic effects of *Clostridium difficile*–derived toxin in animal models established *C difficile* as the major identifiable etiologic agent of AAD with colitis [39].

Reported incidence of AAD varies from 5% to 39% depending on the antibiotic type, and pseudomembranous colitis complicates 10% of these cases [40]. Clindamycin, lincomycin, ampicillin, and cephalosporins have been implicated in most of the reported cases and are the same antibiotics on which oral and maxillofacial surgeons rely heavily. Oral surgeons should therefore be concerned with the potential for outpatients who are prescribed these antibiotics to contract pseudomembranous colitis. In a study of 376,590 antibiotic prescriptions provided to more than 280,000 outpatients over a 4-year period, four cases of acute *C difficile* colitis occurred. The incidence rate was calculated to be 1.6 per 100,000 people exposed to ampicillin, 2.9 per 100,000 exposed to dicloxacillin, and 2.6 per 100,000 exposed to tetracycline [41]. A retrospective cohort study from Harvard Medical School of members of a health maintenance organization (HMO) reported 51 cases of pseudomembranous colitis in 662,500 persons in a year at a rate of 7.7 cases per 100,000 person-years, and 42 individuals (82%) diagnosed and treated exclusively in the ambulatory care setting. Only six patients required hospitalization and all patients were treated successfully. The overall risk rate for community-acquired *C difficile*–associated diarrhea in this study was less than 1 per 10,000 antibiotic prescriptions, and the risk for hospitalization was 0.5 to 1.0 per 100,000 person-years [42]. This report also noted an increased risk with the use of combination antibiotic therapy, especially in combination with cephalosporins. Age-adjusted antibiotic-specific attack rates were at least 10-fold higher ($P<.05$) for nitrofurantoin, cefuroxime, cephalexin plus dicloxacillin, ampicillin/clavulanate plus cefaclor, and ampicillin/clavulanate plus cefuroxime than for ampicillin or amoxicillin alone [42]. These two reports show that the risk for hospitalization from community-acquired antibiotic-induced colitis is very low and that patients who have colitis can be treated adequately on an outpatient basis. Treatment success, however, relies on recognition and early intervention.

Usually the GI symptoms begin 3 to 10 days after starting the antibiotics, but up to 10 weeks may elapse between the start of the antibiotic and the onset of the clinical symptoms. The most common presentation is cramping abdominal pain with profuse, watery, or mucoid, greenish, foul-smelling stool that may contain small amounts of blood. The diagnosis primarily relies on an appropriate history of antibiotic usage. Physical examination findings include fever (temperature may reach 103° F–105°F), abdominal tenderness, and diarrhea. The abdominal pain is most often diffused and cramping but can also manifest as focal pain mimicking an acute abdomen. Evidence of peritoneal signs should immediately raise the possibility of fulminant colitis and toxic megacolon (fever, nausea, vomiting, ileus, rigid abdomen, and, in the most severe cases, rebound tenderness). Cytotoxic assay of the stool for *C difficile* toxins is considered the criterion standard for laboratory diagnosis (the reported sensitivity and specificity for this type of study is high: 67%–100% and 85%–100%, respectively), but it is expensive and takes up 48 hours to complete. Enzyme-linked immunosorbent assay (ELISA) tests are used to detect the presence of toxin A or B in the stool and are cheaper and provide results within an hour. Reported sensitivities range

from 63% to 85%, with specificities of 75% to 100%. *C difficile* produces two toxins, A (enterotoxin) and B (cytotoxin). Toxin A, the tissue-damaging enterotoxin, is the toxin detected by the C. DIFFICILE TOX-A TEST (TechLab Inc., Blacksburgh, Virginia). The C. DIFFICILE TOX A-TEST is a monoclonal antibody-based ELISA and is an alternative to tissue culture assay for detecting *C difficile* toxin in fecal specimens. The test is completed within 1 hour [43].

Oral treatment with antimicrobial agents effective against *C difficile* is the preferred method of treatment. First-line therapy consists of metronidazole 500 mg orally three to four times daily for 10 to 14 days. Metronidazole is an inexpensive drug with a greater than 90% positive response rate [44]. If a patient is pregnant or does not respond to or tolerate metronidazole, vancomycin should be initiated at a dosage of 125 to 500 mg orally four times daily for 10 to 14 days [45].

Paralytic ileus

In paralytic ileus, neurogenic failure or loss of peristalsis occurs in the intestine in the absence of any mechanical obstruction. This effect may range from hypomobility to full paralysis. Some possible causes of postoperative ileus (POI) in the OMFS patient include prolonged use of opiates either during the surgery or in the postoperative phase; metabolic disturbances, particularly those that result in decreased potassium levels; injury or trauma; and pain from another underlying disorder (eg, harvesting bone from iliac crest) or illness. Adverse effects of paralytic ileus are increased postoperative pain, increased nausea and vomiting, delayed resumption of oral intake, delayed postoperative mobilization with increasing risk for pulmonary complications (eg, atelectasis, pneumonia, pulmonary embolism from deep venous thrombosis), and nosocomial infections.

When peristalsis ceases, stagnation occurs in the small and large intestines, producing abdominal cramping, abdominal distention, a reduction or absence of bowel sounds, nausea and vomiting, and the inability to pass gas or stool. Postoperative hypomotility may affect all parts of the GI tract but with different rates in the recovery of normal function. Small intestine function generally normalizes first, often within several hours after surgery. Gastric motility usually returns to normal within 24 to 48 hours postoperatively, but the colon may remain inert for 48 to 72 hours after surgery. Function returns first to the proximal colon and then progresses to the transverse and left colon [46]. Most data support the observation that colonic dysfunction is the limiting factor in the resolution of POI.

Motility of the GI tract is temporarily impaired after most major surgery involving general anesthesia and is characterized by disorganized electrical activity and lack of coordinated propulsion. In the stomach, studies have shown a postoperative period of gastric hypomotility associated with irregular and disorganized electrical activity. Motor activity is similarly disorganized in the small bowel. Normal colonic motility is typically the last to return after surgery. Studies evaluating postoperative colonic motility have frequently found a period of relative hypomotility that is generally associated with random, disorganized bursts of electrical activity [47]. This hypomotility is short-lived, and normal GI function returns quickly after surgery. Anesthetic agents may have a minor effect on decreasing GI motility in the postoperative setting because peristalsis is slowed to some degree by all agents used in the induction and maintenance of general anesthesia. These agents, however, most likely do not play a large role in the pathogenesis of POI, as evidenced by the large number of prolonged nonabdominal surgical procedures performed under general anesthesia without a significant occurrence of POI [48].

Several mechanisms are believed to play a role in causing POI in nonabdominal surgery. One hypothesis is that sympathetic hyperactivity in the postoperative period generates high levels of circulating catecholamines, leading to POI. Plasma catecholamines have been shown to be elevated after surgery [49], and high levels of catecholamines in nonsurgical settings have been associated with inhibiting GI motility. Other theories postulate that neural reflexes involving the sympathetic nervous system play an important role in POI by inhibiting intestinal motility. Another theory is that surgery produces high quantities of endorphins that function like morphine to decrease motility [50].

The first line of treatment is supervised bed rest, continuous nasogastric suction, and bowel rest, where nothing is taken by mouth. Intravenous fluids and electrolytes are administered to maintain adequate hydration. Maintaining an adequate serum potassium level (potassium >4 mEq/L [>4 mmol/L]) by adding potassium as required is especially important. Mild sedation should also be used for patient comfort. Certain drugs can be used to accelerate the resumption of the intestinal function, such as trimebutine maleate and vasopressin.

For the management of pain, ketorolac tromethamine is ideal. This NSAID, which can be administered intravenously, may reduce the duration of POI through its anti-inflammatory actions and through decreasing the postoperative use of opiates for pain control. In

most studies, NSAID administration has improved postoperative bowel in patients experiencing ileus [51].

Malabsorption syndromes

Malabsorption is a broad term that comprises many disease processes. In clinical practice it denotes defects occurring during the digestion and absorption of food nutrients by the gastrointestinal tract. Surgical risks include bleeding secondary to vitamin K deficiency, poor healing secondary to generalized nutritional problems, possible ulcerations of GI mucosa, anemia, and problems with oral medications. Specific malabsorption diseases are celiac sprue, Whipple's disease, short bowel syndrome, lactase deficiency, and bacterial overgrowth (eg, gastric achlorhydria, Crohn's disease, AIDS, motility problems secondary to scleroderma or diabetes).

When a diffuse disorder such as celiac disease (a diagnosis that is doubling every 2 years and may affect up to 1% of the population) affects the intestine, absorption of almost all nutritional elements is impaired. Depending on the disease and its severity, presenting symptoms could include one or more of the following: diarrhea; steatorrhea; weight loss and fatigue; abdominal distention and flatulence; anemia; bleeding disorders; and metabolic defects of bones. Perioperative care focuses on correction of nutritional deficiencies and, when possible, treatment of causative diseases.

Nutritional support involves (1) supplementation of various minerals that may be deficient, such as calcium, magnesium, or iron; (2) caloric and protein replacement; (3) fat replacement with medium-chain triglycerides; (4) supplementation with multivitamins; and (5) vitamin K supplementation if the international normalized ratio (INR) is elevated.

In treating causative diseases, a gluten-free diet helps correct celiac disease; a lactose-free diet helps reduce symptoms of lactose intolerance; antibiotics control bacterial overgrowth; and corticosteroids help treat regional enteritis.

For an urgent oral surgical procedure, an abnormal INR can be corrected with vitamin K, and parenteral nutrition could be used if necessary (see the article on nutrition by Fang, Desai, and Dym in this issue). Prophylactic antibiotics should also be considered.

Organs

Spleen

The four most important functions of the normal spleen are (1) clearance of microorganisms and particulate antigens from the bloodstream; (2) synthesis of IgG (comprises approximately 75% of the immunoglobulins and acts primarily against gram-positive bacteria), properdin (an essential component of the alternate pathway of complement activation), and tuftsin (facilitates the opsonization and phagocytosis that enhances the lysis of bacteria cells); (3) removal of abnormal red blood cells; and (4) embryonic hematopoiesis in certain diseases.

Splenomegaly

Splenomegaly is enlargement of the spleen, and usually occurs as a secondary phenomenon. Although many diseases are associated with an enlarged spleen, splenomegaly is most often related to liver disease, which is very common because of the frequency of alcoholism and hepatitis. Other nonhepatic disorders associated with splenomegaly are infectious mononucleosis, infective endocarditis, malaria, toxoplasmosis, sarcoidosis, amyloidosis, systemic lupus erythematous, hemoglobin disorders (eg, thalassemia, certain sickle cell disorders, congenital Heinz body hemolytic anemia), and neoplasms. To the surgeon, the major risk of splenomegaly is thrombocytopenia.

Approximately 30% to 35% of the circulating platelets normally exist as an exchangeable pool within the spleen, which is the major storage site of platelets. In patients who have splenomegaly, a larger volume of platelets is sequestered, which can lead to thrombocytopenia. In patients experiencing hypersplenism, as much as 90% of the total platelet mass may be found in the spleen [52]. (The term *hypersplenism* is often considered synonymous with *splenomegaly* and refers to the latter in association with a reduction in one or more blood cell counts and resultant hyperplasia of relevant bone marrow tissue.) In most cases the thrombocytopenia secondary to hypersplenism does not cause clinically significant hemostatic defects, and the decrease in platelets is moderate (ie, not falling below 50,000), and usually does not require treatment. (In hypersplenism, the platelet count is usually 50,000–150,000/mL.) However, this decrease should be addressed in selective circumstances, such as preoperative preparation for a surgery [53]. A complete blood cell count should be performed. Elective oral surgery should be postponed if the platelet count is less than 50,000/mm^3, or these patients may undergo transfusion before surgery to raise the count above 50,000/mm^3. However, because of platelet refractoriness (ie, the patient does not have the expected platelet increase after transfusion), the effectiveness of platelet transfusions is significantly decreased in splenomegaly.

Leukopenia is also observed in splenomegaly and is the result of an increase in the marginated granulocyte pool located in the spleen. Sequestration seems to also play a role in the genesis of neutropenia [52]. Prophylactic antibiotics should be considered for patients who have white blood cell counts of 2000 or less because these individuals may be at risk for bacterial infection. Prophylactic antibiotics are mandatory for counts less than 1000.

Patients who have undergone splenectomy

People who do not have spleens are at increased risk for a severe, sometimes life-threatening septicemia called *overwhelming post-splenectomy infection* (OPSI) [54]. Most infections occur within the first 2 to 3 years after splenectomy and the reported mortality rate ranges from 50% to 80% [55] depending on the cause of the disease that necessitated the procedure. The incidence is low in patients who experienced splenic trauma and highest in those who have Hodgkin's disease. Although most (50%–70%) serious infections occur within the first 2 years after splenectomy, patients have experienced serious infections more than 40 years after a splenectomy, indicating that the increased risk is lifelong [56].

The risk for OPSI, however, seems to be small (probably in the range of 1 per 500 person-years of observation) [55] but is not trivial and the consequences are very serious. Up to 50% of cases are fatal despite appropriate antibiotic therapy, and more than half of patients who die do so within 48 hours of admission to the hospital [57]. In one large study the overall cumulative risk for infection severe enough to require hospitalization was 33% at the end of a 10-year follow-up period [56]. Children are especially susceptible because they often have lower levels of specific antibodies against encapsulated organisms [55].

Polysaccharide encapsulated bacteria, such as *Streptococcus pneumoniae*, are responsible for the most serious types of infections seen in patients who have undergone splenectomy. The spleen clears opsonized bacteria from the blood and stores B lymphocytes that respond to polysaccharide antigens. The loss of the spleen, therefore, impairs the antibody response to antigenic challenges from these bacteria and places the individual at an increased risk for infection. Because of the seriousness of OPSI, particularly in children, prophylactic antibiotics are frequently given for an indefinite period. Questions remain regarding the role of prophylactic antibiotics, however, and their use is not universally accepted mainly because scientific evidence supporting their general use is limited [58].

Because most cases of postsplenectomy infection have occurred within the first 2 to 3 years after surgery, several authorities recommend that patients who undergo splenectomy at any age receive prophylaxis for at least this period [59,60]. Another recommendation is that daily antibiotic prophylaxis, typically penicillin V twice daily, be given to children up to the age of 16 years who are asplenic [61]. Because of these recommendations, young patients (<16 years) who have undergone splenectomy may be on long-term antibiotics when they arrive for oral surgery. Within 60 to 90 minutes before tooth extraction, these patients should receive a prophylactic boost with an antibiotic that has a broad spectrum of activity, such as amoxicillin-clavulanic acid or clindamycin in a bactericidal dose. (The long-term penicillin protocol may create β-lactam–resistant strains of oral streptococci, and therefore switching to a different class of antibiotics for prophylactic purposes and relying on clindamycin or ciprofloxacin may be wise.)

Because patients undergoing splenectomy do not have an adequate host immune system, clinicians generally accept that these patients are at increased risk for developing septicemia from tooth extraction–related bacteremia and should therefore be given prophylactic antibiotics before undergoing this procedure [62,63]. These patients should (1) obtain a MedicAlert bracelet or necklace; (2) inform all health care professionals about their asplenic state, including dentists; and (3) take antibiotics before and for 24 hours after any invasive medical procedures, including dental cleanings, oral surgery, catheterization, endoscopy, and other surgeries [62,64].

Summary

The human GI system is very complex and is affected by a wide variety of diseases and abnormal conditions. Starting proximally from the oral cavity, this article discusses commonly encountered and clinically significant entities, with emphasis on assisting the clinician in developing management strategies to reduce the risk associated with GI diseases. Xerostomia, osteoradionecrosis, GERD, and ulcerative diseases that occur in the proximal portion of the GI system and motility disturbances that occur in the distal portion are presented. This article does not discuss the liver and biliary system because they are covered elsewhere in this issue. Lastly, this article addresses suggestions for managing patients who have splenomegaly and have undergone sple-

nectomy. Although other possible diseases and conditions exist, the ones included are those the author considers most important to the practicing oral and maxillofacial surgeon.

References

[1] Helm JF, Dodds WJ, Pelc LR, et al. Effect of esophageal emptying and saliva on clearance of acid from the esophagus. N Engl J Med 1984;310(5):284–8.

[2] Rugg T, Saunders MI, Dische S. Smoking and mucosal reactions to radiotherapy. Br J Radiol 1990;63:554–6.

[3] Johnson JT, Ferretti GA, Nethery WJ, et al. Oral pilocarpine for post-irradiation xerostomia in patients with head and neck cancer. N Engl J Med 1993;329: 390–5.

[4] Marx RE. Osteoradionecrosis: a new concept of its pathophysiology. J Oral Maxillofac Surg 1983;41(5): 283–8.

[5] Marx RE, Johnson RP. Studies in the radiobiology of osteoradionecrosis and their clinical significance. Oral Surg Oral Med Oral Pathol 1987;64:379–90.

[6] Clayman L. Management of dental extractions in irradiated jaws: a protocol without hyperbaric oxygen therapy. J Oral Maxillofac Surg 1997;55:275–81.

[7] Marx RE. A new concept in the treatment of osteoradionecrosis. J Oral Maxillofac Surg 1983;41(6): 351–7.

[8] Fasting S, Gisvold SE. Serious intraoperative problems—a five-year review of 83,844 anesthetics. Can J Anesth 2002;49:545–53.

[9] Warner MA, Warner ME, Weber JG. Clinical significance of pulmonary aspiration in the perioperative period. Anesth 1993;78:59–62.

[10] Engelhardt T, Webster NR. Pulmonary aspiration of gastric contents in anesthesia: survey of anesthesiology. Br J Anaesth 1999;83:453–60.

[11] Harrison GG. Death attributable to anaesthesia: A ten year survey (1967–1976). Br J Anaesth 1978;50: 1041–6.

[12] American Society of Anesthesiologist. NPO guidelines. Available at: http://www.asahq.org/practice/npo/npoguide.html. Accessed January 2005.

[13] Goresky GV, Maltby JR. Fasting guidelines for elective surgical patients. Can J Anesth 1990;37:493–5.

[14] American Society of Anesthesiologist. Sedation guidelines. Available at: http://www.asahq.org/clinical/toolkit/sedmodelfinal.htm. Accessed January 2005.

[15] Koufman JA. The otolaryngologic manifestations of gastroesophageal reflux disease (GERD): a clinical investigation of 225 patients using ambulatory 24-hour pH monitoring and an experimental investigation of the role of acid and pepsin in the development of laryngeal injury. Laryngoscope 1991;101(4 pt 2 Suppl 53): 1–78.

[16] Hill J, Stuart RC, Fung HK, et al. Gastroesophageal reflux, motility disorders, and psychological profiles in the etiology of globus pharyngis. Laryngoscope 1997; 107:1373–7.

[17] Gaynor EB. Gastroesophageal reflux as an etiologic factor in laryngeal complications of intubation. Laryngoscope 1988;98(9):972–9.

[18] Ludemann JP, Manoukian J, Shaw K, et al. Effects of simulated gastroesophageal reflux on the untraumatized rabbit larynx. J Otolaryngol 1998;27(3):127–31.

[19] Tuchman DN, Boyle JT, Pack AI, et al. Comparison of airway responses following tracheal or esophageal acidification in the cat. Gastroenterol 1984;87(4): 872–81.

[20] Mansfield LE, Stein MR. Gastroesophageal reflux and asthma: a possible reflex mechanism. Ann Allergy 1978;41(4):224–6.

[21] Mansfield LE, Hameister HH, Spaulding HS, et al. The role of the vagus nerve in airway narrowing caused by intraesophageal hydrochloric acid provocation and esophageal distention. Ann Allergy 1981;47(6):431–4.

[22] Bauman NM, Sandler AD, Smith RJ. Respiratory manifestations of gastroesophageal reflux disease in pediatric patients. Ann Otol Rhinol Laryngol 1996; 105:23–32.

[23] Morgan GE, Makhail MS, Murray MJ. Respiratory physiology and anesthesia. In: Morgan GE, Mikhail MS, Murray MJ, et al, editors. Clinical anesthesiology. New York: Lange Medical Books/McGraw-Hill; 1996. p. 475–510.

[24] Ng A, Smith G. Gastroesophageal reflux and aspiration of gastric contents in anesthetic practice. Anesth Analg 2001;93:494–513.

[25] Warren JR, Marshall BJ. Unidentified curved bacilli on gastric epithelium in active chronic gastritis. Lancet 1983;8336:1273–5.

[26] Hardin FJ, Wright RA. Helicobacter pylori: review and update. Hosp Physician 2002;38:23–31.

[27] deBoer WA, Tytgat GN. Treatment of Helicobacter pylori infection. BMJ 2000;320:31–4.

[28] Carroll NV, Miederhoff P, Cox FM, et al. Postoperative nausea and vomiting after discharge from outpatient surgery centers. Anesth Analg 1995;80:903–9.

[29] Tramèr MR. A rational approach to the control of postoperative nausea and vomiting: evidence from systematic reviews. Part I. Efficacy and harm of antiemetic interventions, and methodological issues. Acta Anaesthesiol Scand 2001;45:4–13.

[30] Gan TJ. Postoperative nausea and vomiting—can it be eliminated? JAMA 2002;287:1233–6.

[31] Watcha MF, White PF. Postoperative nausea and vomiting: its etiology, treatment, and prevention. Anesthesiology 1992;77:162–84.

[32] Habib AS, Gan TJ. Combination therapy for postoperative nausea and vomiting—a more effective prophylaxis? Ambul Surg 2001;9:59–71.

[33] Scuderi PE, James RL, Harris L, et al. Multimodal antiemetic management prevents early postoperative vomiting after outpatient laparoscopy. Anesth Analg 2000;91:1408–14.

[34] Cechetto DF, Diab T, Gibson CJ, et al. The effects of

propofol in the area postrema of rats. Anesth Analg 2001;92:934–42.

[35] Wiström J, Norrby SR, Myhre EB, et al. Frequency of antibiotic-associated diarrhoea in 2462 antibiotic-treated hospitalized patients: a prospective study. J Antimicrob Chemother 2001;47:43–50.

[36] Freiman JP, Graham DJ, Green L. Pseudomembranous colitis associated with single-dose cephalosporin prophylaxis [letter]. JAMA 1989;262(7):902.

[37] Cummings JH, Pomare EW, Branch WJ, et al. Short chain fatty acids in human large intestine, portal, hepatic and venous blood. Gut 1987;28:1221–7.

[38] Wilcox MH. Gastrointestinal disorders and the critically ill. Clostridium difficile infection and pseudomembranous colitis. Best Pract Res Clin Gastroenterol 2003;17:475–93.

[39] Bartlett JG, Chang TW, Gurwith M, et al. Antibiotic-associated pseudomembranous colitis due to toxin-producing clostridia. N Engl J Med 1978;298:531–4.

[40] Yassin SF. Pseudomembranous colitis: surgical perspective. Available at: http://www.emedicine.com/med/topic2743.htm. Accessed January 2005.

[41] Stergachis A, Perera DR, Schnell MM, et al. Antibiotic-associated colitis. West J Med 1984;140:217–9.

[42] Hirschhorn LR, Trinka Y, Onderdonk A, et al. Epidemiology of community acquired Clostridium difficile-associated diarrhea. Clin Infect Dis 1994;169(1):127–33, 143.

[43] C. DIFFICILE TOX-A TEST: T5001 [product insert]. Blacksburgh, VA: TechLab Inc.

[44] Guerrant RL, Van Gilder T, Steiner TS, et al. Practice guidelines for the management of infectious diarrhea. Clin Infect Dis 2001;32:331–51.

[45] Bartlett JG. Clinical practice: antibiotic-associated diarrhea. N Engl J Med 2002;346:334–9.

[46] Waldhausen JHT, Shaffrey ME, Skenderis II BS, et al. Gastrointestinal myoelectric and clinical patterns of recovery after laparotomy. Ann Surg 1990;211:777–84.

[47] Wilson JP. Postoperative motility of the large intestine in man. Gut 1975;16:689–92.

[48] Holte K, Kehlet H. Postoperative ileus: a preventable event. Br J Surg 2000;87:1480–93.

[49] Smith J, Kelly KA, Weinshilboum RM. Pathophysiology of postoperative ileus. Arch Surg 1977;112:203–9.

[50] Behm B, Stollman N. Postoperative ileus: etiologies and Interventions. Clin Gastroenterol Hepatol 2003;1:71–80.

[51] Ferraz AA, Cowles VE, Condon RE, et al. Nonopioid analgesic shortens the duration of postoperative ileus. Am Surg 1995;61:1079–83.

[52] Kaplan LJ, Coffman D. Splenomegaly. Available at: http://www.emedicine.com/med/topic2156.html. Accessed January 2005.

[53] Pinto AG, Namyslowski J, Pandya P. Severe thrombocytopenia due to hypersplenism successfully treated with partial splenic embolization in preoperative management. South Med J 2005;98(4):481–3.

[54] McMullin M, Johnston G. Long term management of patients after splenectomy. BMJ 1993;307:1372–3.

[55] Brigden ML. Detection, education and management of the asplenic or hyposplenic patient. Am Fam Physician 2001;63:499–506, 508.

[56] Brigden M, Pattullo AL. Prevention and management of overwhelming postsplenectomy infection: an update. Crit Care Med 1999;27:836–42.

[57] Waghorn DJ, Mayon-White RT. A study of 42 episodes of overwhelming post-splenectomy infection: is current guidance for asplenic individuals being followed? J Infect 1997;35:289–94.

[58] Read RC, Finch RG. Prophylaxis after splenectomy. J Antimicrob Chemother 1994;33:4–6.

[59] Barnes JN, Deodhar HA, Marshall RJ. Increased risk of sepsis after splenectomy. BMJ 1993;307:1408–9.

[60] Ellison EC, Fabri PJ. Complications of splenectomy, etiology, prevention, and management. Surg Clin North Am 1983;63:1313–30.

[61] Antibiotic Update. Asplenic patients and immunization. Department of Health. (U.K). CMO's Update 1994;1:3.

[62] DeRossi SS, Glick M. Dental considerations in asplenic patients. J Am Dent Assoc 1996;127:1359–63.

[63] Westerman E. Postsplenectomy sepsis and antibiotic prophylaxis before dental work. Am J Infect Control 1991;19:254–5.

[64] Splenectomy discharge sheet. Ann Harbor (MI): University of Michigan Medical Center. Reviewed June 22, 2004.

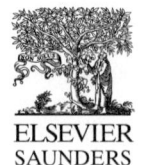

ORAL AND
MAXILLOFACIAL
SURGERY CLINICS
of North America

Oral Maxillofacial Surg Clin N Am 18 (2006) 255–260

Perioperative Management of the Diabetic Patient

Hyon K. Yoo, DDS[a],*, Bethany L. Serafin, DMD[b]

[a]Affiliates in Oral and Maxillofacial Surgery, 989 Reservoir Avenue, Cranston, RI 02910, USA
[b]Department of Oral and Maxillofacial Surgery, Woodhull Medical and Mental Health Center, 760 Broadway,
Room 2C320, Brooklyn, NY 11206, USA

Diabetes is a chronic disease characterized by the body's inability to process blood glucose properly. It is generally classified as either insulin-dependent diabetes mellitus, or *type 1 diabetes mellitus*, and non–insulin-dependent diabetes mellitus, or *type 2 diabetes mellitus*. Type 1 diabetes mellitus is characterized by a defect in insulin secretion by the β cells of the pancreas, usually secondary to autoimmune destruction of those cells [1]. Type 2 diabetes mellitus is characterized by peripheral insulin resistance with an insulin-secretory defect that varies in severity [2]. Diabetes is a common medical condition that affects 6% of Americans younger than 50 years and approximately 10% to 15% of those older than 50 years [3]. Increasing numbers of patients who have diabetes are presenting to the oral surgeon's office for care. Patients who have diabetes have a 50% chance of undergoing a surgical procedure in their lifetime [4].

Type 1 diabetes mellitus

Type 1 diabetes mellitus is characterized by the autoimmune destruction of pancreatic islet β cells, causing the body to lose its ability to secrete insulin. It is sometimes called *juvenile-onset diabetes* because it manifests most commonly in childhood or adolescence. Insulin is synthesized in the pancreatic β cells and functions in various ways, but its primary function is the regulation of glucose metabolism. In addition to its role in glucose metabolism, insulin is used in glycogen synthesis, lipogenesis, DNA synthesis, and growth. In the absence of insulin, glucose cannot be transported into cells and adipose tissue, resulting in hyperglycemia [4]. Hyperglycemia is defined as a fasting glucose level more than 126 mg/dL and can lead to ketoacidosis and severe metabolic abnormalities [5]. Patients who have type 1 diabetes mellitus depend on exogenous insulin because they are unable to produce insulin themselves.

The different types of insulin preparations that are available are rapid-acting (lispro), short-acting (regular, Lente), intermediate-acting (NPH), and long-acting (Ultralente). Standard insulin therapy consists of one to two injections per day using intermediate or long-acting insulin with or without regular or lispro insulin [6]. Intensive insulin therapy refers to multiple (three or more) daily injections, using combinations of insulin, such as regular or lispro insulin three times daily, adjusted before meals, and NPH at bedtime, or through continuous subcutaneous insulin infusion [6]. Calculating insulin dosage still remains empiric [6]. Generally, patients who have type 1 diabetes mellitus typically require an insulin dosage of 0.5 to 1.0 U/kg/d [7].

Type 2 diabetes mellitus

Type 2 diabetes mellitus is found typically in adults older than 35 years of age. It is a complex metabolic disorder resulting from decreased pancreatic insulin secretion and variable contributions of decreased insulin action or insulin resistance in target tissues, mainly muscle and the liver [8]. Obesity and sedentary lifestyle are two known risk factors for

* Corresponding author.
E-mail address: hkydds@medscape.com (H.K. Yoo).

developing type 2 diabetes mellitus. Patients who have type 2 diabetes mellitus often do not need to undergo treatment with oral antidiabetic medication or insulin if they lose weight through successful adherence to a physician-directed weight loss program that includes strict diet control and exercise [2].

The five classes of medications available for treatment of type 2 diabetes mellitus are sulfonylureas, meglitinides, biguanides, α-glucosidase inhibitors, and thiazolidinediones. Sulfonylureas and meglitinides can sometimes cause hypoglycemia, thus they are called *oral hypoglycemic agents*. The other medications target different disease processes and are termed *oral antihyperglycemic agents* [6]. The sulfonylureas and meglitinides increase the release of insulin by the pancreatic β cells to lower the blood glucose level [8,9]. Glyburide, glipizide, and glimepiride are commonly prescribed sulfonylurea drugs, and repaglinide and nateglinide are examples of meglitinides. The biguanides (metformin) reduce the hepatic glucose production in the presence of insulin [10,11]. These drugs also increase anaerobic glycolysis; enhance glucose uptake and use by muscle; and decrease intestinal glucose absorption [6]. The α-glucosidase inhibitors (eg, acarbose and miglitol) interfere with the actions of α-glucosidase in the brush border of the proximal small intestinal epithelium. The α-glucosidase serves to breakdown disaccharides and more complex carbohydrates. Through the competitive inhibition of this enzyme, the α-glucosidase inhibitors delay intestinal carbohydrate absorption and mitigate postprandial glucose excursions [12,13]. Thiazolidinediones (rosiglitazone, pioglitazone) are useful in treating hyperglycemia associated with insulin resistance in type 2 diabetes mellitus and nondiabetic conditions. These agents reduce insulin resistance and improve the peripheral action of insulin, reducing hyperglycemia by increasing the uptake and use of glucose by peripheral tissues and reducing the hepatic glucose production [6].

Diabetes and surgery

Patients who have diabetes present a special challenge to the surgeon and the anesthesiologist. Problems arise in these patients as a result of their inability to maintain a balance between insulin and its counterregulatory hormones [14].

Insulin lowers the blood sugar level by promoting glucose uptake by the muscle and fat cells while decreasing the gluconeogenesis and glycogenolysis of the liver. The blood sugar can be increased by counter-regulatory hormones, such as epinephrine, glucagons, cortisol, and growth hormone. These hormones stimulate gluconeogenesis and glycogenolysis by the liver, increase lipolysis and ketogenesis, and inhibit glucose use by muscle and fat [14].

During surgery and anesthesia, counter-regulatory hormones are released and cause hyperglycemia and increased catabolism as a result of the neuroendocrine stress response. The severity of the hyperglycemia that results depends on the nature of the surgery and complications such as sepsis, hypotension, hypovolemia, and acidosis [15].

Patients who do not have diabetes can maintain their blood glucose level by secreting insulin during a surgical procedure. Patients who have diabetes, however, are unable to respond to the increased blood glucose level during surgery, resulting in hyperglycemia. Patients who have type 1 diabetes mellitus are predisposed to diabetic ketoacidosis (DKA), whereas patients who have type 2 diabetes mellitus are susceptible to hyperglycemic hyperosmolar nonketotic syndrome (HHNK) that may be seen with or without concomitant DKA [14].

Patients who have poorly controlled diabetes are also predisposed to impaired wound healing. Diabetes-induced impaired wound healing is characterized by inhibition of the inflammatory response to wounding, macrophage infiltration, angiogenesis, fibroplasia, reparative collagen accumulation, and wound-breaking strength [16]. Patients who have poorly controlled diabetes are also at increased risk for postoperative infection for several reasons. Phagocytic capabilities of polymorphonuclear leukocytes (PMN) are adversely affected by hyperglycemia [17]. Several PMN defects occur in patients who have diabetes, including impaired migration, phagocytosis, intracellular killing, and chemotaxis [18]. Macrovascular disease and microvascular dysfunction may result in compromised local circulation, leading to delayed response to infection [19].

Other effects of uncontrolled diabetes include increased plasminogen activator inhibitor and abnormal platelet function resulting in abnormal coagulation. Hyperglycemia may also exacerbate ischemic brain injury in elderly patients [20].

Many of these complications can be prevented by a thorough preoperative evaluation and strict control of blood glucose levels during the perioperative period.

Preoperative assessment

Preoperative assessment begins with a physical examination and complete diabetic history. The sur-

geon should contact the patient's physician to determine the current level of diabetes control and the presence of any diabetes-related systemic complications, such as impaired renal function, heart disease, autonomic neuropathy, history of DKA, or HHNK [14].

The surgeon should also determine the patient's medication regimen, including the name of the medication, dosage, and time when the medication is taken. The patient's compliance with the medication regimen should also be investigated.

Cardiac evaluation should include an EKG because patients who have diabetes frequently have hypercholesterolemia, hypertension, macrovascular disease, and neuropathy and therefore have a higher risk for silent ischemia [14]. If any ischemic changes are evident on the EKG, or the patients' history suggests coronary artery disease, a stress test should be performed. A cardiology consultation may also be required.

Renal function should also be evaluated because patients who have diabetes are susceptible to renal failure. Renal workup should include serum urea nitrogen and creatinine levels, and screening for the presence of microalbuminuria and proteinuria.

Hypertension should be identified and treated. If the patient is already taking antihypertensive medication, the medication should be continued throughout the perioperative period.

The autonomic nervous system (ANS) dysfunction may be seen in patients who have diabetes. Any or all of the components of the ANS can be affected, leading to a wide range of disorders. Diabetic autonomic neuropathy is linked to silent myocardial infarction, cardiac dysrhythmias, ulcerations, gangrene, and neuropathy. It is also associated with an increased risk for sudden death. Diabetic autonomic neuropathy may manifest clinically with postural hypotension, resting tachycardia, and lack of heart-rate variability with deep respiration or exercise [21].

Some patients may experience diabetic gastroparesis. History of heartburn or acid reflux when lying supine may indicate delayed emptying of the gastric contents, causing these patients to have an increased risk for vomiting and aspiration during a surgical procedure involving general anesthesia [14].

Preoperative laboratory studies should include a complete blood count and chemistry panel. Chest radiograph is usually not necessary in patients who are otherwise healthy, but if they have any known underlying risk factors, such as smoking, then a chest radiograph must be performed before surgery involving general anesthesia.

Preoperative and intraoperative management of patients who have type 2 diabetes mellitus

Control of type 2 diabetes mellitus with diet alone

After careful preoperative evaluation is performed and it is determined that a patient's diabetes is well controlled by diet modification, the type and extent of the surgical procedure and the nature of the anesthesia must be considered. If the procedure is minor, and a fasting blood glucose measured preoperatively on the morning of the surgery is within an acceptable level ($\leq$ 200 mg/dl) no further modification is necessary [22]. For a major procedure, defined as one requiring general anesthesia for a time in excess of one hour, or if the preoperative blood glucose measurement exceeded 200mg/dl, hourly intraoperative blood glucose monitoring is indicated and administration of insulin is necessary [22].

Because the stress of surgery and anesthesia may contribute to hyperglycemia, previously stable diabetics may require insulin therapy intraoperatively. Whether these patients are managed with small amounts of subcutaneous insulin or intravenous insulin infusion, their management must no longer be considered under the type 2 diabetic protocol. At this point, management should be converted to that of the type 1 diabetic.

Management of type 2 diabetes mellitus with oral hypoglycemic agents only

Generally, oral hypoglycemics are discontinued before surgery. The specific class of medication determines how long it should be withheld before surgery. The first-generation sulfonylureas should be discontinued approximately 3 days before surgery. These long-acting oral hypoglycemics include tolazamide and chlorpropamide. Second-generation sulfonylureas such as glyburide, glipizide, and glimepiride can continue until the morning of the surgery. Thiazolidinediones and metformin should be stopped the night before surgery because of the risk for drug-induced lactic acidosis.

As with diet-controlled diabetes, blood glucose should be monitored preoperatively in diabetes managed with oral hypoglycemic agents, and intraoperative blood glucose levels checked in the same situations.

For minor procedures, a sliding scale of subcutaneous doses of insulin can be used. Emphasis is placed on preventing hypoglycemia. For perioperative hyperglycemia (200–300 mg/dL), 4 to 6 U of

regular human insulin may be administered subcutaneously. For blood glucose levels of 301 to 350 mg/dL, 6 to 8 U of regular human insulin may be given subcutaneously. For a level more than 350 mg/dL, the surgeon may use an insulin infusion to correct the hyperglycemia, or should consider canceling the surgery to stabilize the blood glucose levels and complete a more extensive workup focusing on the cause of the poor control [14]. For patients who required insulin coverage, hourly blood glucose monitoring is recommended. If coverage was not needed, levels may be obtained every 2 to 3 hours intraoperatively [3].

Postoperative management of patients who have type 2 diabetes mellitus

If patients are well controlled preoperatively, oral hypoglycemic agents can be readministered at half the usual dose on the day diet is resumed. Advancement to the patient's full regular medicine schedule can coincide with the patient's return to regular diabetic diet, assuming blood glucose is within acceptable levels. Patients taking metformin should withhold this medication for 3 days after surgery. Patients who have developed postoperative renal failure should not resume metformin until normal renal function is assured.

Patients who have started therapy on insulin coverage and have undergone major surgery or will be hospitalized, transition back to oral therapy must be approached differently. Once the patient begins eating normally, the oral agents are resumed assuming that blood glucose is well controlled. However, the addition of a sliding scale dose of insulin may be needed during the transition period. Patients who have undergone major surgery and have developed complications such as infection are unlikely to return to their same preoperative diabetic status; thus, their insulin therapy regimen may need to be reconsidered and modified.

Preoperative and intraoperative management of patients who have type 1 diabetes mellitus

Patients who have type 1 diabetes mellitus who are undergoing long-acting insulin therapy (protamine zinc insulin, Ultralente, glargine) are generally switched to a regimen of intermediate and short-acting insulin (NPH, lente and regular, lispro, re-

spectively) 1 to 2 days before the procedure [23]. The surgery should be scheduled early in the morning to avoid long NPO periods and patients should have an intravenous line inserted, a dextrose-containing solution started, and blood sugar measured when they arrive at the hospital. Patients undergoing extensive surgery or whose diabetes is poorly controlled may be admitted several days before surgery. Optimization of this patient's condition includes correcting electrolyte imbalances, metabolic abnormalities, and establishing glycemic control.

All patients who have type 1 and those who have type 2 diabetes mellitus that is poorly controlled or who are undergoing major surgical procedures will require insulin preoperatively and intraoperatively to manage blood glucose. Although many insulin regimens exist, experts do not agree on which protocol is ideal for maintaining tight glycemic control.

One regimen involves the use of subcutaneous insulin based on a sliding scale. Despite its advantage of being familiar and convenient, this regimen has been scrutinized in the medical community and is now considered inferior compared with other protocols [23]. One disadvantage of this regimen is that adequate glycemic control is difficult to achieve because of the unpredictable absorption of subcutaneously administered insulin. Another disadvantage is that the sliding scale contributes to increased hyper- and hypoglycemia because the method has an inherent disregard for the patient's insulin sensitivity [3,24]. Administering insulin retrospectively for high blood glucose values also does little to prevent the high blood glucose spikes that tight perioperative glycemic control tries to avoid. Although it is a very common perioperative regimen, sliding-scale insulin therapy alone for type 1 and some type 2 diabetes mellitus is now considered inadequate [3,22,25–27].

An alternative to subcutaneous sliding-scale insulin therapy is a regimen involving the intravenous infusion of insulin, which achieves glycemic control more predictably than through subcutaneous injection [28]. This regimen involves the administration of insulin and glucose intravenously as a variable-rate infusion, which is adjusted according to an algorithm and the patient's hourly glucose readings.

Two methods for maintaining an insulin infusion regimen exist: either the insulin and glucose are infused through separate pumps, or the mixture of glucose, insulin, and potassium in one bag (known as the *GIK regimen*) is delivered by a single system. The GIK regimen is a standard infusion in which glucose as 5% or 10% dextrose, potassium in the form of potassium chloride, and a fast-acting insulin are mixed into one 500-mL bag [3]. This infusion is started at

least 1 hour before surgery and continued throughout the procedure. The blood glucose is checked hourly and adjustments made as the insulin requirements change. This regimen has the advantage of safety; because it is premixed, inadvertent delivery of unopposed insulin or glucose is prevented. The GIK protocol also allows for a physiologic steady-state of glycemic control, thus avoiding extremes in blood glucose levels [3]. The disadvantage, however, is that when insulin requirements change and a new glucose–insulin ratio is desired, a new bag must be mixed.

Another method of insulin delivery through infusion is the modified GIK protocol [29]. One pump delivering dextrose and potassium is infused at a continuous rate and the insulin is titrated and delivered by a syringe driver or piggybacked tubing according to the patient's blood glucose level. This method allows insulin delivery to be adjusted without a new bag needing to be mixed. Regardless of which delivery method is used, rates are adjusted to maintain blood glucose levels between 120 mg/dL and 180 mg/dL [22].

Postoperative management of the patient who has diabetes mellitus requiring insulin

Insulin injection or infusion should be maintained during the postoperative period until the patient resumes normal oral intake. Patients who will undergo maintenance on a liquid diet would benefit from continued insulin infusion until their normal diabetic diet is reinstituted. Patients who have type 1 diabetes mellitus and are fasting still require insulin at a basal rate, and sliding-scale subcutaneous insulin injections alone will not be adequate to meet that requirement. Blood glucose levels should be monitored hourly for the duration of the infusion. Serum potassium levels should be measured postoperatively and then daily until normal diet is resumed.

In patients who were previously non–insulin dependent but who had undergone conversion to insulin therapy in the perioperative period require close monitoring during the transition period. Until oral hypoglycemic therapy can be fully reinstituted, short-acting insulin before meals can be used in combination with a long-acting insulin for basal requirements.

In the patient who has type 1 diabetes, subcutaneous insulin can be reinstituted before the first solid meal. The intravenous insulin infusion can be stopped 1 to 2 hours later and the patient can resume their normal insulin therapy [25].

Insulin, glucose, and fluids

The goal of intraoperative management of the patient who has diabetes should be to maintain blood glucose within a narrow range throughout the surgery because of the devastating effects of hyper- or hypoglycemia. Insulin administration may be considered for all patients who have diabetes, whether a type 1 or type 2, because they are generally insulin-deficient. One exception is the patient who has well-controlled type 2 diabetes mellitus who is undergoing a short surgical procedure. The stress of surgery and anesthesia, which increases insulin requirements in all patients, compounds the problem of relative insulin deficiency [4].

Because one of the goals during preoperative management of patients who have diabetes is to prevent protein catabolism, glucose infusion with insulin coverage is administered. An intravenous infusion of a solution containing 5% dextrose at 125 mL/h reduces catabolism in patients who have maintained an NPO status [3].

Fluid management is very important in the intra-operative management of patients who have diabetes, and is determined partially by the duration of the procedure and modified according to patient restrictions. The perioperative administration of fluid can help prevent excessive hyperglycemia and, more importantly, hypoglycemia. For patients who undergo minor procedures who are anticipated to return to normal oral fluid intake within hours after surgery, D5 ½ NS is acceptable at 100 ml/h. When fluid restriction is necessary, the physician may consider using 10% dextrose at 50 ml/h. Losses must be replaced by non–lactate- and non–dextrose-containing solutions to avoid contributing to hyperglycemia [30].

Summary

Diabetes is a common medical condition that affects many patients who seek oral and maxillofacial surgical care. These patients present various challenges to the perioperative management team. Careful preoperative planning, detailed preoperative assessment, and meticulous perioperative monitoring are essential in managing patients who have diabetes and will undergo surgical procedures.

References

[1] Votey S, Peters A. Diabetes mellitus, type 1—a review. Available at: http://www.emedicine.com/emerg/topic133.htm. Accessed December 15, 2004.

[2] Votey S, Peters A. Diabetes mellitus, type 2—a review. Available at: http://www.emedicine.com/emerg/topic134.htm. Accessed December 15, 2004.

[3] Pace B, Cheung R. Perioperative management of the diabetic patient. Available at: http://www.emedicine.com/med/topic3165.htm. Accessed December 15, 2004.

[4] Alberti KGMM, Thomas DJB. The management of diabetes during surgery. Br J Anaesth 1979;51: 693–710.

[5] Report of the Expert Committee on Diagnosis and Classification of Diabetes Mellitus. Diabetes Care 1998;21(Suppl 1):S5–19.

[6] Barnett P, Braunstein G. Diabetes mellitus. In: Andreoli T, Carpenter C, Griggs R, et al, editors. Cecil essentials of medicine. 5th edition. Philadelphia: WB Saunders Company; 2001. p. 590–3.

[7] Hirsh IB. Type 1 diabetes mellitus and the use of flexible insulin regimens. Am Fam Physician 1999; 60(8):2343–52, 2355–6.

[8] Inzucchi S. Oral antihyperglycemic therapy for type 2 diabetes: scientific review. JAMA 2002;287(3):360–72.

[9] Luna B, Feinglos MN. Oral agents in the management of type 2 diabetes mellitus. Am Fam Physician 2001; 63(9):1747–56.

[10] Stumvoll M, Nurjhan N, Perriello G, et al. Metabolic effects of metformin in non-insulin-dependent diabetes mellitus. N Engl J Med 1995;333:550–4.

[11] Johansen K. Efficacy of metformin in the treatment of NIDDM: meta-analysis. Diabetes Care 1999;22:33–7.

[12] Goke B, Herrmann-Rinke C. The evolving role of alpha-glucosidase inhibitors. Diabetes Metab Res Rev 1998;14(Suppl 1):S31–8.

[13] Lebowitz HE. $\alpha-$Glucosidase inhibitors as agents in treatment of diabetes. Diabetes Rev 1998;6:132–45.

[14] Plodkowski RA, Edelman SV. Pre-surgical evaluation of diabetic patients. Clin Diabetes 2001;19:92–5.

[15] Marks JE, Hirsch IB. Surgery and diabetes. In: Deforms RA, editor. Current management of diabetes mellitus. St. Louis (MO): Mosby Year Book; 1998. p. 247–54.

[16] Qiu JG, Chang TH, Steinberg JJ, et al. Single local instillation of Staphylococcus aureus peptidoglycan prevents diabetes-induced impaired wound healing. Wound Repair Regen 1998;6(5):449–56.

[17] Drachman RH, Root Jr RK, Wood WB. Studies on effect of experimental nonketotic diabetes on antibacterial defense – I. Demonstration of a defect in phagocytosis. J Exp Med 1966;124:227–40.

[18] Valerius NH, Eff C, Hansen NE, et al. Neutrophil and lymphocyte function in patients with diabetes mellitus. Acta Med Scand 1982;211:463–7.

[19] Goodson III WH, Hunt TK. Wound healing and the diabetic patient. Surg Gynecol Obstet 1979;149: 600–8.

[20] Haag BL. Presurgical management of the patient with diabetes. In: Leahy JL, Clark NG, Cefalu WT, editors. Medical management of diabetes. New York: Marcell Dekker; 2000. p. 631–9.

[21] Vinik AI, Erbas T. Recognizing and treating diabetic autonomic neuropathy. Cleve Clin J Med 2001;68: 928–44.

[22] Dagogo-Jack S, Alberti K. Management of diabetes mellitus in surgical patients. Diabetes Spectrum 2002; 15:44–8.

[23] Christiansen DL, Schurizek BA, Malling B, et al. Insulin treatment of the insulin-dependent diabetic patient undergoing minor surgery. Continuous intravenous infusion compared with subcutaneous administration. Anaesthesia 1988;43:533–7.

[24] Queale WS, Seidler AJ, Brancati FL. Glycemic control and sliding scale insulin use in medical inpatients with diabetes mellitus. Arch Intern Med 1997;157:545–52.

[25] Marks JB. Perioperative Management of Diabetes. Am Fam Physician 2003;67:93–100.

[26] Schade DS. Surgery and diabetes. Med Clinics of North America 1988;72:1531–43.

[27] Mokshagundam SPL. Perioperative management of diabetes mellitus. Crit Care Nurs Q 2004;27(2):135–47.

[28] Hirsch IB, McGill JB. Role of insulin in management of surgical patients with diabetes mellitus. Diabetes Care 1990;13:980–91.

[29] McAnulty GR, Robertshaw HJ, Hall GM. Anaesthetic management of patients with diabetes mellitus. Br J Anaesth 2000;85(1):80–90.

[30] Thomas DJB, Alberti KGMM. The hyperglycemic effects of Hartmann's solution in maturity onset diabetics during surgery. Br J Anaesth 1978;50:185–8.

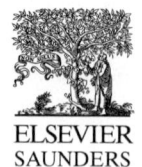

ELSEVIER
SAUNDERS

Oral Maxillofacial Surg Clin N Am 18 (2006) 261 – 273

ORAL AND
MAXILLOFACIAL
SURGERY CLINICS
of North America

Early Perioperative Care of the Acutely Injured Maxillofacial Patient

Orville D. Palmer, MD, MPH, FRCSC[a,b,*], Vaughn Whittaker, MD[c],
Carolyn Pinnock, MBBS, DM[d,e]

[a]Division of Otolaryngology, Head and Neck Surgery, Department of Surgery, Harlem Hospital Center, 506 Lenox Avenue,
New York, NY 10037, USA
[b]Department of Otolaryngology, Columbia College of Physicians and Surgeons, New York, NY USA
[c]Department of Surgery, Harlem Hospital Center, New York, NY USA
[d]Bustamante Hospital for Children, Kingston, Jamaica
[e]Department of Surgery, University of the West Indies, Kingston, Jamaica

Maxillofacial trauma involves injury to the facial soft tissue or its bony structure. It is commonly associated with multiple system injuries and occurs in 33% of severely injured trauma victims brought into emergency rooms [1]. The most common mechanisms of injury are blunt or crush injuries caused by personal assault and motor vehicle accidents [2,3]. These injuries often are associated with other serious injuries in as many as 54.8% to 70.2% of victims [2]. These concomitant injuries include cranial, spinal, and upper and lower body injuries [4,5].

Patients who have maxillofacial injuries are first and foremost trauma patients who must be seen and assessed by the trauma team, and the care must be multidisciplinary [6]. At the time of injury, patients should be transported immediately to the closest and most appropriate facility, preferably a confirmed trauma center [7]. Adequate prehospital stabilization includes maintaining the airway with immobilization of the cervical spine, providing effective oxygenation, controlling external hemorrhage, and starting fluid resuscitation. The trauma center or receiving facility must be informed of patient arrival so that the appropriate team can be mobilized and

be on standby [7]. Patients must be triaged with special consideration given to the early securing of the airway. Advanced trauma life support guidelines are helpful, but patients may deteriorate rapidly if inappropriate attempts at intubation are made. An otolaryngologist should be summoned as soon as possible if a patient is suspected of having significant laryngeal or tracheal injury. Patients who were unrestrained in a motor vehicle (including motorcycles) are more likely to suffer uncommon laryngeal and tracheal injuries. A high index of suspicion is necessary for early detection.

Early referral to an ophthalmologist to evaluate for injuries to the eye, orbital wall, and its adnexae is important [8]. A complete ocular examination should be performed [2]. A neurosurgeon is consulted if there are associated head injuries, traumatic cerebrospinal fluid (CSF) leaks, and complicated skull fractures [9]. Various other specialties are included as dictated by the injury profile of the patient.

Review of advanced trauma life support protocol

Universal infection control precautions must be stressed while caring for these patients. The initial evaluation is performed following the advanced trauma life support protocol. After efficiently obtaining the vital signs, a primary survey is undertaken using the "ABCDEs" of trauma care. Only after a

---

* Corresponding author. Division of Otolaryngology, Head and Neck Surgery, Department of Surgery, Harlem Hospital Center, 506 Lenox Avenue, New York, NY 10037.
E-mail address: odp3@columbia.edu (O.D. Palmer).

1042-3699/06/$ – see front matter © 2006 Elsevier Inc. All rights reserved.
doi:10.1016/j.coms.2006.02.001

patient is stable will a more detailed secondary survey follow to assess injuries and plan for definitive care [8]. The aim of the "ABCDEs" of trauma care is to identify life-threatening injuries and resuscitate vital functions. During the early evaluation, an individual with multiple facial trauma (MFT) should be given special considerations because of the increased risk to the airway and highly sensitive neurologic structures.

"ABCDEs" of trauma care

A Airway maintenance with protection of the cervical spine

B Breathing and ventilation

C Circulation and hemorrhage control

D Disability and neurologic status

E Exposure/environmental control: completely undress the patient but prevent hypothermia [9]

Airway management with cervical spine protection

Supplemental oxygen must be provided to all trauma patients. Airway patency must be assessed rapidly for foreign bodies and mandibular, laryngeal, or tracheal fracture (bruising and deformity). In a patient who has maxillofacial trauma, one must have a high index of suspicion for laryngeal fracture or incomplete upper airway transaction because these injuries are uncommon and, when associated with multiple other injuries, are often missed on initial assessment [10]. The airway should be secured while cervical immobilization is ensured using devices such as collars and supports or manual inline immobilization, when necessary. The cervical spine must be immobilized until radiologic confirmation of normalcy is attained [11]. Chin lift and jaw thrust are used initially to achieve the task of airway control. If this does not render the airway patent, a nasopharyngeal airway may be used. In an unconscious, drunk, obtunded, or severely injured patient, airway integrity is of utmost importance. Patients who have severe head injury and altered mental status as evaluated by the Glasgow Coma Score of 8 or less require a definitive airway by either nasal or oral endotracheal intubation. As a general principle, a definitive airway should be established if there are any doubts about a patient's ability to maintain airway integrity. If laryngeal or tracheal injury is suspected, intubation should be performed in the presence of an otolaryngologist whenever possible. Frequent reassessment of airway patency is critical because a patient who has maxillofacial injuries is always at risk for progressive airway obstruction [9].

A subgroup of these patients requires management with a tracheostomy or other surgical airway. The indications are discussed later.

Breathing and ventilation

Rapid assessment of the mechanics of ventilation is the next step in the primary survey. During this phase, it is important to differentiate an airway problem from a ventilatory problem. Ventilatory effort and chest excursion are assessed and wounds noted. Inspection of the chest wall may reveal bruises, which suggest rib fractures, or paradoxical movement, which suggests a flail chest segment. An opened wound may suggest a tension pneumothorax, which must be treated immediately upon detection. The presence of air or fluid in the pleural cavity usually can be detected by percussion and auscultation.

Pulse oximetry is a useful adjunct for monitoring hemoglobin saturation and the effectiveness of ventilatory efforts. As with airway patency, frequent re-evaluation of breathing is important to detect any deterioration in clinical status [9].

Circulation and hemorrhage control

In any trauma patient, hypotension is most likely caused by blood loss, and rapid restoration of circulating volume may prevent death. Rapid clinical assessment of the hemodynamic status of a patient is performed by looking at the level of consciousness, skin color, and pulse [9]. Hemodynamic compromise is characterized by altered mental levels of consciousness, ashen gray skin of the face, pale extremities and mucosa, and rapid thready pulses that are absent peripherally and weak centrally. An adequately perfused patient is alert and pink and has full, slow, and regular pulse. Rapid volume replacement is essential to avoid complete circulatory collapse. The placement of two large-bore intravenous catheters should be established early, ideally during the prehospital phase of resuscitation. At the initial vasculatory access, blood should be drawn for the standard laboratory investigations, including type and screen and β-human chorionic gonadotropin for all women of childbearing age. The initial volume replacement should be performed with crystalloids. If a patient remains unstable or more than half the estimated blood volume has been infused, then blood should be infused. Type-specific blood is ideal, but O-negative blood can be used when it is not available.

The patient who has maxillofacial trauma can have profound bleeding, which may produce significant blood loss and circulatory collapse. The head

and face have an extensive blood supply from the common carotid and subclavian arteries, which are branches off the aortic arch on the left and the brachiocephalic trunk on the right, respectively. The common carotid terminates in the internal and external carotids. The external carotid terminates in the superficial temporal and maxillary arteries. The maxillary artery is divided into three parts (in relation to the lateral pterygoid muscle), each with five branches. The external carotid supplies the face via the facial artery through its superior and inferior labial arteries. The internal carotid supplies the intracranial structures. The ophthalmic artery (from the internal carotid) sends supraorbital and supratrochlear arteries to the forehead [3,12]. Direct pressure is the most effective means for immediate control of active bleeding in MFT. Most nosebleeds and bleeding from the ear are venous (slow) and do not require immediate control measures. Brisk arterial bleeding from the nose or ears is unusual and requires urgent specialist assessment.

Control of major maxillofacial bleeding

Minor nasal or oral bleed is a common feature of facial bone fractures. In most instances, soft tissue bleeding subsides after the suturing of orofacial lacerations, and only rarely does exploration for a source of bleeding become necessary. Occasionally, however, a major bleed may require nasal or intraoral packing for control during the early management of patients who have MFT. When this occurs the two common sources of bleeding are the maxillary artery at the level of the pterygopalatine fossa, which manifests as a bluish discoloration and an obvious bulging of the buccal mucosa caused by hematoma, and the common carotid at the level of the skull base. Localizing the source of bleeding usually can be achieved by clinical examination only, but angiography always should be considered when in doubt. After controlling the bleed with local, nasal, and oral packing, a maxillary artery bleed can be controlled with transantral sphenopalatine hemoclips. In instances in which a more expeditious approach is needed, ligation of the maxillary artery can be achieved by incising the buccal mucosa adjacent to the ipsilateral maxillary tuberosity and ligating the main trunk before it enters the pterygopalatine fossa. Internal carotid bleed usually can be controlled by intra-arterial balloon occlusion. When this approach is not successful, a combined middle cranial fossa and infratemporal fossa approach to the skull base for bypass or ligation may be necessary.

Disability (neurologic evaluation)

Head injuries with underlying central neurologic deficits are often associated with maxillofacial trauma. Resulting deficits may vary from having no clinical manifestations to deep coma. Initial rapid assessment of the level consciousness in the trauma patient is available with the use of the AVPU method [9]:

A Alert
V Responds to vocal stimuli
P Responds only to painful stimuli
U Unresponsive to all stimuli.

The Glasgow Coma Score is a more detailed and reliable method of assessing patient level of consciousness and has good prognostic value for predicting early hospital mortality (81.9% predictive value). The APACHE III (82.4% predictive value) provides prognosis of late mortality and functional outcome [13].

Neurologic status must be evaluated frequently and continuously until it is certain that neurologic damage is not progressive. Subtle changes may be a clue to ongoing neurologic injury, such as a case of a bleed in which a patient was initially lucid. Any alterations in the level of consciousness should prompt immediate re-evaluation of a patient's oxygenation, ventilation, and perfusion status. (It also may be affected by alcohol or drugs.) Once hypoxia and hypovolemia are excluded, the alteration should be considered to be the result of trauma to the central nervous system until proven otherwise. Early involvement of a neurosurgeon can be life saving.

Exposure

A patient should be completely undressed even if it seems that the trauma involves only the maxillofacial region. Many instances of life-threatening injuries being missed by narrowly focusing on the maxillofacial region have been reported. An undressed individual should be warmed using blankets or heaters. All infused fluids should be warmed. Injuries identified by the primary survey may be life threatening and should be treated rapidly and efficiently while aggressively resuscitative measures are used to ensure that a patient has an optimal chance of survival.

Secondary survey

A patient undergoes secondary survey after the primary survey (ABCDEs) is completed, resuscita-

tion is well established, and vital signs are returning to normal. This survey includes a focused history, head-to-toe physical examination, and frequent re-evaluation of vital signs. Initial radiologic investigations are performed during this survey. The history focuses on current or past medical information that may influence immediate treatment options and looks at the mechanism of injury, which gives clues into the expected pattern of injury. The "AMPLE" pneumonic is the recommended guide for this brief but important history taking [9].

A Allergies
M Medications currently used.
P Past illnesses/pregnancy
L Last meal
E Events/environment related to the injury.

Head and neck examination in maxillofacial trauma

The entire scalp, head, face, and neck should be examined during the secondary survey. Special considerations for the examination of the eye, ears, nose/midface, and neck must be made in the trauma patient who has damage to the maxillofacial region.

Examination of the eye

Periorbital edema may limit eye examination, but it should evaluated for

Visual acuity
Pupillary size
Hemorrhage of the conjunctiva and fundi
Penetrating injury
Contact lenses (remove before edema occurs)
Dislocation of lenses
Ocular entrapment

The ophthalmology service should be contacted early if there is any suspicion of ocular/visual injury.

Examination of the nose and midface

Patients who have fracture of the midface are at risk for fracture of the cribriform plate, and gastric intubation should be performed from the oral route. Minor nasal or oral bleed is not an uncommon feature of facial fractures. Inspection of the oral cavity may reveal a hematoma, which suggests major arterial injury.

Cervical spine assessment

Cervical spine injury occurs in 2% to 3% of trauma patients and is missed in up to 10% of patients [11]. Delay in diagnosis or unwarranted manipulation of the injured spine can increase neurologic morbidity and mortality to as much as 3% to 25% [11,14–16]. Radiologic investigations are the hallmark for evaluating spinal injuries, but normal radiologic examinations in the presence of neck pain, tenderness, and neurologic deficit do not rule out cervical spine injury [17,18]. Clinical judgment of spinal injury has a diagnostic accuracy of only 50% [10], and plain radiographs only improved the accuracy of diagnosis to 52% from pooled figures of a meta-analysis [19]. A common approach in many hospital emergency departments is to use a plain radiographic series, which consists of lateral, anteroposterior, and odontoid views [16]. CT has a greater sensitivity and specificity for diagnosing cervical spine injuries, especially when used as an evaluating tool.

Guidelines from Santa Barbara Cottage Hospital for the evaluation of the cervical spine are as follows:

1. Any patient without clinical evidence of neurologic injury, alcohol, drug intoxication, altered mental status, or distracting injury undergoes cervical spine evaluation by clinical examination in the trauma room, and the spine is cleared if physical examination evaluation is negative.
2. Any patient who does not meet criteria to have the spine clinically cleared (eg, continued neck pain, altered mental status) undergoes CT scanning with 3-mm cuts of the entire cervical spine with reformats of sagittal images.
3. If a patient has a normal CT scan but neurologic deficit is present, an MRI is obtained.
4. If a patient is not evaluable secondary to coma, the CT is without abnormality, and the patient is moving all four extremities upon arrival to the emergency department, the cervical spine is cleared and spinal precaution removed.
5. If a patient is in coma or under neuromuscular blockade and there is no observed movement of the lower extremities, he or she is kept in spinal precautions until such movement is observed or until MRI scan is obtained.

CT scanning using these protocols for cervical spine injury had a sensitivity of 99% and specificity of 100%, with a 0.04% risk of missing injuries. It had a positive predictive value of 100% and negative predictive value of 99% [20].

Maxillofacial trauma is considered a distracting injury when assessing cervical spinal integrity, and as many as 3% to 6.7% of patients with MFT have an underlying cervical spinal injury [13,21]. In suspicious cases of possible spinal injury, CT is also the best choice for ruling out cervical spinal injury in a patient with MFT. The cost benefit analysis of CT scanning of the cervical spine versus plain radiography shows a distinct advantage for CT scanning. There is convincing evidence that spiral CT of the cervical spine as an initial screening tool for moderate- to high-risk patients seen and treated in urban trauma center reduces the incidence of paralysis and institutional costs [22].

The body

Examination of the chest, abdomen, perineum, and musculoskeletal system in the secondary survey should be performed with a high index of suspicion based on the mechanism of injury. A patient must be examined front and back and log-rolled to ensure spinal stabilization, and all appropriate radiologic and endoscopic investigations must be obtained at that time. The leader of the trauma team must ensure that re-evaluation of vital signs and physical findings, complete physical examination, appropriate investigations, and appropriate urgent referrals to specialist services be coordinated and executed while patient stability is maintained. Pain control measures also must be implemented once the patient is stable.

Management of cerebrospinal fluid leak/fistula (rhinorrhea, otorrhea, paradoxical rhinorrhea)

CSF leak occurs in 4.6% of patients who have maxillofacial trauma [23]. Leaks result from a skull fracture with an associated dural tear. Within the anterior cranial fossa, fracture of the frontobasal skull (usually the cribriform plate) may present with CSF rhinorrhea [2]. In the middle cranial fossa, fracture of the temporal bone may result in otorrhea [24]; paradoxically, the CSF may track along the Eustachian tube and result in what is referred to as "paradoxical" rhinorrhea. Management of CSF leaks is influenced by injuries within other organ systems that may delay intervention and the presence of concomitant maxillofacial injuries, which may influence surgical access [2].

Investigations are used to (1) confirm the presence of CSF in the fluid seen and (2) identify the site of the leak (bone and dura).

Is this cerebrospinal fluid?

The presence of β_2-transferrin (tau protein) in the leaking fluid is the most sensitive test to detect the presence of CSF, because it is found only in the CSF, perilymph, and vitreous humor. Caution must be exercised in patients who have cirrhosis who may have abnormally elevated β_2-transferrin levels in the blood, which could lead to a possible false-positive result [13,25]. Less sensitive tests, such as fluid versus blood glucose levels or the halo sign, are of limited use. The halo sign is present when nasal secretions on bed linens or dressings form a halo, which occurs when blood-stained CSF spreads onto an absorbent surface. The blood (darker) forms a ring/halo around the CSF (lightly stained center). Mixture of blood with tears or saliva can give the same effect (false positive).

Investigations to determine the localization of injury

High-resolution, fine-slice (1 mm) CT scanning with multiplanar reconstruction is the standard imaging method for identifying bony and dural points of injury. Bony defects are easily detected, but the dural defect is more difficult to identify, particularly with an inactive tear (no clinical leak). MRI has been useful for the evaluation of CSF fistula with no clinical evidence of leaking. The studies are complementary [26]. In a difficult to localize CSF leak, metrizamide CT cisternography may be helpful.

Management of cerebrospinal fluid leak/fistula

More than 99% of CSF leaks secondary to trauma resolve within a week of conservative management [23]. Conservative management involves continuous lumbar CSF drainage (ventricular drainage in some cases), bed rest, carbonic anhydrase inhibitor, and the use of antibiotic prophylaxis. Antibiotic prophylaxis is especially useful if a patient is immunocompromised or has indwelling drains or when gross soilage/contamination has occurred [3]. The use of prophylactic antibiotic is considered by some clinicians to be unwarranted, however, because of the poor penetration of uninflamed meninges and the possibilities for developing resistant strains [27]. It should be avoided unless clinically warranted by a dirty wound or gross contamination of an open fracture. Head elevation is an adjunct in conservative management.

Distinct indications for surgical management of traumatic CSF fistulae are midline fractures, bone displacement >1 cm, compound, comminuted, largely

extended, and depressed fractures [2], involvement of the cribriform plate, encephalocele, myelocele, hematoma, open trauma, severe bone derangement, and continued CSF leak for more than 1 week with conservative management. If surgical intervention is undertaken for the repair of associated maxillofacial fractures, then closure or repair of the CSF leak at the time of surgery is indicated. The approach to surgical management of CSF leak depends on the results of localization studies and the regions of the fractured skull.

Timing of surgery depends on patient stability, the extent of injury, and the presence of concomitant injuries that may require urgent operative interventions. Patients may warrant emergency intervention if extensive pneumocephalus, significant intracranial hematoma, or gross open craniofacial disruption trauma is present. Delay is warranted in cases of cerebral edema and raised intracranial pressure (ICP) that results from severe head injury.

The main sequelae of a CSF leak are meningitis and pseudomeningocele. There is a higher rate of recurrent CSF leak in patients managed conservatively compared with patients treated surgically [2].

Frontobasal fistulas

Approach to the frontobasal fracture can be extracranial or transcranial

The extracranial approach can be via the ethmoid or frontal paranasal sinuses or directly through the nose (transnasal approach). The main advantage of the extracranial approach is the decreased risk of seizures in the long-term. The use of nasal endoscopy has revolutionized the transnasal approach and minimized scarring and iatrogenic disfigurement of the face. This procedure tends to be limited to smaller, well-localized fistulas and may not be suitable for patients who have MFT with open trauma or severe destruction of the nose or paranasal sinuses. The transcranial approach provides superior access and is used in more significant CSF rhinorrhea with encephalocele or myelocele.

Temporal bone fistulas

For temporal bone fracture, the transmastoid craniotomy approach, middle fossa approach, and combined transmastoid–middle fossa approach are the common surgical techniques used. Posterior defects are approached via a transmastoid approach [10,15], which is technically easier and has fewer associated risks and lower complication rates. There

is quicker recovery time and less long-term risk of epilepsy, which accompanies the intracranial technique [28]. Defects in the tegmen are approached by the middle fossa craniotomy [28].

The advantage of the transmastoid approach is that it gives good access to the posterior cranial fossa; defects in this area can be sealed well with a low complication rate and a low incidence of postsurgical epilepsy. The disadvantage, however, is the inaccessibility to anterior tegmen defects without significant ossicular displacement. Recurrence rates seem to be higher with this approach [28].

The middle cranial fossa approach offers superior access to the anterior tegmen down to the petrous apex and enables easier graft placement at the time of fistula repair. The disadvantages are longer recovery time, increased risk of epilepsy, and relative inaccessibility to posterior fossa fistulae [29].

Management of laryngeal injuries

Laryngeal injury is an uncommon injury. It occurred in 0.04% of trauma cases in one series [30] and is often linked with other life-threatening injuries. It is associated with loss of airway and immediate death at the time of incident. The larynx functions to maintain airway patency and produce speech. It is well protected by virtue of its location and composition. The bony structures of the mandible and sternum offer protection superio-inferiorly, particularly when the head is flexed and the sternocleidomastoid muscles protect this vital organ laterally.

The elastic properties of the laryngeal cartilages allow some degree of deformity without fracturing the framework, including the thyroid cartilage, cricoid, and tracheal ring. This elastic framework is at increased risk for disruption in elderly persons (because of calcification) and in victims of high-velocity trauma.

The most common mechanisms of injury to the larynx are a road traffic accident during which a driver's extended neck impacts on the steering wheel and a motorcycle accident in which the rider suffers from a clothesline-type injury [31]. Seatbelt harness injury of the larynx has been described, but the use of seat belts and airbags most likely decreases the risk of serious laryngeal injuries [31]. High-velocity sports, such as cycling, motorcycle racing, ice hockey, and martial arts, are also associated with laryngeal trauma [32,33]. Assault accounts for a small number cases.

Clinical indicators of laryngeal injury include hoarseness, localized pain, dyspnea, subcutaneous

emphysema, and hemoptysis. In the multi-trauma patient who has MFT, laryngeal fractures are often missed in the primary assessment because other injuries, such as to the head and cervical spine, draw attention from the larynx [31]. Late presentation and delayed management can result in higher risk of complications, including difficult decannulation, permanent tracheostomy, and a poor or absent voice. A high index of suspicion is important in patients who have MFT.

Methods used to secure the airway in patients who have MFT with suspected or confirmed laryngeal trauma depend on airway patency at the time of assessment. If a patient has a patent airway and laryngeal injury is suspected, then appropriate investigations can be undertaken while closely monitoring the airway and oxygenation. If a patient has failure of airway patency, then an emergency tracheostomy must be performed. Flexible laryngoscopy/anterior commisuroscopy also should be performed when feasible. Patients who have with multiorgan injuries and laryngeal injury who require emergency surgery should have a tracheostomy for safe and effective airway management.

The use of endotracheal intubation and laryngeal mask airway is not recommended for patients who have laryngeal trauma. Attempt at endotracheal intubation may worsen pre-existing injuries and possibly cause further tears or cricotracheal separation [31].

Laryngeal mask airway

This device plays a definite role in severe cervical injury in which neck flexion is limited because it can be placed with the neck in the neutral position. It is also helpful in patients with maxillofacial trauma in whom the anatomy is distorted or there is visual impairment with blood and secretions [31]. There is controversy regarding its use as a primary airway device or as an adjunct to fiberoptic intubation in trauma patients, however. Failure rates as high as 30% have been noted in elective cases. The use of a laryngeal mask airway may result in worsening of laryngeal injury and cause neural injuries, most commonly to the hypoglossal [34], lingual [35–38], and recurrent laryngeal nerves [39,40]. The associated distortion of anatomy caused by underlying laryngeal damage may lead to inadequate ventilation because of distal obstruction and an inadequate seal around the laryngeal inlet with air leak, insufficient oxygenation, and aspiration with a laryngeal mask airway.

New proposal

For patients who have laryngeal trauma, we recommend that intubation should be performed in the presence of an attending otolaryngologist. An anterior commisurescope should be used to assess fully the airway and guide the intubation in a direct, fully visualized and controlled fashion. It is our experience that sedation is helpful in these patients. This tool plays a dual role of being diagnostic for the laryngeal injury and therapeutic in securing the airway. Mucosal injury, hematoma, and distortion of anatomy because of cartilaginous fracture can be detected. Information gained from this approach to intubation may obviate the need for further investigation and allows for early planning of subsequent operative or nonoperative intervention. Definitive management must be individualized for patients.

Investigations

CT scan plays a definite role in stable patients who have clinical evidence of laryngeal injury without airway compromise (Figs. 1 and 2). It is not used in unstable patients unless direct visualization was not possible at the time of intubation, but it can be added if CT scanning of the head is being performed. Esophagoscopy is important in the initial evaluation of these patients. In experienced hands, a carefully performed esophagoscopy is a valuable tool

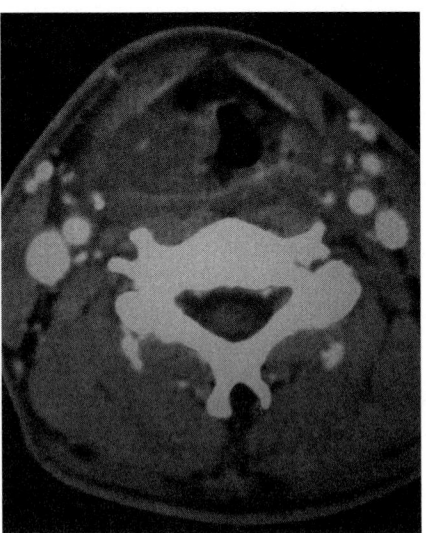

Fig. 1. Paraglottic hematoma.

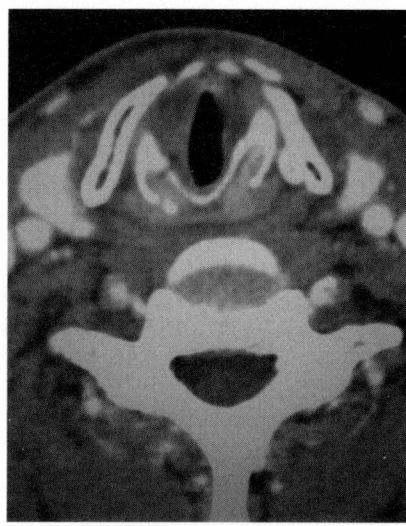

Fig. 2. Comminuted thyroid fracture and cartilage.

in completing an evaluation in patients who have upper airway injury.

Management goals

The main goals are vascular control (hemostasis and the evacuation of hematoma) and restoration of laryngeal anatomy (evacuation of deforming hematoma and covering denuded cartilage). Management of laryngeal injury should seek to restore the skeletal framework and epithelial lining and maintain the functions of airway patency and speech. Minor laryngeal injury, such as nondeforming hematoma and undisplaced laryngeal fracture, may be managed conservatively or with microendoscopes. More significant injuries, such as displaced laryngeal cartilage, are best managed through open exploration.

Surgical considerations

Mucosal lacerations not only are closed but also the mucosa must be approximated to the underlying perichondrium by way of absorbable sutures. Traditionally, cartilaginous fractures were reduced and fixed with wire or sutures. The use of miniplates offers rigid fixation and decreased hospital stay and have proved to be well tolerated [41–43].

The cricoid cartilage is the only complete cartilaginous ring in the larynx, and mucosal or cartilaginous injuries frequently lead to stenosis. Cricoid

injury can be treated successfully by stenting. Preformed laryngeal stents are available from various manufacturers. A cut endotracheal tube that fits through the vocal cords with modifications for sutures at its upper end is acceptable, however. Stents are fixed externally with nonabsorbable sutures and should be removed endoscopically between 2 and 4 weeks postoperatively.

Tracheostomy and alternatives

In the presence of massive bleeding, significant swelling, and disruption of the anatomy in the upper airway from fractures of the facial bones and larynx, tracheostomy is the most reliable method of securing an airway in patients who have maxillofacial trauma. This life-saving procedure is not without complications, however, and as such, its role and indications are constantly being re-evaluated. Other alternatives to tracheostomy include the judicious use of the endotracheal intubations and cricothyroidotomy.

Tracheostomy is performed in 0.9% to 12% of patients with facial trauma [6,10,18,25,32,44]. Most tracheotomies are performed for midface fractures 92% [18]. Other indications include

Upper airway obstruction
Bilateral condylar fractures associated with symphyseal fracture that decreases tongue support
Severe midface fractures (Le Fort type) and injury associated nasal or mandibular fracture
Edema of the larynx and glottis
Gross retropositioning of the maxilla
Suspected cervical spine injury
Maxillomandibular fixation in patient in need of reintubation
Multiple laceration of the floor of the mouth and tongue
Chronic lung disease or respiratory problems that necessitate constant suction of airway secretions
Head injury that necessitates prolonged ventilatory support
Cricothyroidotomy on arrival to the hospital
Operator convenience in fracture management

Tracheostomies have been reported to incur a morbidity rate of 14% to 45% and mortality rate of 1.6% to 16% [44]. Complications include pneumothorax, hemorrhage, infections, and recurrent laryngeal nerve injury.

Endotracheal intubation

Orotracheal and nasotracheal intubations are reasonable alternatives to tracheostomy in stable patients who have midface fractures. Nasotracheal intubation in patients without nasal bone fractures has been shown to offer adequate airway protection during surgery to repair midface fractures. This may be followed by orotracheal intubation after repair [44].

Cricothyroidotomy

The most common indications for cricothyroidotomy are clenched teeth (inability to open the mouth), blood or vomit obscuring visualization of the upper airway, severe maxillofacial injuries, inaccessibility because a patient was trapped in the acute setting, and failed/contraindicated endotracheal intubation [45,46]. In summary, tracheostomy is the gold standard in securing a difficult and complex airway in maxillofacial trauma [47], but alternative procedures may be used in select patients.

Ophthalmic considerations in maxillofacial trauma

Maxillofacial trauma is associated with ophthalmologic injuries in as many as 20% of patients. This severity is linked to the nonuse of seatbelts, which increases the risk of blindness with MFT from 2% to 20% [48]. Blindness occurs in 0.5% to 3% of cases of midfacial fracture [48], and there is a high correlation between the severity of maxillofacial injury and ocular injury leading to blindness. Traumatic blindness is caused by injury to the eyeball, optic nerve, or visual pathways. Optic nerve injury can be direct or indirect. Direct nerve injury involves nerve compression with resultant ischemic optic neuropathy that can be caused by retrobulbar hemorrhage, perineural edema, vascular spasm, or thrombosis [49]. Perineural edema is the most common cause of optic nerve injury. Indirect optic nerve injury, as described by Walsh and Hoyte [50], is that which occurs with no initial ophthalmologic or external signs with a traumatic cause.

Early diagnosis of visual impairment is linked directly to preventing visual loss. There always should be a high index of suspicion of eye injury with MFT, particularly when a history of nonuse of seatbelts is obtained. When visual loss is delayed or progressive, the prognosis for recovery is better than for immediate visual loss. The use of serial examination of function cannot be overstated [49,51]. Early input by an ophthalmologist is important to rule out injury to the conjunctiva, globe, and optic nerve. Optic nerve injury should be assessed clinically by visual acuity, visual field, pupillary reflex, and fundoscopic examination and visual evoked response [49]. Visual evoked potentials are performed using light-evoked potentials if a patient is unconscious or unable to cooperate. In an alert, cooperative patient with at least 10% visual acuity, pattern-evoked potentials are obtained [52].The degree to which a patient is examined is based on the degree of injury. High-resolution CT scan is the examination of choice in patients with suspected ocular injury and orbital cavity and bony injuries. Perineural edema, retrobulbar hematoma, and associated fractures can be detected [48].

Management of optic nerve injury may be conservative (high-dose steroids) or operative (decompression). Kline and colleagues [49] proposed the following algorithm regardless of the method of injury in the absence of clear-cut transection of the optic nerve:

- If there is loss of vision, then there is no intervention.
- If there is a delay in the development of visual loss or progressive loss on serial examination, then surgical exploration and decompression of the optic nerve are indicated.
- In ischemic ophthalmic retinopathy caused by retrobulbar hematoma, perineural edema, or orbital apex syndrome, reversible neuropathy caused by edema, contusion, and compression of the nerves, then high-dose (megadose) steroid is used as an adjunct to surgical management.

If vision is restored on high-dose steroids and subsequent loss of acuity occurs when steroids are tapered or discontinued, then surgical decompression is indicated [51]. Other studies suggest concomitant use of high-dose steroid (methylprednisone, loading dose 30 mg/kg IV over 15 minutes then 5.4 mg/kg/hr IV infusion for 23 hours) and surgical decompression.

A transethmoidal approach to surgical decompression of the optic nerve is popular and straightforward. Intranasal endoscopy is a useful adjunct in selected cases and offers the advantages of decreased morbidity, preservation of olfaction, rapid recovery time, a more acceptable cosmetic result, and less operative stress on patients. The procedure is contraindicated in patients with complete disruption of the optic nerve or chiasm, complete atrophy of the optic nerve, and carotid cavernous sinus fistula. Patients who undergo craniotomy for any reason can have optic nerve decompression performed at the same time [52].

Retrobulbar hematoma requires urgent decompression using lateral canthotomy with cantholysis. Patients who are unfit for general anesthesia should be decompressed under local anesthesia by means of lateral canthotomy and inferior cantholysis. For more stable patients, lateral brow incision and orbital decompression through a pterional approach are used. The transethmoidal transantral approach is a more familiar approach, however [53].

Acute repair over a silastic stent should be considered in the obviously transected lacrimal duct system. Injury to the lacrimal canalicular system usually has a delayed presentation, however (2–3 weeks after the acute traumatic event). Patients present with epiphora. The Schirmer test can be used to assess for true epiphora, basal secretion, and stimulated tear production in the affected eye. Jones dye tests I and II can help to determine the level of lacrimal system disruption. It is recommended that early repair be performed over a silastic stent. Definitive repair may include dacrorhinocystostomy.

Acute head injury and fluid management

One in three patients with multiple trauma has associated cerebral injury, which is a leading cause of mortality in trauma patients [54]. Patients with midface and orbital blowout fractures have a 21.9% and 23.8% chance of concomitant neurologic injury, respectively [8]. Secondary ischemic injury caused by reduced cerebral perfusion pressure and inadequate ventilation is more common than primary traumatic cerebral injury. Adequate oxygenation and hemodynamic stability are vital for controlling this preventable injury. The degree of cerebral injury sustained can be assessed with the simple AVPU system or the Glasgow Coma Score. Frequent re-evaluation is key to detecting deterioration in neurologic function.

Early fluid resuscitation of the multitrauma patient with head injury must achieve restoration of circulating volume and the efficient correction of shock, which avoids secondary ischemic insult to the brain. Efforts also are geared toward controlling increased ICP that may occur later [54]. The infusion of normal saline (0.9%) or Ringer's lactate is often used to resuscitate trauma patients. The volume required to restore circulating volume (4–6 L) may worsen ICP by enhancing brain edema, however. Colloids (type-specific blood or O-negative blood when type-specific is not available) should be infused once more than half a patient's estimated blood volume must be given.

Standard fluid therapy includes the use of mannitol, which acts as a diuretic. It acts as an osmotic agent that dehydrates normal and abnormal brain. Its hemodynamic profile includes improving preload and cerebral perfusion pressure and reducing ICP through cerebral autoregulation. Other actions include reduction of blood viscosity. Its shortcomings include hypovolemia and induction of hyperosmotic state. Monitoring should keep osmolality less than 320 mOsm/kg [55].

The literature also supports the use of hypertonic saline [54,55]. The hemodynamic profile of hypertonic saline includes improved cerebral perfusion pressure, cardiac index, and pulmonary artery occlusion pressure. It also includes significant reduction in ICP [56]. Once hemodynamic stability has been achieved, ICP should be assessed (clinical and investigations: ICP monitoring); acute raised ICP should be managed by CSF drainage and head elevation to 30°. Hyperventilation is not used because it may worsen brain injury in some patients (cerebral vasoconstriction, cerebral hypocapnea). Rebound CSF acidosis and vasodilation occur when eucapnia is restored [56].

The key to managing a patient who has head injury is preventing secondary brain injury from hypoxia, hypovolemia, and increased ICP. In managing a patient with acute head injuries, the Glasgow Coma Score is an important monitoring tool.

Facial bone fractures

The diagnosis of facial fractures is based on history and physical examination and is confirmed with radiographs. Plain facial radiographic views are still used to delineate most facial fractures when CT scan is not available. Axial and coronal CT scans, however, give far superior information in suspected comminuted fractures, posterior wall of frontal sinus fractures, and orbital apex fractures (Figs. 3 and 4). CT reconstruction views are rarely needed, although they may be useful in cases with significant fracture displacement or comminution. MRI plays a limited role except in the evaluation of orbital and intracranial pathology. Nasal bone fractures, which may be simple or open, deserve special mention. History and physical examination are of importance in determining whether to operate. Radiographs have no place in the decision-making process regarding management of simple nasal bone fractures [57]. Simple displaced nasal fractures seen within the first 4 to 6 hours, open fractures, or fractures associated with gross deformity are treated with immediate surgery. Others are reassessed in 3 to 4 days

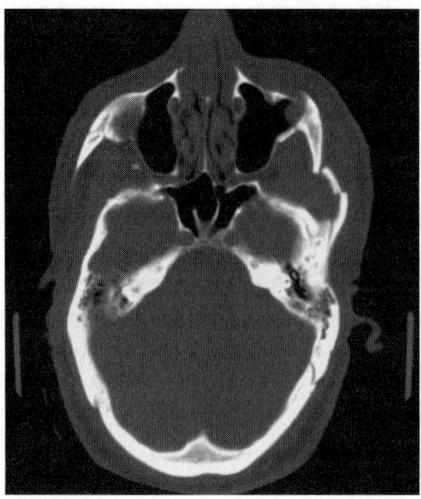

Fig. 3. Displaced fracture of ZMC complex and zygomatic arch.

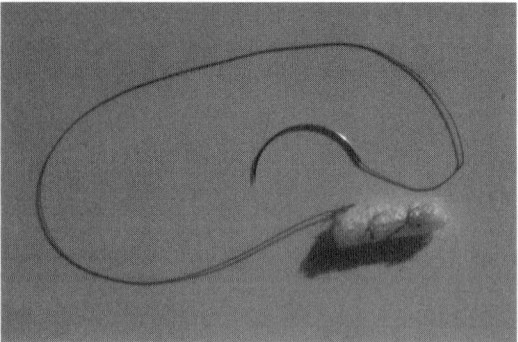

Fig. 5. Surgicel roll intranasal splint with sutures for transnasal percutaneous placement.

when acute edema has subsided. Attempts are made to reduce the fractures within the first 10 days in adults and 7 days in children. The nasal bones are manipulated and splinted under local or general anesthesia. Where there is a deforming septal fracture, septoplasty is performed Internal splinting may be performed using rolled Surgicel (Fig. 5), which is held in place under the nasal bone with transnasal percutaneous absorbable sutures taped to the skin with Steristrips. External splinting with

Plaster of Paris or other synthetic material is important [57].

Summary

Initial management of the airway is of prime importance in a patient who has sustained multitrauma and has suffered maxillofacial trauma. Loss of facial skeletal support, soft tissue swelling, intraoral and oropharyngeal bleeding, dislodged teeth, or loose dentures can lead to airway obstruction. A high index of suspicion is necessary to recognize less common cervical spinal, ocular, and laryngeal injuries. The guiding principles of the advanced trauma life support management apply to all injured patients. Injury to the maxillofacial region may be masked by other distracting system injuries, such as chest, abdominal, or musculocutaneous. A methodical system of surveillance must be applied in every trauma patient to effect favorable outcome in all cases.

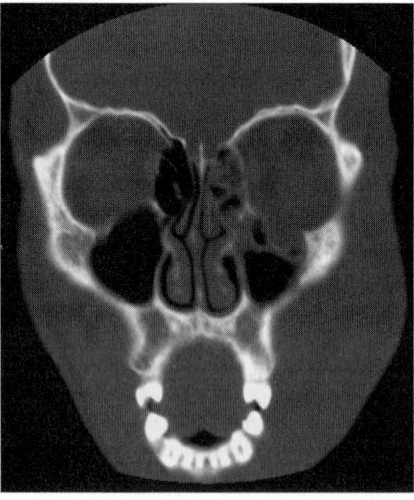

Fig. 4. Left orbital blowout fracture.

References

[1] Hayter JP, Ward AJ, Smith EJ. Maxillofacial trauma in the severely injured patients. Br J Oral Maxillofac Surg 1991;29(6):370–3.

[2] Shere JL, Boole JR, Holtel MR, et al. An analysis of 3599 midfacial and 1141 orbital blowout fractures among 4426 United States Army soldiers 1980–2000. Otolaryngol Head Neck Surg 2004;130:164–70.

[3] Haug RH, Prather J, Indresano AT. An epidemiologic survey of facial fractures and concomitant injuries. J Oral Maxillofac Surg 1990;48(9):926–32.

[4] Hussain K, Wijetunge DB, Grubnic S, et al. A comprehensive analysis of craniofacial trauma. J Trauma 1994;36:34–47.

[5] Oikarinen KS. Clinical management of injuries to the maxilla, mandible, and alveolus. Dent Clin North Am 1995;39:113–31.

[6] Gassner R, Tuli T, Hachl O, et al. Cranio-maxillofacial trauma: a 10 year review of 9543 cases with 21 067 injuries. J Craniomaxillofac Surg 2003;31:51–61.

[7] Rocchi G, Caroli E, Belli E, et al. Severe craniofacial fractures with frontobasal involvement and cerebrospinal fluid fistula: indications for surgical repair. Surg Neurol 2005;63:559–64.

[8] Al-Qurainy IA, Dutton GN, Ilankobvan V, et al. Midfacial fractures and the eye: the development of a system for detecting patients at risk for eye injury. A prospective evaluation. Br J Oral Maxillofac Surg 1991;29(6):368–9.

[9] Krantz BE. Initial assessment and management. In: Advanced trauma life support program for doctors. 6th edition. 1997. p. 21–46.

[10] Lundy LB, Graham MD, Kartush JM, et al. Temporal bone encephalocele and cerebrospinal fluid leaks. Am J Otol 1996;17:461–9.

[11] Banit DM, Grau G, Fisher RJ. Evaluation of the acute cervical spine: a management algorithm. J Trauma 2000;49:450–6.

[12] The head. In: Agur AM, editor. Grant's atlas of anatomy. 9th edition. Baltimore: Williams & Wilkins; 1991. p. 493.

[13] Cho DY, Wang YC. Comparison of APACHE 111, APACHE 11 and Glasgow Coma Scale in acute head injury for the prediction of mortality and functional outcome. Intensive Care Med 1997;23(10):77–84.

[14] Young JS, Northrup NE. Statistical information pertaining to some of the most commonly asked questions about CSI. Sci Dig 1979;Spring:111.

[15] Bohlman HH. Acute fractures and dislocations of the cervical spine: an analysis of three hundred hospitalized patients and review of the literature. J Bone Joint Surg Am 1979;61:1119–42.

[16] Lanani Z, Bonanthaya KM. Cervical spine injury in maxillofacial trauma. Br J Oral Maxillofac Surg 1999;37(3):245.

[17] Bachulis BL, Ling WB, Hynes GD, et al. Clinical indications for cervical spine radiographs in the traumatized patients. Am J Surg 1987;153:473–7.

[18] Benson DR. Emergencies in the vertebral column. In: Travis TC, Warner CG, editors. Emergency medicine: a comprehensive review. 2nd edition. Rockville (MD): Aspen Publishers; 1987. p. 143–62.

[19] Holmes JF, Akkinepalli R. Computed tomography versus plain radiography to screen for cervical spine injury: a meta-analysis. J Trauma 2005;58(5):902–5.

[20] Sanchez B, Waxman K, Jones T, et al. Cervical spine clearance in blunt trauma: evaluation of a computed tomography-based protocol. J Trauma 2005;59(1):179–83.

[21] Hackl W, Hausberger K, Sailer R, et al. Prevalence of cervical spine injuries in patients with facial trauma. Oral Surg Oral Med Oral Pathol Oral Radiol Endod 2001;92(4):370–6.

[22] Grogan EL, Morris Jr JA, Dittus RS, et al. Cervical spine evaluation in urban trauma centers: lowering institutional costs and complications through helical CT scan. J Am Coll Surg 2005;200(2):160–5.

[23] Bell RB, Dierks EJ, Homer L, et al. Management of cerebrospinal fluid leak associated with craniomaxillofacial trauma. J Oral Maxillofac Surg 2004;62(6): 676–84.

[24] Hanson MB. Skull base: CSF otorrhoea. 2003. [E-medicine]. Available at: http://www.emedicine.com/ent/topic242.htm. Accessed November 11, 2005.

[25] Naidich TP, Moran CF. Precise anatomic localization sphenoethmoidal cerebrospinal fluid rhinorrhoea by metrizamide CT cisternography. J Neurosurg 1980;53: 222–8.

[26] Gammal ET, Sobol W, van Wadlington R, et al. Cerebrospinal fluid fistula: detection with MR cisternography. AJNR Am J Neuroradiol 1998;19:627–31.

[27] Greig JR. Antibiotic prophylaxis after CSF leak lacks evidence base. BMJ 2002;325(7371):1037.

[28] Stenzel M, Preuss S, Orloff L, et al. Cerebrospinal fluid leaks of temporal bone origin: etiology and management. ORL 2005;67:51–5.

[29] Dutt SN, Mirza S, Irving RM. Middle cranial fossa approach for the repair of spontaneous cerebrospinal fluid otorrhoea using autologous bone plate. Clin Otolaryngol 2001;26:117–23.

[30] Gussack GS, Jurkovich GJ, Luterman A. Laryngotracheal trauma: a protocol approach to a rare injury. Laryngoscope 1986;96(6):660–5.

[31] Hwang SY, Yeak SCL. Management dilemmas in laryngeal trauma. J Laryngol Otol 2004;118:325–8.

[32] Hanft K, Posternack C, Astor F, et al. Diagnosis and management of laryngeal trauma in sports. South Med J 1996;89:631–3.

[33] Rejali SD, Bennett JD, Upile T, et al. Diagnostic pitfalls in sports related to laryngeal injury. Br J Sports Med 1998;32:180–1.

[34] Stewart A, Lindsay WA. Bilateral hypoglossal nerve injury following the use of the laryngeal mask airway. Anesthesia 2002;57:264–5.

[35] Ahmad NS, Yentis SM. Laryngeal mask airway and lingual nerve injury. Anaesthesia 1996;51:707–8.

[36] Gaylard D. Lingual nerve injury following use of the laryngeal mask airway. Anaesth Intensive Care 1999; 27:668.

[37] Brain AI, Howard D. Lingual nerve injury associated with laryngeal mask us. Anaesthesia 1998;53:713–4.

[38] Majumder S, Hopkins PM. Bilateral lingual nerve injury following the use of the laryngeal mask. Anesthesia 1998;53:184–6.

[39] Lowinger D, Benjamin B, Gadd I. Recurrent laryngeal nerve injury caused by a laryngeal mask airway. Anaesth Intensive Care 1999;27:2002–5.

[40] Sacks MD, Marsh D. Bilateral recurrent laryngeal nerve neuropraxia following laryngeal mask insertion: a rare cause of serious upper airway morbidity. Pediatr Anaesth 2000;10:435–7.

[41] Woo P. Laryngeal framework reconstruction with miniplates. Ann Otol Rhinol Laryngol 1990;99:772–7.

[42] Pou AM, Shoemaker DL, Carrau RL, et al. Repair of laryngeal fractures using adaptation plates. Head Neck 1998;20:707–13.

[43] De Mello-Filho FV, Carrau RL. The management of laryngeal fractures using internal fixation. Laryngoscope 2000;110:2143–6.

[44] Taicher S, Givol N, Peleg M, et al. Changing indications for tracheostomy in maxillofacial trauma. J Oral Maxillofac Surg 1996;54:292–5.

[45] Wright MJ, Greenberg DE, Hunt JF, et al. Surgical cricothyroidotomy in trauma patients. South Med J 2003;96(5):465–7.

[46] Jacobson LE, Gomez GA, Sobieray RJ, et al. Surgical cricothyroidotomy in trauma patients: analysis of its use by paramedics in the field. J Trauma 1996;41(1): 15–20.

[47] Boyd S. Discussion changing indications for tracheostomy in maxillofacial trauma. J Oral Maxillofac Surg 1996;54:295–6.

[48] Ashar A, Kovacs A, Khan S, et al. Blindness associated with midfacial fractures. J Oral Maxillofac Surg 1998;56:1146–50.

[49] Kline LB, Morawetz RB, Swaid SN. Indirect injury of the optic nerve. Neurosurgery 1984;14:756.

[50] Walsh FB, Hoyte WF. Clinical neuro-ophthalmology, Vol. 3. Baltimore: Williams & Wilkins; 1969. p. 2380.

[51] Anderson RL, Panje WR, Gross CE. Optic nerve blindness following blunt forehead trauma. Ophthalmology 1982;89:445.

[52] Luxenberger W, Stammberger H, Jebeles J, et al. Endoscopic optic nerve decompression: the Graz experience. Laryngoscope 1998;108(6):873–82.

[53] Gerbino G, Ramieri GA, Nasi A. Diagnosis and treatment of retrobulbar haematomas following blunt orbital trauma: a description of eight cases. Int J Oral Maxillofac Surg 2005;34(2):127–31.

[54] Berger S, Schurer L, Hartl R, et al. Reduction of post-traumatic intracranial hypertension by hypertonic/hyperoncotic saline/dextran and hypertonic mannitol. Congress of Neurological Surgeons 1995;37(1):98–108.

[55] Munar F, Ferrer AM, deNadal M, et al. Cerebral hemodynamic effect of 7.2% hypertonic saline in patients with head injury and raised intracranial pressure. J Neurotrauma 2000;17(1):41–51.

[56] Dunn LT. Raised intracranial pressure. J Neurol Neurosurg Psychiatry 2002;73:i23–7.

[57] Mondin V, Rinaldo A, Ferlito A. Management of nasal bone fractures. Am J Otolaryngol 2005;26(3):181–5.

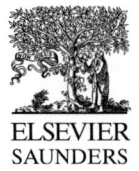

ELSEVIER
SAUNDERS

Oral Maxillofacial Surg Clin N Am 18 (2006) 275–281

ORAL AND
MAXILLOFACIAL
SURGERY CLINICS
of North America

Index

Note: Page numbers of article titles are in **boldface** type.

Changing Your Address?

Make sure your subscription changes too! When you notify us of your new address, you can help make our job easier by including an exact copy of your Clinics label number with your old address (see illustration below.) This number identifies you to our computer system and will speed the processing of your address change. Please be sure this label number accompanies your old address and your corrected address—you can send an old Clinics label with your number on it or just copy it exactly and send it to the address listed below.

We appreciate your help in our attempt to give you continuous coverage. Thank you.

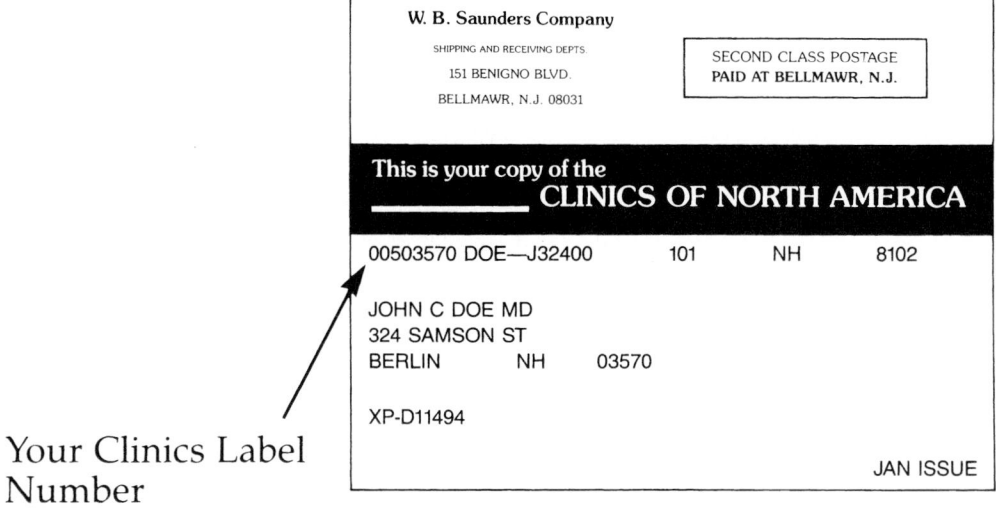

Your Clinics Label Number
Copy it exactly or send your label
along with your address to:
W.B. Saunders Company, Customer Service
Orlando, FL 32887-4800
Call Toll Free 1-800-654-2452

Please allow four to six weeks for delivery of new subscriptions and for processing address changes.

DISCOVERY LIBRARY
LEVEL 5 SWCC
DERRIFORD HOSPITAL
DERRIFORD ROAD
PLYMOUTH
PL6 8DH